AIDS, BEHAVIOR, AND CULTURE

AIDS, BEHAVIOR, AND CULTURE

Understanding Evidence-Based Prevention

Edward C. Green

and

Allison Herling Ruark

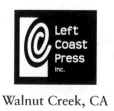

Walnut Creek, CA

LEFT COAST PRESS, INC.
1630 North Main Street, #400
Walnut Creek, CA 94596
http://www.LCoastPress.com

ISBN 978-1-59874-478-1 hardcover
ISBN 978-1-59874-479-8 paperback

Library of Congress Cataloging-in-Publication Data:
Green, Edward C. (Edward Crocker), 1944-
  AIDS, behavior, and culture : understanding evidence-based prevention / Edward C. Green and Allison Herling Ruark.
     p. cm.
  Includes index.
  ISBN 978-1-59874-478-1 (hardcover : alk. paper)—
  ISBN 978-1-59874-479-8 (pbk. : alk. paper)
1. AIDS (Disease)—Prevention. 2. AIDS (Disease)—Social aspects.
3. HIV infections—Prevention. 4. HIV infections—Social aspects.
I. Ruark, Allison Herling. II. Title.
  RA643.8.G736 2010
  362.196'9792—dc22

                              2010025900

Printed in the United States of America

♾™ The paper used in this publication meets the minimum requirements of American National Standard for Information Sciences—Permanence of Paper for Printed Library Materials, ANSI/NISO Z39.48–1992.

Cover design by Andrew Brozyna
Cover illustration © Steven Brooke Studios

Contents

ACKNOWLEDGMENTS

Most of this book was written while we were working at the AIDS Prevention Research Project, which was supported by the John Templeton Foundation, at the Harvard Center for Population and Development Studies. We wish to thank our team members from the AIDS Prevention Research Project (Daniel Halperin, Tim Mah, and Jennifer Goldsmith), the John Templeton Foundation, the Harvard Center for Population and Development Studies, and our Harvard Faculty Advisory Committee. We also wish to thank a number of individuals for intellectual input and/or moral support, in alphabetical order: Emily Chambers, Jim Chin, Paul DeLay, Nicole D'Errico, Cedza Dlamini, Melissa Farley, Norman Hearst, Janice Hogle, Estie Hudes, Phoebe Kajubi, Moses Kamya, Doug Kirby, Laurie Krieger, John Lozier, Suzanne LeClerc-Madlala, Ray Martin, Tom Merrick, Elaine Murphy, Vinand Nantulya, Neill Orr, David Patient, Bill Roberts, Sam Ruteikara, Rand Stoneburner, Jim Shelton, Cathy Watson, and Bill Weintraub. Discussions with these friends and colleagues certainly made this a better book, but they do not necessarily agree with or endorse everything written here.

We wish to especially thank H. Russell Bernard and Jennifer Collier of Left Coast Press for recognizing the significance of this book and for being such pleasant people to work with in bringing it to press. Russ Bernard has provided extraordinary support and guidance to Green for over 30 years. And special thanks to Carole Bernard for copy editing above and beyond the call of duty.

Finally, we are grateful for the invaluable support shown by friends and family members (particularly our spouses, Suzie McLaughlin and Joel Ruark) throughout this endeavor.

ABBREVIATIONS AND ACRONYMS

AA	Alcoholics Anonymous
ABC	Abstain, Be faithful, or use Condoms
AARG	AIDS and Anthropology Research Group
AIDSCAP	AIDS Control and Prevention Project
ANC	Antenatal clinic
ART	Antiretroviral therapy
ARV	Antiretroviral drug
CDC	[U.S.] Centers for Disease Control
DHS	Demographic and Health Surveys
FBO	Faith-based organization
FGD	Focus group discussion
FRELIMO	Frente de Libertãçao de Moçambique
GEMT	Gambinete de Estudos de Medicina Tradicional
HRC	Harm Reduction Coalition
HIV	Human immunodeficiency virus
IDI	In-depth interview
IDU	Intravenous drug use or users
IMAGE	Intervention with Microfinance for AIDS and Gender Equity
INPUD	International Network of People who Use Drugs
IPV	Intimate partner violence
MARP	Most-at-risk population
MCP	Multiple and concurrent partners
MSM	Man (or men) who has sex with men
NA	Narcotics Anonymous
NEP	Needle exchange program
NGO	Non-governmental organization
NIH	[U.S.] National Institutes of Health
PACHA	[U.S.] Presidential Advisory Council on HIV/AIDS
PEPFAR	[U.S.] President's Emergency Plan for AIDS Relief (Emergency Plan)
PLHIV	Person living with HIV
PMTCT	Preventing mother-to-child transmission

PSI	Population Services International
RCT	Randomized controlled trial
SOMARC	Social Marketing for Change
STI	Sexually transmitted infection
TASO	The AIDS Support Organization
TOP	The Omari Project
UNAIDS	Joint United Nations Programme on HIV/AIDS
UNDP	United Nations Development Programme
UNFPA	United Nations Population Fund
UNGASS	United Nations General Assembly Special Session on HIV/AIDS
UNICEF	United Nations Children's Fund
UNIFEM	United Nations Development Fund for Women
USAID	U.S. Agency for International Development
VCT	Voluntary counseling and testing
WHO	World Health Organization

INTRODUCTION

Perhaps no other health issue in the modern era has attracted as much controversy as HIV/AIDS, and perhaps no aspect of HIV/AIDS has been as contested as the question of how to prevent its spread. Indisputably, most prevention efforts have failed. In the first 25 years of the global pandemic, some 32 million people have died and another 33 million are currently infected. Although global HIV prevalence peaked more than a decade ago and is no longer rising, an estimated 2.7 million people are newly infected each year. In the countries of southern Africa and in high-risk subpopulations throughout the world, prevalence has stabilized at very high rates and the epidemic is far from over. A massive global effort has succeeded in putting approximately 5 million people on life-saving antiretroviral drugs (ARVs), but the international community seems to have reached the limit of its willingness to pay for such treatment, even as nearly 3 million more people are infected every year.

Two-thirds of those who need treatment today are not receiving it, and this gap seems destined to grow, especially in the context of the current global economic crisis. In a March 2009 survey by the World Bank and UNAIDS, 11% of the 71 countries surveyed reported that the economic crisis had already affected antiretroviral treatment programs, and another 31% expected such an impact by the end of 2009 (World Bank, UNAIDS 2009). In a July 2009 letter to *The Lancet*, Dr. Peter Mugyenyi, founder of Uganda's largest treatment center, pleaded: "The global financial crisis cannot justify a return to the bleak pre-PEPFAR[1] days when limited drug supplies forced us . . . to choose which desperately ill patients live and which ones die. Already, funding constraints are forcing health clinics to stop enrolling new patients in antiretroviral treatment" (p. 292).

It is often said that we cannot treat our way out of the AIDS pandemic; the only solution to the global crisis is to stop the flood of new infections. Prevention must be the mainstay of any response to AIDS, but nearly 30 years into the pandemic we seem to be no closer to effective prevention globally.[2] Yet in the midst of prevention's bleak track record, there are some successes to be found and, we believe, lessons to be learned. In the growing list of countries in which the transmission of HIV has declined, behaviors have fundamentally changed, usually in response to very simple messages. These successful responses have often been community based, low cost, low tech, and culturally grounded. Rather than relying on foreign technology, products, or expertise, they have been built on the knowledge, institutions, and cultures of affected communities.

If involvement in this type of AIDS prevention sounds like a job for anthropologists, well, we believe that it is. We propose that the tools and perspective of anthropology are quite suited to the task of working from within other cultures. Anthropologists should be at the forefront of demanding a new approach to HIV prevention globally that does not depend on Western "expertise," technologies, and ideas, but rather builds on the expertise and resources extant in other cultures. Unfortunately, anthropologists have often missed opportunities to apply the tools and principles of their discipline to solving the complex problems of AIDS, specifically prevention.

We write this book for all who are interested in applying anthropological methods to AIDS prevention because we believe that an anthropological perspective is desperately needed. HIV is transmitted by behaviors that are deeply embedded in human cultures, so solutions will also be fundamentally cultural. As we will show, effective responses to HIV prevention have arisen out of local societies, often apart from (or even in spite of) HIV prevention programs and agendas of Western donors. We argue that many of the HIV prevention programs devised by the West have been deeply out of sync with the values and realities of the groups in which they have been implemented. Once we start seeing HIV prevention from within the framework of other cultures rather than from within the confines of ours, and start listening to the solutions they propose, we may get somewhere in HIV prevention.

For example, understanding factors that contribute to multiple and concurrent sexual partners (MCP) in east and southern Africa—whether men's institutionalized control over women and economic resources, or increasing freedom from social control mechanisms embedded in family, village life, and/or religion—might contribute new insights about how these behaviors might be influenced. An understanding of indigenous theories of AIDS and other sexually transmitted illnesses might point to other key insights in preventing AIDS. For example, indigenous beliefs that sex with strangers, with women who might be menstruating, with widows prior to a cleansing ceremony, or with those who belong to one's extended kin group in exogamous systems might serve as deterrents to casual sex, and perhaps to having concurrent sexual partners (Green 1999a).

As with any contagious disease driven by behavior, especially one as intimate and complex as sexual behavior, there are biological, epidemiological, sociological, psychological, and, of course, cultural dimensions to tease out and consider. As Marshall and Bennett observed in 1990, anthropologists have the opportunity to make a unique contribution to AIDS preventive efforts, not least because of our holistic perspective. We are well positioned to study sexual behavior and its determinants, such as norms, beliefs, mores, values, prevailing social controls, and so on. Yet the fundamental problem of AIDS prevention, in our view, is that we are *not actually expected to* deal with the drivers of this particular pandemic; at best, we only *pretend* to do so.

Underlying all the fine-sounding words written and spoken at global AIDS conferences seems to be a belief—at least among Western AIDS professionals—that we are not really going to change basic sexual or drug-injecting behaviors nor should we really try. Many feel that it is our basic human right to seek pleasure without being denied or constrained by public health do-gooders, and certainly not by judgmental, stigmatizing, moralizing religious zealots. The core Western value of sexual liberation discourages any real interference with sexual behaviors. We promote technologies to *reduce* the risk, while doing or saying little about *avoiding* or *eliminating* the risk. Our position in this book is that both approaches have a role to play, but objectively or epidemiologically, the latter has more impact.

Unfortunately, much of the global AIDS response continues to center around biomedical and other nonbehavior-based strategies. Rather than addressing the basic behavioral and social factors that lead to risk, global AIDS prevention has relied on a variety of technologies and products. For sexually transmitted epidemics (which account for the great majority of infections worldwide), the standard prevention approach for most of the AIDS pandemic has been a three-pronged approach of condom promotion (especially through social marketing), voluntary counseling and testing, and treatment of the curable sexually transmitted infections (STIs). There is strong evidence that these approaches are *not* working, particularly in the population-wide, hyper-epidemics of Africa.[3] Anthropologists in particular should not be surprised that a single formula would not be appropriate and effective for all people everywhere. Even within a particular society, there should be targeting based on age, gender, behavioral risk factors, and occupation, among other considerations. Yet, after all the rhetoric around AIDS, condoms and testing are essentially what global AIDS prevention consists of.

In the face of discouraging results from existing HIV prevention technologies, many are pinning their hopes on new HIV prevention technologies or new applications of existing technologies, no matter how far-fetched such strategies may be. Anthony Fauci, director of the National Institute of Allergy and Infectious Diseases and one of the top U.S. AIDS scientists, avoided any discussion of sexual behavior (or any behaviors at all) in a 2009 *Washington Post* opinion piece on HIV prevention. He instead called for "three bold new approaches to controlling the HIV/AIDS pandemic," each of which would require massive investment in HIV testing and treatment (in other words, in drugs and technology). Unfortunately, none of these strategies have yet been proven effective or even feasible. Two involve greatly increasing the number of people on expensive, toxic ARV drugs and the time spent on such drugs—both of which strategies are fraught with ethical as well as practical challenges. It is perhaps a sign of the deep despair within the HIV prevention community that such expensive and potentially hazardous strategies are even being discussed, much less felt to be the most promising ideas on the horizon.

What *has* been shown to work in bringing down HIV infection rates? As we will discuss, there are not only different modes of HIV transmission but also different patterns of epidemics, which *require different strategies* to prevent new infections. Much of this book will focus on the generalized epidemics of sub-Saharan Africa, particularly east and southern Africa, where the primary mode of transmission is heterosexual sex. (A generalized epidemic is one in which HIV spreads in the general population, rather than among certain high-risk groups.) The available evidence suggests that, so far in these generalized epidemics, *only* male circumcision and reduction in number of sexual partners seem to impact HIV infection rates at the population level. Reduction in partners is now recognized as the primary factor explaining HIV declines in Uganda, which has experienced the greatest HIV prevalence decline of any country in Africa or, indeed, anywhere in the world (Green 2003; Green et al. 2006; Shelton et al. 2004; Stoneburner and Low-Beer 2004). Partner reduction is associated with prevalence decline in eight or nine other countries in Africa as well (Green et al. 2009). No other factor, including levels of condom use or numbers of people tested, has been associated with all cases of HIV prevalence decline in generalized epidemics (Buve et al. 2001; Caraël and Holmes 2001; Shelton et al. 2004).

An AIDS prevention strategy for these generalized epidemics that arises from evidence (rather than consensus or hope in future scientific breakthroughs) would therefore place primary emphasis on discouraging multiple partner sex of any sort: casual, concurrent, commercial, and condom "protected." Unfortunately, this has not been the case. In 2006, a meeting of HIV prevention experts convened by the Southern Africa Development Commission (SADC) in the southern Africa region (a region that accounts for nearly half of the world's HIV infections) concluded that "high levels of multiple and concurrent sexual partnerships by men and women with insufficient consistent, correct condom use, combined with low levels of male circumcision are the key drivers of the epidemic in the sub-region" (SADC 2006: 5). Those at the meeting recommended as the first two key priorities reducing multiple and concurrent sexual partnerships and rolling out voluntary male circumcision. Nevertheless, as a group of AIDS researchers observed recently (two years after the SADC meeting), "the largest donor investments are being made in interventions for which evidence of large-scale impact is increasingly weak, whereas much lower priority is given to interventions for which the evidence of potential impact is greatest" (Potts et al. 2008:750). There is a clear disconnect between science and the reality of prevention efforts in terms of far too little funding for interventions that emphasize fundamental changes in sexual behavior (e.g., partner reduction and mutual fidelity).

We are advocating for HIV prevention approaches based on the best available evidence, which is that risk of HIV infection increases with number of sexual partners (for men and women) and that concurrent partners (those who overlap in time) may be particularly risky. We are certainly far from alone in such a view. For instance, a "common ground" statement, published in the British medical journal *The Lancet* in 2004 and signed by over 150 global HIV prevention experts, stated the following HIV prevention priorities:

> When targeting young people, for those who have not started sexual activity the first priority should be to encourage abstinence or delay of sexual onset. . . . When targeting sexually active adults, the first priority should be to promote mutual fidelity with an uninfected partner as the best way to assure avoidance of HIV infection. . . . When targeting people at high risk of exposure to HIV infection (i.e., engaging in commercial sex, multiple partnerships, anal sex with high-risk partners, or sex with a person known or likely to be infected with HIV or another sexually transmitted infection), the first priority should be to promote correct and consistent condom use, along with other approaches such as avoiding high-risk behaviours or partners. (Halperin et al. 2004:1913)

An evidence-based approach to HIV prevention would also follow standard public health logic and practice by emphasizing primary prevention or risk avoidance, instead of just risk reduction, which has been the emphasis of most donors and HIV programs to date. This is particularly important when it comes to HIV transmission among high-risk groups such as sex workers, men who have sex with men (MSM), and intravenous drug users (IDU). The global AIDS community has adamantly pursued a harm reduction approach when it comes to reducing HIV risk in such groups, despite evidence that the success of such an approach is often limited. (For our purposes, harm reduction will be regarded as a more specific type of risk reduction.) We are not arguing against a harm reduction approach in all cases, but rather that if there is the option of risk avoidance—of avoiding inherently risky behaviors altogether—real resources should be put into offering this choice to those at high risk.

In advocating for an emphasis on behavior change in generalized epidemics we are not arguing for shifting attention and resources away from those at high risk, including the powerless, oppressed, exploited, raped, and abused. We are saying that it is inaccurate to characterize all people this way. Some resources clearly must be targeted to high-risk groups, and some resources must be directed to what survey and epidemiological evidence show are the majority of people. To target only those at high risk is to effectively ignore most of the population. Targeting both minority (high-risk) and majority populations need not result in diminished quality or even quantity of prevention resources going to either group. Reducing the risk of HIV infection for *all* people is the only truly compassionate and ethically sound response.

Fortunately, the fight against AIDS has become more evidence based in the last few years. AIDS experts and programs are increasingly willing to focus on changing sexual behaviors (especially in the context of concurrent partnerships) and consider tactics such as mobilizing faith-based organizations (FBOs) and indigenous resources (e.g., traditional healers and chiefs in an African context) if that will result in measurable reduction of risk behaviors. For example, there is a growing international consensus that unique patterns of concurrent sexual relationships in southern Africa have contributed to that region's hyper-epidemics and that changing these patterns requires an engagement with culture and social norms that has up until now been largely missing from AIDS prevention. We also note an increasing willingness in the AIDS community to grapple with the complex ways in which HIV takes root within cultures, even if the epidemiological evidence leads us along paths we might not expect when it comes to gender, wealth, and power.

Let us be clear: In our call for a change in HIV prevention priorities we are not speaking from a moralistic or values-driven point of view, but simply talking about what increases or decreases the likelihood of HIV infection. We recognize that sexuality is a deeply value-laden issue, whether someone holds a value of sex only within heterosexual marriage or is a proponent of poly-partnering and no restraints on sexual behavior. We are not arguing that people should not hold values regarding sexuality, or that there should not be conversations about the moral-ethical aspects of sexuality. (Certainly we should not be value-neutral on such subjects as rape or seduction of children.) What we are suggesting is that people with divergent personal views and values about sexuality should be able to reach a common understanding of what the epidemiological evidence shows about sexual behavior and HIV risk and achieve consensus on sound HIV prevention priorities.

It is more than unfortunate that the American culture wars, which center on debates such as condoms versus abstinence education in U.S. schools, have become the template for discourse (at least in the United States) about what might be best for HIV prevention around the world. Evidence-based HIV prevention has been a casualty of such ideological battles, but public health priorities for AIDS prevention should be based on public health arguments, namely what will best reduce new HIV infections and create the most health for the most people. We hope this book can contribute to debunking the notion that the debate over AIDS prevention can be reduced to something that falls neatly between the fault lines of liberals versus conservatives and will show that there is ample common ground to be found, if we will only honestly examine the evidence.

Successful HIV prevention will require a fundamentally different approach than what has, for most of the epidemic, been accepted as best practice. Ideology, inertia, and the financial self-interest that has have grown up around a robust and ever-expanding AIDS-related industry have largely set the HIV prevention agenda, causing even experts (including anthropologists) to miss clear evidence. In our view, anthropologists ought to be more aligned with advocates for simple, low-cost, sustainable, and culturally tailored solutions and less aligned with the multi-billion dollar industry of biomedical research and pharmaceutical companies, hospitals, and clinics. We ought to be more willing to "speak truth to power" (an old Quaker call to action) and more ready to challenge Western-driven approaches to AIDS. It is time to put financial, political, and ideological interests aside and adopt approaches to AIDS prevention that make public health and anthropological sense—and that work.

Chapter 1 addresses the basic question of what anthropology has to offer to AIDS prevention, arguing that anthropologists have many tools with which to understand sexual behavior in cultural context and contribute to an evidence-based, culturally grounded approach to AIDS prevention. We present an overview of anthropology's study of sexuality and discuss the contribution of prominent figures such as Mead, Freud,

Foucault, and Kinsey. Finally, we offer a framework for understanding anthropologists' work in AIDS (along with illustrative examples), that of four roles operating within four distinct paradigms.

Chapter 2 draws on Green's previous work on indigenous theories of disease, including how it applies to HIV/AIDS. Green's work in collaborating with African indigenous healers in HIV prevention during the 1990s is presented as a case study.

Chapter 3 presents a brief history of the global response to AIDS and discusses how some of the actors, agendas, and historical peculiarities of this response created a Western-driven approach to HIV prevention that was not well suited to the generalized epidemics that were emerging in Africa. A clash of values has repeatedly erupted between Western AIDS programs and the societies in which they operate, which continues to hamper effective prevention.

Chapter 4 discusses the need for a primary prevention/risk avoidance approach to HIV prevention. Global AIDS prevention has almost exclusively employed a risk reduction approach, often under the rubric of human rights. We argue that human rights cannot be the only lens through which to view HIV prevention.

Chapter 5 further discusses the topic of primary prevention, with a focus on the three high-risk groups of MSM, IDU, and sex workers. We argue that the harm reduction measures that are being pursued with these populations are far from ideal and are in many settings failing from an HIV prevention point of view. We further argue that a primary prevention/risk avoidance approach is urgently needed both to reduce the spread of HIV and to offer people the alternative of giving up high-risk behaviors such as prostitution or drug use that may continue to cause harm even *if* HIV risk is reduced.

Chapter 6 explains the basic epidemiology of HIV transmission in generalized epidemics, including the biological basis for cutting-edge areas of prevention, particularly male circumcision and reducing multiple and concurrent partnerships. This chapter also describes the failure of standard prevention measures such as counseling and testing, STI treatment, and condom promotion in generalized epidemics.

Chapter 7 presents case studies of behavior change and HIV decline in Uganda, Kenya, Zimbabwe, and other countries.

Chapter 8 demonstrates that the relationship between HIV prevention and structural factors such as poverty, gender inequality, and war is often more complicated than it is assumed to be and that addressing such structural factors does not necessarily result in effective HIV prevention.

Chapter 9 addresses the complex issue of gender, marriage, and HIV risk. We discuss such questions as whether violence fuels HIV, whether marriage is a risk factor and for whom, and what sero-discordant couples can do to reduce risk.

Chapter 10 discusses what a truly endogenous approach to AIDS prevention in Africa would look like and presents a case study of how such an approach is being investigated in four countries of southern Africa.

Finally, in the Conclusion we note some encouraging signs of movement toward more evidence-based HIV prevention, particularly in Africa's hyper-epidemics, and summarize the key lessons we believe should guide evidence-based HIV prevention.

NOTES

1. PEPFAR is the U.S. government's President's Emergency Plan for AIDS Relief, launched in 2003 by President George W. Bush.
2. This is not for want of trying: Between 1998 and 2007, donor funding for HIV/AIDS rose from 5.5% to nearly half of all aid for health, according to data from the Development Assistance Committee of the Organization for Economic Cooperation and Development, which tracks donor aid (cited in Shiffman et al. 2009:S45–S48).
3. STI treatment as an HIV prevention strategy has been somewhat deemphasized as the lack of evidence for it has been acknowledged, although costly trials to test STI treatment strategies are ongoing.

Chapter 1

AN ANTHROPOLOGICAL APPROACH TO AIDS PREVENTION

Anthropology as a discipline focuses on culture as a complex, adaptive system. Culture, in the famous words of E. B. Tylor in 1871, is "that complex whole which includes knowledge, belief, art, law, morals, customs and any other capabilities and habits acquired by man as a member of society." There have been many definitions of culture since Tylor's, including some that emphasize cognitive, linguistic, and communicative aspects to a greater degree. In the 1980s, postmodernist anthropologists questioned the entire concept of culture, arguing that it is not as uniform and static as traditional definitions had implied. But Tylor's classic definition has held up over time as being general, descriptive, and inclusive, even if contemporary anthropologists might use more cognitively oriented definitions.

Anthropology offers a holistic view of behavior, society, and culture—of complex issues in their entirety—that transcends disciplines. Anthropologists today are trained in quantitative survey methods, but our discipline arose through a method almost unique to anthropology, that of qualitative participant-observation research. This type of research required that the researcher live with the people under investigation, under the same conditions that they do. For example, while Green was conducting his PhD research in the early 1970s, he lived in a thatch hut in a Maroon village in the Amazon rain forest, conducting fieldwork in the Saramaka language.

Anthropology prides itself on taking a comparative view, one that avoids ethnocentrism, or viewing unfamiliar behaviors and institutions through the eyes of one's own traditions. According to the principle of cultural relativism, we strive to not judge the behavior and social patterns of others, particularly in societies different from our own, by the standards of our own culture. We analyze each culture on its own terms and in most matters strive to suspend value judgments. Of course, this cultural relativism does not necessarily mean *moral* relativism, and we are not suggesting that anthropologists should suspend value judgments on matters, for instance, such as rape and violence.

In the early years of the discipline, anthropologists deliberately sought to study cultures as different from their own cultures as possible. That meant studying hunting and gathering bands, tribally organized minority peoples, or disempowered peasants during the colonial and postcolonial eras. As anthropologists immersed in the lives of non-Western people, we typically underwent a profound transformative process whereby we came to see the world through the eyes of people whose culture was very different from ours. Because our fieldwork was "on the ground" and involved intense interpersonal interaction and sharing the hardships of subsistence, we could not fail to see the injustices faced by the people with whom we lived. For example, postindependence governments often pressed ahead with modernization with little consideration for tribal rights over large tracts of rainforest (or other resources), leading to trampling of land rights and human rights among minority populations. As anthropologists, we developed empathy and sympathy for these "Fourth World" peoples (a term referring to minorities in the Third World) and often found ourselves fighting for protection and justice for the underdog.

This was sometimes called advocacy or action anthropology, a form of applied anthropology in which anthropological tools are used to solve problems that face a people or a community of study, or, more broadly, to achieve specific social and policy goals. Anthropologists developed an inclination to criticize and challenge prevailing political authority, as well as conventional wisdom, which often meant criticizing a Western or European perspective. At times, we identified and exposed the economic self-interests of elite groups such as multinational corporations, when their interests and actions were at odds with the well-being of minority or otherwise disempowered groups.

This type of total immersion fieldwork in an alien culture for one or two years—once the norm—is becoming less common. Qualitative methods are still a hallmark of anthropology, and among qualitative methods, long-term participant observation has perhaps been the gold standard. Qualitative methods are well suited to studying sensitive or complex subjects, such as human sexual behavior or drug addiction. These methods are particularly useful when we don't know much about the subject area or when the information sought is of a sensitive nature. In the first case, we would not know what questions to ask in a survey, let alone how to ask them. Nor would we have a framework for understanding the resulting answers. Second, information may relate to private, highly personal behavior such as sexual intercourse or bodily excretion, or to something illegal, such as drug use. In such a case, surveys would also be unlikely to elicit accurate (valid) information.

For example, to gain knowledge about crack cocaine addicts and their subculture, anthropologists have "hung out" on the street and in crack houses, immersing themselves in the subculture and befriending the addicts, part-time users, dealers, and criminals caught up in this lifestyle. *Crack Pipe as Pimp*, edited by Mitch Rattner (1993) and providing accounts from anthropologists in cities across the United States, provides a good example of this type of powerful, gripping inside account. Anthropologist Jack Weatherford, well known for his ethnography of the U.S. Congress (1985), worked as a clerk in a pornography shop in Washington, DC, to learn about the particular subculture surrounding pornography (1986). He was accepted into the subculture in part because he was willing to provide some addicts with "clean" urine of his own, so that the addicts could pass tests intended to detect drug use. Anthropologists such as Terri Leonard and Deborah Pellow brought ethnographic methods to the study of another high-risk group: commercial sex workers and their clients, both in the United States and in Africa (Leonard 1990; Pellow 1977).

THE CHECKERED HISTORY OF ANTHROPOLOGY'S STUDY OF SEXUALITY

Some anthropologists argue that the discipline of anthropology was slow to take on sexual behavior as a significant or even valid domain of research. Anthropology's relationship to the study of sexual behavior has been complex and contradictory, and neither particularly courageous nor paradigm-shifting (Davis and Whitten 1987; Vance 1991). This may be partly because of a dubious legacy that anthropology has had to live down, which began with explorers and missionaries who told tales of unrestrained sexuality in Africa and other exotic locales. For instance, Richard Burton (an explorer regarded by many contemporaries as an anthropologist) wrote descriptions of African sexual practices to titillate the imaginations of prudish, sexually repressed Victorian readers—descriptions that anthropologist Quentin Gausset (2001) suggested might be better called ethnopornography.

It was sometimes difficult to distinguish anthropological accounts of sexual behavior from those of missionaries, explorers, or other amateur ethnographers. Leading anthropologists gave the world titles such as *The Sexual Life of Savages* (Malinowski 1929). Such works soon became something of an embarrassment, especially as once-remote tribal peoples become more urban and educated, sometimes earning PhDs in anthropology and studying Western cultures.

As anthropologist Carol Vance wrote in 1991, the prevailing cultural view was that "sexuality is not an entirely legitimate area of study, and that such study necessarily casts doubt not only on the research but on the motives and character of the researcher" (p. 875). Fear of being confused with ethnopornographers or of having prurient interests inhibited anthropological studies of sexual behavior from the 1950s to the early AIDS pandemic, some 30 years later. Although there have been major advances since 1991, the study of sexuality is still somewhat ill defined, at least in part because it transcends disciplinary boundaries.

To paraphrase a review of anthropological contributions to studies of sexuality, these include the social construction of sexuality (whether or not in antipathy to biomedical constructs) and of gender, identity, and sexual institutions such as prostitution. Sexuality may refer to behavior or to identity including biological identity (maleness or femaleness). Wider definitions, including those used by anthropologists, include the social foundation of sexual behavior, institutions, and structures. A third focus incorporates both orientation and preference (homosexuality, bisexuality, etc.) as well as passion, desire, and sexual response (Manderson et al. 1999).

With the rise of the AIDS pandemic, anthropologists were suddenly in demand to help gather accurate information on sexuality to explain why HIV was spreading so quickly in certain populations and parts of the globe. According to Gausset (2001), citing Fasin (1999):

> The state of "anthropological emergency," and the desire to save lives lowered the level of ethical, theoretical and methodological self-control of the researchers. . . . Like the first studies of African sexuality, it was once again the "exotic, traditional, irrational and immoral practices" that were the focus of the research. (p. 511)

To the extent that they have done fieldwork in the area of sexuality, most anthropologists have historically followed what is called the "cultural influence model." This model "acknowledges cross-cultural variation in the expression of sexuality," but "the manifestation of sexuality and its assumed biological impetus and ultimate reproductive function is generally viewed as universally consistent" (Parker and Easton 1998). Traditional anthropology has viewed key elements of sexual behavior as culturally universal (Vance 1991), yet has also documented great variability in behavior, supplying a comparative perspective that becomes essential, for example when dealing with AIDS (Parker and Easton 1998; Vance 1991). Another strength of the cultural influence model has been its use of the tools of relativism and cross-cultural variability to "question the uniformity and inevitability of Western sexual norms and mores" (Parker and Easton 1998).

Conventional anthropology also emphasizes the roles of culture and learning in shaping sexual behavior and attitudes, such as in rites of passage that initiate adolescents to adulthood and appropriate gender roles and identities. Anthropologists have long provided ethnographic accounts of societies in which sexual customs are markedly different from those in the West. Within the cultural influence model, the core of sexuality is reproduction. Thus, marriage, pregnancy, reproduction, childbearing, child rearing, menstruation, and menopause were all given due attention, but there was little investigation of nonreproductive sexuality or erotic pleasure-seeking, nor did theoretical constructs develop in this area (Vance 1991:879). Although culture is thought to shape sexual expression in the form of behavior, norms, and customs, within the cultural influence model, the foundation of sexuality (known as the sex drive or sex impulse) is assumed to be universal and biologically determined (Vance 1991:878).

In recent years, social construction theory has largely replaced the cultural influence model among anthropologists and virtually all who study sexuality. Social construction theory challenges the notion that biology determines sexual identity and behavior and criticizes the cultural influence model for being essentialist and holding that certain phenomena such as sex roles are natural and inevitable (Irvine 1990, cited in Delamater and Hyde 1998). Within social constructionism, the idea of an objectively knowable truth does not exist; Knowledge is seen as an artifact constructed through social interpretation and the subjective or emic influences of a particular group, and hence influenced by values, language, and culture in general. Social constructionism holds that identity based on sexuality is an *achieved* status and is molded by specific historical and cultural settings (including language and discourse) rather than a biologically determined inherited status. Sexual identity is plastic and malleable, and gender roles are performed following recognizable "cultural scripts" (Parker and Gagnon 1995).

In much recent anthropological research on sexual behavior, emphasis has shifted to the social organization of sexual interactions, to these sexual scripts found in different social and cultural settings, and to the complex relations between meaning and power and how they constitute sexual experience. Foucault's pioneering work has led to a focus on the investigation of diverse "sexual cultures" and how they are perceived (Parker and Easton 1998) and hierarchically arranged.[1] Nonacademic activists have been the primary force behind the development of social construction theory, and feminist theory and activism have greatly influenced both social construction theory and anthropologists operating within the sexual liberation paradigm.

Considering the overwhelming evidence of diversity of women's roles cross-culturally, historically, and generationally, feminist theory also contests the implicit biological determinism in Western constructs of sexual behavior and gender differences, thereby validating social construction theory:

> The existence of cross-cultural variation contradicts the notion of universal gender roles and uniform female sexuality. This attention to the cultural variability of gender roles inspired an analytical reconfiguration of the categories of sexuality and gender, fueled by the struggle for reproductive rights. (Parker and Easton 1998)

Even with the advent of social constructionism, some anthropologists have criticized their discipline for being slow to discard essentialist views of sexuality. Vance, writing in 1991, warns against a return to the cultural influence model as the "commonsense, anthropological approach to sexuality." She observes:

> The recent development of a more cultural and non-essentialist discourse about sexuality has sprung not from the centre of anthropology but from its periphery, from other disciplines (especially history) and from theorizing done by marginal groups. The explosion of exciting and challenging work in what has come to be called social construction theory during the past 15 years has yet to be felt in mainstream anthropology. (p. 865)

But nonessentialist thinking about sex roles began much earlier, with the "founding mothers" of anthropology, Margaret Mead and Ruth Benedict. Mead and Benedict, in addition to being pioneers in anthropology, also struggled to make room for women in the university and scientific establishment. Benedict was in feminist rebellion against patriarchal systems at Columbia University and she soon enlisted Mead in her efforts. Both were students of Franz Boas, considered the father of American anthropology; Boas, for his part, was determined to challenge biological determinism, the prevalent thinking of his day, by showing how much of human life is shaped by culture. Mead and Benedict also planted other seminal ideas in the field of anthropology, such as notions that sex roles are simply social inventions and are not determined by biology.

In her 1928 classic *Coming of Age in Samoa*, Mead popularized the idea of sexual freedom, especially for young females, famously claiming that the Samoans enjoyed lives of free love and pre- and extramarital liaisons without the burden of shame, guilt, or sexual jealousy. *Coming of Age* was tremendously popular, and, even after Mead's death 50 years later, was still selling 100,000 copies a year (Dalrymple 2000). The unsubtle subtext to Mead's work was that adolescent sexual behavior (and sexual behavior generally) should not be controlled, and that attempts to do so were antipleasure and would have negative effects. Such a message was embraced by many who felt that Western culture was repressed and that fewer sexual constraints would lead to the end of guilt, shame, jealousy, anxiety, frustration, hypocrisy, and confusion. When the first panel on gay issues was held at the 1974 American Anthropological Association meeting in Mexico City, Margaret Mead served as one of the discussants and was described as "at her best . . . there with her transsexual secretary, relatively open about her bisexuality, [and] absolutely tremendously supportive" (Amory n.d.).

The quality and validity of the fieldwork for which Mead is best known was later called into serious question by careful, longer term research that found that Samoan teenage girls were actually about as sexually liberated as girls in Victorian England. Anthropologist Derek Freeman, beginning with his 1986 book *Margaret Mead and Samoa: The Making and Unmaking of an Anthropological Myth* (and continuing through two additional books), challenged virtually all of Mead's findings on empirical grounds.[2] He found and interviewed some of Mead's key informants, one of whom (Fa'apua'a Fa'amu) testified that she and another Samoan woman, both young women at the time, had made up stories for Mead, according to the common Samoan practice of hoaxing known as *taufa'ase'e*. According to Fa'amu, Mead "failed to realize that we were just joking and must have been taken in by our pretences" (Freeman 1986:viii). As a result of investigation by Freeman and others, many anthropologists today regard Mead's fieldwork in Samoa to have little or no scientific value. But that work marked the beginning of a revolution in understanding the impact of culture, and Mead's portrayal of Samoa found fertile ground (in anthropology and beyond) among people who wanted to believe in a society without sexual inhibitions, jealousy, or constraints to sexual expression.

We should remember that Mead (and Benedict) had no data on sexual behavior to go by and that in the 1920s there was little appreciation of the influence of culture. They lived in an age when Freud's ideas about the power of libido operating at an unconscious level were gaining popularity in the academic world and among educated people. Herbert Marcuse would further develop Freud's idea (presented in *Civilization and Its Discontents*) that the all-powerful sex instinct is unnaturally repressed by society, with Marcuse making the case that society can and should overthrow this repression and free Eros (the god of love). On the other hand, Freudian diagnostic language was used to label virtually all exceptions to heterosexual norms and behavior as pathological, which interfered with objective appraisal of variance in sexual cultures (Herdt 1999).

The developing sexual liberation paradigm also owed much to philosopher Michel Foucault and sex researcher Alfred Kinsey, whose ideas have had far-reaching impacts. Foucault seems to have believed that we once lived in a blissful, polymorphously perverse world of innocence, without divisive categories of homo- and heterosexual (as if such divisions were invented in Foucault's 18th-century France). A recent sociology textbook adopts Foucault's notion that the classification of homosexual is a recent invention, stating that "Michel Foucault *showed* that before the 18th century, the notion seems barely to have existed" (Giddens and Duneier 2000:450; emphasis added). Scholars continue to cite Michel Foucault's *History of Sexuality* as if he were a scientific authority who had done systematic studies. Yet he was a gay man consigned to the margins of French society at a time when homosexuals had to hide their sexual identity. We can be entirely sympathetic to Foucault yet acknowledge that he had an axe to grind against a homophobic world, a fact that certainly compromised his objectivity when it came to his Eurocentric study of sexuality.

Kinsey's personal persuasions also made him less than objective as a researcher. James H. Jones's 1997 biography of Kinsey describes him as a bisexual who experimented in masochism and engaged in sex with his research staff, and Kinsey deliberately sought outliers in his studies of sexual behaviors, recruiting men in prisons, group sex parties, and gay hang-outs. His research violated what has become the fundamental rule of survey research: Use a randomly selected sample, at least if you plan to generalize your results to whole populations (such as the United States).

Although the lack of rigor of Kinsey's research methods is now acknowledged, Kinsey's research is nonetheless defended by a number of contemporary sexologists and anthropologists (Parker et al. 2004:366). A recent article in *Annual Review of Sex Research* states that "Kinsey started this huge project before modern sampling methods had been devised" (Bankcroft 2004:23), as if this disclaimer conferred validity on Kinsey's results. In their textbook *Perspectives on Human Sexuality,* anthropologists, Anne Bolin and Patricia Whelehan describe Kinsey's "scientific rigor" and "concern for representativeness" (2004:32). A current sociology textbook implies that Kinsey was right in believing it impossible "to persuade a randomly selected group of Americans to answer deeply personal questions about their sexual behavior" (Giddens and Duneier 2000:449). This text then offers as fact Kinsey's dubious findings that "no more than half of all American men are completely heterosexual, judged by their sexual activities and inclinations after puberty" and "37% of men had had at least one homosexual experience to the level of orgasm" (p. 450).

Many anthropologists remain dedicated not just to a defense of Kinsey's research, but also to a Kinseyan view of human sexuality. People and societies are deemed "sex positive" or "sex negative," based on the litmus test of their acceptance of the free expression of virtually all forms of sexual expression. For instance, Bolin and Whelehan write of a particular *"sex positive* Polynesian culture in which premarital sex is the norm" (2004:226). Those who do not embrace sufficiently "liberated" sexual norms are labeled "sex negative" or accused of having a phobia (such as homophobia or erotophobia). Andreas Philaretou has described erotophobia as a type of "antisexualism," which is "aimed at discouraging individuals from aspiring toward a more liberal, naturalistic, and expressive erotic and sexual ethos" (2006:293).

Anthropologists such as Margaret Mead, researchers such as Kinsey, and gay intellectuals such as Foucault built on a momentum developed by Freud, Marcuse, and others and helped spark the sexual revolution and a radical reshifting of the way that the academic establishment and society as a whole regarded sexuality. Their "findings" may have been highly suspect according to the standards of empirical research, but this mattered little as Western culture—or the zeitgeist—was ready for a radical change in sexual norms, values, and behavior. This change was spurred by high mobility, the advent of automobiles, and increasing urban anonymity. The advent the availability of effective contraception and treatment for sexually transmitted infections removed much of the risk of pregnancy and disease from sexual intercourse. Casual sex came to be regarded as safe, liberating, fun, freely available, and something that members of modern consumer cultures felt much freer to consume. Divorce rates rose. Lesbians and gays came out of the closet and fought for and earned their civil liberties. Sexology, erotics, queer theory, and the anthropology of sexuality came out of the academic closet, so to speak, and moved from the margins of scholarship more into the mainstream, in the process forming alliances with feminist theory and the feminist movement, reproductive health and family planning, feminism, postmodernism, and other progressive academic and social movements. Sexual liberation had become a force to be reckoned with.

ANTHROPOLOGISTS' AIDS WORK IN THE CONTEXT OF FOUR PARADIGMS

Anthropologists have been involved in studying AIDS from the very beginning of the pandemic and have contributed in so many diverse ways that at least one typology has developed to categorize and help explain these contributions. George C. Bond and Joan Vincent have suggested that since the advent of the AIDS pandemic nearly 30 years ago, anthropologists have assumed three basic roles within AIDS prevention, those of *handmaiden, cultural expert,* and *political economist.*[3] This typology is useful in bringing the diverse contributions of anthropologists into a framework that links roles with paradigms (sets of assumptions, or meta-narratives of thought and discourse). In light of the material covered in the last section, we expand the three roles suggested by Bond and Vincent to include a fourth, that of anthropologist as *sexologist*, operating within what we call the sexual liberation paradigm.

Thus, the four roles and their respective paradigms are:

1. anthropologists as handmaidens, within the biomedical paradigm;
2. anthropologists as cultural experts, within the community paradigm;
3. anthropologists as political economists, within the structural violence paradigm; and
4. anthropologists as sexologists, within the sexual liberation paradigm.

Bond and Vincent do not present the first three roles as equivalent types. They see them as progressing in a historical sequence and moving toward more enlightened thinking and effective engagement with AIDS. They see the first role type, that of *handmaiden*, as being less valuable and implying servility without independent or critical thought or perhaps even political awareness. Political economists, on the other hand, are seen as the most useful of the types.

All four roles have been there virtually from the beginning of the AIDS pandemic and they are all still very much present. Further, virtually all anthropologists have endorsed the biomedical approach to AIDS prevention (which has relied on condoms, testing, and drugs), even if they have *also* assumed other roles. A third point is that anthropologists (and others) might operate at the boundaries of this typology, cross boundaries, or contribute in two or more different types of roles. As in any typology, boundaries are inexact and the somewhat idealized types identified and characterized represent arbitrary cutoffs along a continuum. Finally, we believe that these paradigms are often unduly influenced by politics and ideology. The latter two roles (that of political activist and sexologist) in particular lend themselves to social and political activism and are driven by the belief that society must address inequalities or become more accepting of various forms of sexual expression and diversity to adequately address AIDS.

We look next at the way anthropologists have contributed as handmaidens, cultural experts, political economists, and sexologists to the fight against AIDS.

Anthropologists as Handmaidens within the Biomedical Paradigm

Before the advent of AIDS, anthropologists had already begun to lend their perspective, skills, and insights to health planning and delivery in non-Western countries (and among minority groups within Western cultures as well). When Green began consulting with or in connection with the United States Agency for International Development (USAID) in 1980, that important source of funding in international health had already began to require social soundness analyses of projects in certain parts of the world, such as sub-Saharan Africa. This meant that someone trained in anthropology or a closely allied field would review a project in the design phase to generally ensure "wide and significant participation of the poor in the development process," and specifically:

> (1) the compatibility of the activity with the sociocultural environment in which it is to be introduced (*its sociocultural-feasibility*); (2) the likelihood that the new practices or institutions introduced among the initial activity target population will be diffused among other groups (*i.e., the "spread effect"*); and (3) the *social impact* or distribution of benefits and burdens among different groups, both within the initial activity population and beyond. (USAID n.d., emphasis in the original)

This was for projects in all sectors, not only health, and it was one of several areas in which an increasing number of anthropologists began working with USAID and other major donors, as well as with the civil society groups they funded, during the 1970s and 1980s.

When global AIDS efforts emerged in the mid-1980s, a number of anthropologists were already involved in large-scale family planning and reproductive health programs and surveys of sexual behavior. This group, which included Edward Greeley, Priscilla Reining, Brooke Schoepf, Edward Green, and many others, thus had a head start in research in the new field of global AIDS (Gowan and Reining 1988). One area in which their skills were put to use was in the dynamic and relatively new field of social marketing, which brought together Madison Avenue marketers with experts in family planning and contraception.[4] USADI had become so interested in social marketing by 1985 that it launched a $21 million global program to promote contraceptives for family planning, called Social Marketing for Change (SOMARC). Researchers working under the SOMARC contract conducted some of the first studies of sexual behavior in connection with AIDS in developing countries, mostly concerning the promotion of condom use. Green served on the SOMARC Advisory Board in 1984 (albeit as something of a token anthropologist), drawing on resources such as the Human Relations Area Files and advising about the need to understand sexual behaviors and related subjects (such as gender relations and fertility beliefs) from several different levels, from the individual to the peer group, to family lineage, society, and culture.[5]

As the AIDS pandemic evolved, there was ever-greater reliance on social marketing and allied methods of family planning to get condoms distributed to as many people as possible. As social marketing became mainstream, market research methods such as focus group discussions became standard in public health and even anthropology. Those in the business marketing professions felt that they had developed market research techniques that could quickly teach marketers and advertisers what they needed to know about the consumer habits of various target audiences, typically stratified by socioeconomic factors. They reasoned it was simple to apply this formula to marketing contraceptives to Africans or Asians, and generally paid little attention to the occasional anthropological viewpoint that culture differences are more profound than consumer habits and brand name preferences for condoms. To the extent that behavior was considered or studied at all, the focus was on such things as consumer preference or purchasing aspects of behavior.

In Green's experience, anthropologists were involved in the new field of AIDS prevention mostly as adjuncts (or handmaidens) to social marketing programs or as researchers who were tasked with designing and implementing qualitative studies to evaluate condom marketing programs or provide formative research. Few anthropologists (or anyone else) took a step back to take a comprehensive, critical look at basic assumptions of AIDS prevention such as the reliance on technology and commodities and focus on marketing of products rather than understanding sexual behavior. There seemed to be an unspoken assumption that it was inappropriate or unrealistic to expect fundamental changes in sexual behavior, and neither social marketers nor others working in HIV prevention exhibited much interest in how to work in culturally sensitive ways to discourage risky behaviors.

Besides condom promotion, there are other components of AIDS prevention in which anthropologists have played a key role as handmaidens. For example, by the mid-2000s, enough research had been done on the protective effects of male circumcision that major AIDS organizations were gearing up to develop interventions that encouraged voluntary male circumcision. Robert Bailey, Edward Green, Daniel Halperin, and Priscilla Reining were among the first researchers in any field to study the relationship between the practice of male circumcision and HIV infection and prevalence (Green et al. 1993). Halperin and Bailey published an influential summary of evidence in *The Lancet* in 1999, and Bailey conducted one of the three landmark and policy-shifting randomized controlled trials showing that male circumcision is highly effective in reducing risk of HIV acquisition for adult men in Africa and perhaps elsewhere. Green's research and activism related to Uganda's behavior-based HIV-prevention approach, with significant help from Daniel Halperin, led to the adoption of the ABC policy (Abstain, Be Faithful, Use Condoms) by USAID (December 2002) and by PEPFAR a few months later, for African generalized epidemics. These are two examples of anthropologists having a significant influence on U.S. and global HIV/AIDS policy and programming.

The handmaiden role of serving biomedicine is probably the easiest to caricature. Anthropologists carry out surveys and focus groups at the behest and direction of medical authorities, often as part of multidisciplinary efforts. In the handmaiden role, we are asked to keep our focus within the terms of reference and not ask broader questions like: "Why are these particular people sick? Why do poor people get certain diseases more often that wealthier people?"

Bond and Vincent note the shortcomings of this role in the context of Uganda's first decade of anthropological involvement in AIDS. In an epidemic that was almost exclusively heterosexually transmitted, anthropologists were asked to do targeted research (i.e., on particular behaviors of a particular group) but were rarely asked to review existing treasure troves of anthropological literature on Ugandan cultures and behaviors, suggesting that the funding agencies were unaware of this literature (Bond and Vincent 1997:87). But anthropologists have made major contributions to biomedical research, including those (such as Bailey's circumcision trial) that have had a major impact on AIDS prevention priorities, and the term "handmaiden" probably does not do justice to them.

Anthropologists as Cultural Experts within the Community Paradigm

As *cultural experts,* anthropologists have been called on to explain what cultural factors might drive the wildly divergent AIDS epidemics seen in different parts of the world. This work could be said to operate within the *community paradigm,* because the focus is on cultural context of a particular society or community. Had anthropologists been less consigned to being handmaidens and more in the position of being decision-makers, they might have more effectively used the tools and resources of anthropology as cultural experts.

For example, a great deal of ethnographic research related to sexual and related behaviors in the context of various cultures already existed at the beginning of the AIDS pandemic, and anthropologists might have more systematically surveyed and synthesized this research to guide AIDS prevention efforts that did, after all, have to operate within the context of various cultures. Ironically, it was two demographers (not anthropologists) who first attempted such a review of sexuality literature. John and Pat Caldwell concluded that a relative lack of moral and institutional constraints on sexual practices in sub-Saharan Africa, particularly among women, along with weak marriage ties and a legacy of polygamy, resulted in a pattern of sexual permissiveness in sub-Saharan Africa. In their view, this sexual permissiveness went a long way toward explaining why HIV prevalence was so high in Africa (Caldwell et al. 1989). These conclusions have been quite controversial. Some anthropologists have questioned the empirical basis of the findings of the Caldwells and colleagues arguing, for instance, that in sub-Saharan Africa sexual behavior was quite socially regulated, especially for women (Le Blanc et al. 1991; Denis 2006).

Whether the Caldwells' conclusions are justified or not, we argue that there has not been enough attention given to the various cultural factors that underlie sexual behaviors and the spread of HIV within populations. The kind of controversy stirred up by the conclusions of Caldwell and colleagues is perhaps just the kind of robust debate we need about the relationship between culture and HIV—not just among Western researchers, but including members of these cultures. On the other hand, we believe that when culture has been considered in the context of HIV, it has often been solely in a negative light, as something to blame. There has been an often unexpressed attitude among many Western AIDS experts that non-Western cultural practices were dangerous, dysfunctional, retrograde, and problematic when it comes to the spread of HIV/AIDS. In Chapter 2, we will explore a more "culture-positive" view of culture and AIDS, including examples of how many cultural practices can provide a positive basis from which to address AIDS.

The fact that the AIDS field has been plagued by ethnocentric thinking and mistaken assumptions about sexual behaviors in non-Western cultures is somewhat understandable considering how early research unfolded. For example, early in the African epidemics, some studies conducted among highly *non*-representative men and women, such as truck drivers, fishermen, traders, and sex workers, showed very high numbers of sexual partners. These data were assumed to be representative and it was therefore concluded that just as among MSM in the West, African heterosexual HIV transmission could be blamed on high numbers of sexual partners (Kocheleff 2006; Packard and Epstein 1991). Researchers also erred in assuming that African epidemic patterns were similar to those in other parts of the world and that homosexuality and drug use were likewise key risk factors in Africa (Kocheleff 2006).

The epidemic spreads of HIV in Africa has been particularly blamed on male sexuality; African men have been stereotyped as hypersexual and possessing unrestrained sexuality (Gausset 2001:511). They have also been accused of indulging in practices such as widow inheritance (marriage of a widow to her dead husband's brother), sex with much younger women or even rape of babies, large numbers of sexual partners, and circumcision and scarification rituals practiced on a large scale with the same knife. These practices have some factual basis in some African populations, but the attention they have received as drivers of AIDS in Africa has been out of proportion to their epidemiological importance, whereas the more important but mundane practices that spread AIDS (as well as positive and protective cultural practices) are relatively ignored. The combined corrective contributions from anthropologists as cultural experts have not been sufficient to present an alternative narrative script to the stereotype of the sexually irresponsible African man engaging in exotic and dangerous cultural practices.

Within the AIDS field, men are depicted as "playing marginal and somewhat villainous roles" in the narratives of women, according to several basic scripts (Bingenheimer 2010). Husbands leave wives in the village work and live elsewhere, often acquiring a girlfriend in their new place of residence and simultaneously failing to provide for the wife at home. Poor rural or urban women are forced to engage in transactional sex to feed themselves and their children, and the men with whom they have sexual relationships put them at risk of HIV infection (often refusing to use condoms). Adolescent girls are similarly put at risk by men (likely to be HIV infected and unlikely to submit to condom use) when they exchange sex for money or gifts from an older male "sugar daddy," to provide for basic needs or school fees, or to elevate their social status through acquiring consumer goods (Bingenheimer 2010; Luke 2003). These scripts describe the reality of many women's lives, but we would challenge the extent to which they have become *the* narrative of women's experience, along with the assumption that African women are powerless and therefore individual behavior change is a luxury that they simply cannot afford.[6] These issues will be taken up in more detail in Chapter 9.

In studying sexual cultures, anthropologists have also focused on norms of female sexual behavior, based on the assumption that women's sexual conduct is more tightly controlled and that men operate with relative freedom. Studies of premarital sexuality also have mostly focused on women, reflecting the fact that the cultural management of female sexuality tends to be stricter and more observable (e.g., out-of-wedlock pregnancy) than is control of male sexuality prior to marriage in most societies. According to one summary of the anthropological literature on sexual behavior, there seem to be few rules in most societies that operate to control male sexuality prior to marriage—in fact, male sexual inexperience by the time of marriage may be considered a liability—and within the institution of marriage there is less control of men than of women (Manderson et al. 1999). Another view is that men perhaps do not operate with quite the degree of sexual freedom often attributed to them and that (according to the author of a study of men's sexual partnerships in 15 African countries) men, like women, operate within "traditional mechanisms of social control" (Bingenheimer 2010).

In 1988, Francis Conant pointed out that sexual relations everywhere are constrained by culturally based expectations on the part of individuals as well as by the rules and institutions governing relationships between groups. In his words,

> Thus the topics relevant to AIDS begin but by no means end with normative patterns of gender acquisition and sexual maturation, and reproductive and non-reproductive sexual behavior. If HIV is mainly or even only sexually transmitted, a number of different topics are involved: kinship restrictions on sexual behavior, rules of exogamy and endogamy regulating marriage, belief systems, perceptions of health and disease, and support systems for the care of the desperately sick and dying. There are whole sets of behaviors that initially appear only remotely connected to sexual behavior but are nonetheless there as constraints on, or inducements to, particular patterns of sexuality, gender behavior and gender relations. In dealing with AIDS we are not just dealing with sex; we are dealing with lifeways and complex culture patterns. (p. 198)

In a chapter in the same volume, Green (1988) stressed the need to understand African cultures to find ways to influence sexual and related behaviors, observing that having many wives or sex partners tends to bring high status for men, but "a good deal of female behavior in Africa can be viewed as economic survival and adaptation to patterns of male dominance" (p. 180). Green also suggested that promoting reduction in numbers of sexual partners should be the key intervention in Africa and that partner reduction must be accompanied by empowering African women to be able to refuse unwanted sex. Daniel Halperin (Halperin and Allen 2000) conducted early research of approaches to AIDS prevention that focused on changing sexual behavior, including targeting multiple and concurrent sexual partnerships. Suzanne Leclerc-Madlala's work on transactional and intergenerational sex helped focus attention on the special vulnerability of young women in southern Africa and the need for behavior change programs that are informed by local cultural logics for prestige and economic advancement (Leclerc-Madlala 2001, 2003, 2008).

Anthropologists also lent their skills as cultural experts to understanding the behavior of groups at high risk in concentrated epidemics, including intravenous drug users (IDUs). The February 1987 *Anthropology Newsletter* published an RFP (request for proposals) calling for anthropologists interested in "research on intravenous drug-using subcultures, influence of social and cultural factors on intravenous drug abuse, identification of factors associated with the progression from nonuse to casual use to compulsive intravenous use . . . to better understand the contribution role of IDU to HIV incidence and prevalence."

Anthropologists such as Philippe Bourgois, Merrill Singer, and Michael Agar have been at the forefront of AIDS prevention among IDU and the ethnography of addicts. Agar had written ethnographies of heroin users prior to the emergence of AIDS, and AIDS-related IDU research reports began to appear, such as a study in Miami that used ethnographic methods to study syringe sharing, use of shooting galleries, drug sharing between syringes, accidental punctures, and related behavior of IDUs (Page et al. 1990). Despite the anthropological contribution toward the understanding of drug-using behaviors, there was little focus on modifying drug-related risk behaviors.

Anthropologists as Political Economists within the Structural Violence Paradigm

Several decades into the AIDS pandemic, as prevention interventions have seemed to produce so few results, there has been a move away from individual-centric understandings of the epidemic toward an understanding of AIDS as fueled by structural factors such as poverty, lack of education, gender inequality and other forms of discrimination, and broad-level political and economic forces. Even before the advent of AIDS, critical anthropologists like Merrill Singer and Hans Baer focused on the links between disease and structural factors or forces, from a neo-Marxist, critical, and world systems theoretical perspectives. Critical medical anthropology is committed to praxis, to the merger of theory with social action to fight for the rights of the working-class, indigenous peoples and peasants, sexual minorities, and other oppressed groups (Baer et al. 2003:ix) and against "imperialist expansion and bourgeois cultural hegemony" (Baer 1997:1568). According to Baer and Singer, health systems in the capitalist world are exploitative and driven by profit-seeking, with little regard for the health or well-being of workers or the polluted and often dangerous environments in which they live and work.

In the era of AIDS, anthropologists have functioned as *political economists* or indeed *political activists*. Political economy–oriented anthropologists like Paul Farmer and Jim Yong Kim have argued that *structural violence*—namely, societal "structures" such as racism, sexism, and other inequalities—causes direct and indirect harm to individuals and should be the principal perspective through which to understand AIDS (Farmer 1996).

Within the structural violence paradigm, sexual risk taking is seen as just one more manifestation of poverty and structural inequalities. The poor don't need condoms as much as they need money, power, and collective bargaining muscle. Exploitative systems need to be challenged and injustice redressed, and this takes precedence over, for example, an approach that focuses on changing risky sexual behaviors. For anthropologists adopting the role of political economists, it makes little sense to try to understand or prevent AIDS in South Africa without fully taking into account structural inequalities caused by apartheid.

The structural violence paradigm has shed much-needed light on the macro-economic and other forces that underlie many diseases around the world, and Farmer and Kim have been among the strongest advocates for making antiretroviral treatment for AIDS available to the poor. As we will discuss in Chapter 8, however, the assumptions made by the structural violence paradigm about the relationship between structural factors (such as poverty) and HIV largely do not hold true, particularly in Africa. We believe that the structural violence paradigm cannot fully explain the spread of HIV, nor will doing away with structural inequalities end the AIDS pandemic, either in poor countries or rich ones.

In our opinion, AIDS prevention efforts have largely failed not primarily because people are at the mercy of structural factors (although we do not mean to dismiss the influence of these factors), but because we have not pursued the right prevention policies aimed at changing cultural forces and individual behaviors. Within certain parts of the public health community, there has been an extreme reaction against notions of individual psychology, choice, or self-control. Women particularly are often depicted as victims of circumstances beyond their own control. As we will discuss in later chapters, the reality is somewhat more complicated. And in the most successful AIDS response ever, that of Uganda during the late 1980s and early 1990s, there was a strong emphasis on what *individuals* themselves could do to change (or maintain) behavior, and they were empowered to do these things so as *not* to become HIV infected.

Further, although anthropologists operating within the structural violence paradigm provide a valuable perspective, their approach does not adequately capitalize on anthropology's comparative advantage—i.e., a rich understanding of the local cultural context. A structural violence paradigm, therefore, risks ignoring an important level of anthropological analysis—the local culture (Ramin 2007:127). Paul Farmer's influential book *AIDS and Accusation*, based on his ongoing fieldwork and clinical experience (as an anthropologist and physician) in Haiti during the 1980s, argues that the spread of AIDS in Haiti was not because of "cultural factors" such as Voodoo beliefs and practices. Rather, the underlying cause was socioeconomic factors such as crippling poverty, the lack of an adequate biomedical health-care system, and exposure to a sex tourism trade that catered to Americans.[7] We agree with Farmer that in looking for explanations for the spread of AIDS, culture should not be made the scapegoat, but a purely structural explanation does little to explain how culture might be related (in various and by no means all negative ways) to the unique epidemiology of AIDS in Haiti.

Anthropologists as Sexologists within the Sexual Liberation Paradigm

The sexual liberation paradigm grew out of the sexual revolution of the 1960s and 1970s, in which gay activists, feminists, and others sought equal rights and recognition (legal and societal), and rejected "heteronormative," traditional sexual morality. As previously discussed, the sexual revolution can trace its roots back to Mead and Benedict, who asserted that sexual constraints were mere social constructions (and therefore optional); to Freud, who associated conservative sexual mores with being neurotic, uptight, and guilt-ridden about sexuality; and to Kinsey, who pulled back to the curtain to reveal (or allege) that mainstream sexual morality was little more than hypocrisy.

But this was in the West. Many regions of the world have yet to have a comparable sexual revolution, and many societies and cultures remain bastions of sexual conservatism. As sexual mores change around the world (sometimes quite rapidly), anthropologists may be able to serve as cultural brokers and help mitigate the clash of values, beliefs, norms, and expectations. They should certainly be at the forefront of brokering or mediating between the *culture* of donor organizations and that of recipient groups or countries and pointing out the lack of AIDS interventions geared toward majority, largely rural, more sexually conservative populations. Yet anthropologists in the sexual liberation vein often view sexual conservatism as problematic and approach cultural resistance to sexual liberalism with a battering ram and a firm conviction that such cultures need to be "liberated" from antiquated moral values regarding sex.

Douglas Feldman and Ralph Bolton, two anthropologists with long experience in AIDS, have been major proponents of the sexual liberation paradigm as well as influential voices in the AIDS and anthropology community. The cause of sexual liberation has strongly influenced discourse about AIDS in at least one public forum, the AIDS and Anthropology Research Group (AARG). Feldman contributed the following comment to an online AARG discussion forum, in response to an African woman who had written "[L]et us take responsibility for every soul that will perish because of our great teachings about the condom":

> Unlike gibbons and some other mammals, humans are not naturally monogamous. Some major religions make polypartnering (having sex with several partners) a sin in order to promote monogamy. However, there is nothing intrinsically wrong with polypartnering. . . . The ideology of the sexual revolution which occurred in North America and Western Europe during 1965–75 was very important in breaking down the Victorian morality of the past, allowing people to become more sexually free. I believe this was a positive change in human growth, and we should not use the

HIV/AIDS crisis as an excuse to revert back to a monastic view of sex. We need to be more sex positive, and encourage people to feel they can become open to sexual experiences with different people. There is nothing wrong with sex with different partners. The problem is not the sex, but the failure to prevent unwanted pregnancies and sexually transmissible diseases. Responsible polypartnering requires condoms and birth control as a given at all times. We need to teach those who engage in the joys of polypartnering how to effectively protect themselves from potential dangers.[8]

Feldman has long been a champion of the idea that such a version of multi-partner, "sex positive" living is not only desirable but also available to those who use condoms properly. Gay journalist Gabriel Rotello, feminist (and current executive director of the International AIDS Society) Robin Gorna, and others have called this idea or approach to AIDS "the condom code." The condom code grew out of the gay community's resolve to act as if having a fatal virus doesn't make a difference in their sex lives (Gorna 1996; Rotello 1997). A number of anthropologists have called for supplying and delivering condoms as the main solution for Africa, as, for example, in a paper Douglas Feldman presented at the 2004 Society for Applied Anthropology meeting entitled "Creating a Viable AIDS Program for Africa: Condoms, Condoms, and More Condoms" (Feldman 2004). As will be discussed in Chapter 6, an ever-growing body of evidence that condoms have failed to curb HIV infections in Africa should cause even the most ardent condom supporter to question such a prescription, at least for that continent.

The sexual liberation paradigm holds a core belief that nothing should interfere with sexual freedom, including the threat of AIDS. Bolton has equated promotion of partner reduction with an attack on gays themselves: "Promiscuity was a key feature of gay culture as it evolved as it evolved, and attempts to extirpate promiscuity could be interpreted as an attack on gay culture and gay liberation" (1992:168). Similarly, psychologist Walt Odets famously argued that "[W]e are not addressing the human needs of the gay community by offering—or insisting upon—biological survival as an exclusive and adequate purpose for human life. . . . The reduction of HIV transmission can only be the *secondary* task because it must be built on the foundation of lives experienced as worth the trouble" (Odets 1994:1). For Odets, mere biological survival is clearly not the primary goal.

Yet we should not assume other societies share this view that survival is subordinate to sexual freedom. As anthropologists, we should recognize that in many parts of the world, sexual freedom is not a core cultural value, especially compared to survival in the face of a deadly disease. Sexual liberation is something that Africans (and members of other cultures) should decide for themselves.

The anthropologist-sexologist is in an awkward position. It is a fundamental tenet of anthropology to remain neutral about our subject matter. If the subject is something we cannot help but have our own strong views about, we are trained to suspend our personal norms, values, and ideas and simply report our findings. But when the subject is sex, this has been easier said than done. Many anthropologists have been unable to refrain from making value judgments about sexual behavior or from seeing the world through their own cultural lens. Perhaps because our own sexuality or sexual orientation is so linked to our core personal identities, most of us have very strong opinions about what is acceptable, normative, and healthy when it comes to sex. Many anthropologists seem uncomfortable with any restraints or constraints on sexual behavior, reflecting a worldview informed by the West's sexual revolution of the 1960s. We fail to see that our approach to prevention is out of sync with cultures that are still largely constrained by social or religious controls and traditional norms.

One reason for highlighting the sexual liberation paradigm is that a great many anthropologists who were pioneers in the emerging AIDS field and contributed to the development, perpetuation, and defense of the dominant biomedical AIDS prevention paradigm come right out of this tradition. The pervasive message of AIDS prevention arose as a direct result: Look to technology for answers and leave sexual behavior and sexual freedom alone. In a way that is inimical to the foundations of anthropological methodology, there has been little discussion among anthropologists of the sexual and drug-using behaviors that drive the spread of HIV or of how to work in culturally grounded ways to discourage these behaviors. Anthropologists have been wary of AIDS prevention approaches that conflict with the core Western value of sexual liberation. But whatever our personal values about sex, anthropologists have a particular obligation to respond objectively to diverse cultural values and beliefs about sexuality in non-Western cultures.

We are not arguing against a sexual liberation approach to AIDS from a moralistic point of view, only pointing out that it is ill suited to a country like Swaziland, which has been devastated by AIDS and which has the dubious honor of having the world's highest HIV prevalence. As Leclerc-Madlala has observed, indigenous Swazi (and Zulu) leaders and elders have attempted to revive the practice of virginity testing specifically because of a perceived existential threat to the survival of their people in the face of AIDS (Leclerc-Madlala 2001). Their common-sense and logic took them in an opposite direction from demanding more sexual freedom or license. Whatever outsiders to the cultures might think of virginity testing (something even anthropologists have had a hard time assessing or discussing outside a Western, feminist framework), we must let other cultures decide how values of sexual liberation do (or do not) fit into their own context.

Multiple and concurrent sexual partnerships are widely recognized as fueling the AIDS epidemic in Swaziland, and a 2007 UNDP Swaziland report frankly referred to premarital, extramarital, and multiple concurrent partner sex as "negative sexual practices" (UNDP 2007:4). Although this phrase might strike some in the West as judgmental, in our view it is simply a self-evident and honest statement that certain sexual behaviors are highly efficient in transmitting the AIDS virus and should therefore be discouraged not to promote any particular morality or lifestyle, but to promote health and the saving of lives. We need to let epidemiology—the basic facts of what leads to HIV infection and what does not—guide our prevention priorities, rather than letting prevention become bogged down in the politics of culture wars and competing visions of what constitutes healthy and normative sexuality.

Anthropologists as sexologists, along with others in the sexual liberation paradigm, have made important contributions to ensuring human rights and fighting discrimination and marginalization, particularly for sexual minorities and other vulnerable groups. Part of this push for rights is the movement to demand (and win) AIDS treatment for those who cannot afford to pay for it. The sexual liberation paradigm has also included a strong push for risk reduction measures, particularly for groups at high risk of HIV infection such as MSM and sex workers, and risk reduction practices such as condom use and clean needles have contributed to reducing the spread of HIV in some settings. (The contribution of risk reduction will be discussed in more detail in Chapter 5.)

Joining Paradigms to Epidemiology

As noted in the beginning of the chapter, in practice there is often considerable overlap between these paradigms, and most anthropologists (and others) working in HIV/AIDS probably borrow various perspectives and tools from these paradigms, at various times. Each paradigm offers useful perspectives, and we do not believe that any one is wholly sufficient on its own.

We *do* argue that whatever other perspectives (as cultural expert, political economist, or sexologist) an anthropologist brings to the matter of AIDS prevention, what we know about epidemiology must guide our conclusions about prevention. When we refer to the need to let epidemiological evidence guide prevention, we are not arguing for further medicalization of AIDS, which often is used to mean valuing treatment over prevention. There has been too much medicalization of AIDS already.

We want to *behaviorize* AIDS, if we might be permitted a neologism. Anthropologists should do what they do best, which is study culturally patterned sexual and related behaviors and then apply this knowledge in the service of reducing sickness and death. But we must also integrate this cultural perspective into what epidemiological research has taught us about AIDS.

We have noted that anthropologists have often resisted accepted epidemiological evidence, as if that evidence threatens other types of knowledge that they value. In our conversations with anthropologists or in online fora such as the AARG, some seem uncomfortable with the concept of risk groups or even risk behaviors, including evidence that HIV infection rates are closely associated with number of partners, lack of male circumcision, and other behavioral factors. They seem to fear that identifying key risk behaviors or risk groups will stigmatize and blame certain individuals or groups, while making other groups feel that they are not at risk. The message of much of HIV prevention has become, "We are all at risk of AIDS." This has a nice, egalitarian ring ("We are all in this thing together"), but it is simply not true. With the exception of a handful of generalized epidemics, in most places in the world the great majority of people are actually at very low risk. Differences in epidemiological patterns, cultural settings, and risk factors are real, calling for a fine-tuned and epidemiologically informed approach to prevention.

Anthropologists have been known to challenge that there is a difference between types of epidemics, such as between "African AIDS" (or generalized epidemics) and epidemic patterns which have come to be called concentrated epidemics. Maryinez Lyons called African AIDS a biomedical construct or paradigm "which, like all accepted scientific models, has been powerful in its influence and difficult to dislodge" (1997:133). She quotes a now-dated source, which asserts: "There is a widespread myth that AIDS in Africa, and the way it is transmitted, is somehow different from AIDS in developed countries. . . . African AIDS is transmitted in exactly the same way as AIDS in other societies (Duh 1991:53)." In fact, patterns of transmission are quite different in the hyper-epidemics of southern Africa.

During a 2009 discussion on the AARG listserv, a number of anthropologists posted comments that showed they had little interest in the epidemiological evidence for either sexual behavior change or male circumcision, two interventions that are strongly supported by existing evidence and increasingly being accepted by major donors as critical in African hyper-epidemics.[9] One anthropologist commented that randomized controlled trials (long the gold standard of scientific evidence and research) were not necessarily any stronger or weaker than any other type of evidence. Other participants in the discussion did not seem to accept data that consistently show that wealth and mobility are key risk factors in Africa and that AIDS is *not* more prevalent among the poor. For example, one contributor argued for greater investment in poverty reduction for AIDS prevention, suggesting that behavioral approaches are passé (even as addressing sexual behaviors is becoming a top priority in the world's most severe epidemics in southern Africa):

> The people I know who are working on interventions aren't giving ABC [abstain, be faithful, use condoms] much attention these days and the focus is moving toward poverty reduction and social empowerment. . . . If all the money spent on western interventions and ABC campaigns had gone into genuine poverty reduction programs that empower and strengthen civil society (in the public sphere sense of critical social theory rather than through NGOs) we would probably be looking at a very different picture right now.[10]

NOTES

1. This refers to the manner in which "different sexual practices, expressions, identities, and communities are ranked, from the most normative and socially approved to the most stigmatized and despised" (see Miller and Vance 2004:6).
2. Freeman conducted fieldwork in Samoa off and on for 40 years, learned the Samoan language, and was given a chiefly title that allowed him to attend the chiefly assemblies, giving him far more exposure to Samoan life than Mead had ever enjoyed.
3. The same typology is used by Brodie Ramin (2007).
4. Social marketing attempts to use commercial marketing techniques to promote products that are desirable from a public health viewpoint, such as contraceptives or oral rehydration salts. The basic idea is to market the product through existing wholesale and retail channels to reach the maximum number of "consumers." The product tends to be sold at a relatively low, subsidized price at first, but some degree of program cost recovery is possible because the product is sold, not given free.
5. The Human Relations Area Files are a searchable data base of ethnographic data on sexual behavior in diverse cultural settings, housed at Yale University, New Haven, Connecticut.
6. This was a theme repeated throughout an otherwise useful 11-country conference on acknowledging African culture: The HIV/Culture Confluence: Changing the River's Flow: Possibilities and Challenges in Programming, April 12–13, 2010, Johannesburg, South Africa (SAFAIDS).
7. For a contrast between two distinct approaches to AIDS and engaging indigenous medicine (i.e., Edward Green's and Paul Farmer's), see Steinglass 2001.
8. This posting was made sometime before 2003 and was reposted by Green in a discussion on the AARG listserv on April 1, 2003 (found at http://groups.

creighton.edu/aarg/prevention.html [accessed April 1, 2010]). In a reply to the listserv, Feldman stated about his earlier posting that "I wouldn't change a word of it today (although I now prefer the term multipartnering instead of polypartnering)" (AARG).

9. We have noticed an increased civility in online AARG discussions compared to previous years, and there is more tolerance now for a diversity of viewpoints.

10. Comment posted on AARG listserv, March 31, 2009.

Chapter 2

SEX, CULTURE, AND DISEASE

Beginning in the 19th century, a number of explorers, adventurers, missionaries, and amateur anthropologists produced highly ethnocentric, sensational, moralizing accounts of native sexual behavior. By the 1950s, some anthropologists who did long-term fieldwork in Africa had developed a different position. Writing of the Zulu, Max Gluckman observed:

> [O]ld records on the Zulu . . . indeed affirm that they were a "moral" people among whom divorce, adultery, and illegitimacy were rare. Chastity was highly valued, and was part of the ethical code enforced by the age set regimental organization which was directly under the king. Regiments could only begin to marry when the king gave them permission as a set to marry a younger age set of girls, who by this time would be well in their twenties. (1956:181)

More recently, the advent of AIDS has renewed interest in exotic sexual practices that purportedly spread AIDS. These include: sex and marriage at very young ages (especially for girls); polygyny and multiple sexual partners; inheritance of widows whose husbands had died of AIDS; circumcision and scarification rituals that might spread HIV through contaminated cutting instruments; rape and coercion of women and girls, including by "sugar daddies"; beliefs that sex with a virgin, even a baby, could cleanse one of AIDS; extremely high STI rates; and reports that some men were actually proud to have an untreated STI (De Bruyn et al. 1995). A 10-country research report on multiple and concurrent sexual partnerships in southern Africa refers to "culture and social norms" such as polygamy, widow inheritance, female subordination, and postpartum sexual taboos, all of which are depicted as drivers or exacerbators of the hyper-epidemics of southern Africa (Jana et al. 2008). The report did not mention positive cultural practices that might mitigate the spread of HIV. Thus, even good studies fall back into the habit of seeing African culture only in a negative light almost any time that AIDS and African cultural practices are discussed together.

As one researcher writes about Uganda, "Early researchers were look-ing for things to blame, and identified African cultural practices as cul-prits" (Gausset 2001:511). The list of possible culprits has run the gamut from practices that seem to be more the stuff of urban legend than reality (e.g., having sex with a virgin as a cure for AIDS[1]) to those that undoubt-edly are significant contributors to the spread of HIV (e.g., multiple and concurrent sexual partners) (Epstein 2007). The implied or stated solution to soaring HIV transmission rates has been to stamp out seemingly dan-gerous cultural practices, like dry sex, polygyny, coming-of-age rituals, and widow inheritance, and to bring the law down on sugar daddies.

Even if doing so might reduce HIV transmission, we must remem-ber that some of these interventions may appear to Africans to be yet another example of cultural hegemony, of white Americans advising black Africans to renounce their heritage. Africans have also noticed that public health programs do not normally target for annihilation *Western* cultural practices that spread HIV, but instead offer far less draconian solutions, such as safer sex and clean needles. In the West, anyone who proposes that people give up anal sex, sex work, or drug use will be assumed, at least in public health and AIDS circles, to be a religious or cultural conservative and homophobe, rather than to be promoting a public health solution.

Clearly, not all cultural practices are positive or neutral when it comes to HIV/AIDS; some must be reexamined and modified if the struggle against AIDS is to be won. Yet African cultures also have many pro-tective practices and platforms from which to build an effective AIDS response. These positive elements are less often acknowledged and dis-cussed, much less brought into AIDS prevention.

Reflecting on the differences between Western and African attitudes toward sickness and healing, Godfrey Tangwa of the University of Yaounde, Cameroon, writes that in traditional African society, medicine was divorced from commerce and that "the resources of the immediate community were always mobilised on behalf of a seriously ill person" (2005:179). When it came to selling goods, the seller would take into account the poverty and need of the buyer, and if the item was needed by a sick person the price was often very cheap or free. Tangwa notes that, in contrast, Western commerce is based on the laws of supply and demand (i.e., the more a product or service is needed, the more expensive it becomes). He observes:

> The response to the HIV/AIDS pandemic in Africa has so far ignored im-portant traditional African values and attitudes toward disease and com-merce. These values and attitudes are significantly different from the lib-ertarian, market-driven, profit-oriented values and practices of important

sectors of the Western world. To deal with this epidemic, the world should consider respect for, and possibly even adoption of those African values.

There are also conspiracy theories to contend with, such as those that blame whites for inventing AIDS and injecting it into blacks. These might be especially potent in and around South Africa, where for years key figures in the Mbeki government denied the causal role of HIV and claimed the West was blaming the victim. Other parts of the legacy of apartheid also nurtured conspiracy theories, such as the realities (revealed in the Truth and Reconciliation Commission) that black women would sometimes get sterilized without their knowledge or consent and that some white scientists tried to manufacture drugs in their laboratories to destroy black fertility (Carton 2006).

We argue for a "culture-positive" approach to behavior change and HIV prevention, meaning that we look for the opportunities African culture provides for developing effective behavior change communication strategies. HIV prevention programs are often implemented as if African culture and leadership structures were nonexistent or merely a series of obstacles to overcome before achieving an effective, human rights-based set of HIV prevention interventions. Programs involving collaboration with indigenous or traditional healers, in HIV prevention as well as in primary health care, child diarrheal disease, and family planning, have been largely successful (Janzen and Green 1999a, 2003; Oyeneye 1985; Warren 1982).

INDIGENOUS THEORIES OF DISEASE

Anthropologists generally hold that etiology (the cause attributed to illness) is the key to understanding indigenous theories of illness as well as the prevention and treatment practices associated with those theories. Many Western observers have described African etiology as mostly supernatural or personalistic and assumed that by and large, Africans believed AIDS to be the result of witchcraft (Ankrah 1992; Bond and Vincent 1997; Miller and Rockwell 1988). There is a widespread belief among health professionals, including AIDS donors and organizations, that African medicine is a system that is irreconcilable with ours (Foulkes 1992; Velimirovic 1984; Ventevogel 1992). Many African physicians are especially critical of those with whom they compete for patients. According to one: "Most of it [traditional medicine] is based on superstition, meaningless pseudo-psychological mumbo-jumbo, which is positively harmful" (Motlana quoted in Freeman and Motsei 1990). When Africans do not quickly embrace whatever is offered them from the alien system, they are criticized for being stubborn or backward.

Western biomedicine is often promoted as if there were no medical system already in place, as if Africa were a *tabula rasa*. In fact, Africa possesses an extensive indigenous system of treatment and healing for physical maladies; it is generally accepted that about 80% of the people of sub-Saharan Africa rely on traditional healers for treatment of all conditions, even if many also visit hospitals (Bannerman et al. 1983). Research suggests that traditional healers see and attempt to treat many or most STIs in southern Africa, if not in all of Africa (Good 1987; Green 1999a; Nzima 1995). Healers also provide "vaccinations" and participate in ritual scarification, using razor blades for both, a practice that has made healers targets of HIV awareness and prevention campaigns as there may be a risk of HIV transmission through blood if razor blades are reused and not properly cleaned.[2]

The perceived association between African health beliefs and witchcraft has been used as an excuse *not* to take prevailing beliefs or practitioners into consideration when developing health programs because doing so might encourage witchcraft beliefs and retard acceptance of mature, rational thought. But what if African health beliefs are *not* primarily witchcraft related? Green has provided documentation that shows, looking at the diseases that account for the greatest morbidity and mortality, that indigenous and biomedical etiologic models are *not* very different, in some fundamental and important ways.[3] Etiologic beliefs regarding contagious illnesses—including AIDS and other STIs—tend to be naturalistic, empirically based, and nonsupernatural. This suggests that there *is* a basis for collaboration between biomedical and indigenous healers.

In African traditional medicine, diseases are believed to be caused by contact between people (including but not limited to sexual intercourse) who are considered to be in a state of contamination or pollution, by tiny insects or worms (paralleling the concept of germs), or by wind or air that carry disease. Pollution occurs through contact with potent bodily fluids that can be considered polluted. Code words such dirt, impurity, contamination, heat, darkness, "shadow of death" (the impurity that comes from death and is carried by a widow prior to a purification ceremony), and bad blood are commonly used to describe pollution mechanisms. Contamination or pollution can occur through contact with death, funerals, or menstrual blood, or through sexual contact with wives who have been "protected" from extramarital sex through sorcery (e.g., *likhubalo* among the Swazi and Zulu) (Green 1999a; Murdock 1980). A number of indigenous syndromes with genito-urinary symptoms are explained by traditional healers as relating to contamination with impure sexual fluids such as menstrual blood, impure blood from a partner who has had many other partners, or the "shadow of death."

A second type of contagion is described as worms or tiny or invisible insects that are transmitted from a sick person to a non-sick person through contact such as sexual intercourse (Green 1999a). Diseases not classified biomedically as sexually transmitted, such as tuberculosis and certain types of child diarrhea, might also be believed to result from illicit sex (Green 1994; Pateguane 1983). A third contagion belief is sometimes called "illness in the air" or "wind illness" in African languages. Tuberculosis, malaria, colds, flu or asthma, or even measles are believed to spread by inhalation of unclean dust carried by the wind, because only air or wind has sufficiently widespread contact with people to cause outbreaks (Green 1999a; Imperato and Traoré 1979). Harriet Ngubane (1977) regarded this category of airborne illness as a type within a broader category of environmental dangers.

Green found that especially in the early years of the pandemic, some Africans believed that the new disease of AIDS was caused by witchcraft. Other anthropologists have also documented these ideas. There was also a widespread belief early on that AIDS was solely a disease of whites and homosexuals. In researching AIDS and STI beliefs in countries including Nigeria, Liberia, Swaziland, South Africa, Zambia, Uganda, Malawi, Tanzania, and Mozambique, Green found that as education about HIV began to spread in Africa, there was increasing reliance on indigenous, etiologic theories of known, familiar STIs. AIDS then came to be considered just one of a number of STIs, even if it was known to be more serious than the others. The pattern of understanding AIDS in naturalistic terms seems to have become widespread in sub-Saharan Africa by the end of the 1990s (Green 1999a).

We suggest there can be at least a partial fit between indigenous and biomedical models of STI (and AIDS). Both models agree that the cause of sexually transmitted illness is impersonal (not supernatural or personalistic) or due to ritual or taboo violation. In either case disease is related to conditions that may be modifiable, such as avoiding contamination or pollution with an unseen agent of illness that can be sexually transmitted through sex with strangers, with partners who are too young or too old, with those who are married to other partners, with women during menstruation or women during a mourning period and prior to purification rituals, or with partners with "bad blood" from having other partners. For example, a discussion among traditional healers in South Africa representing diverse ethnic groups[4] discussed ways to prevent locally recognized STIs. These included taking traditional medicine (usually orally before engaging in risky sex); sticking to one or few sexual partners; avoiding sex with risky partners (i.e., those who have had many other partners, or sex with strangers); and avoiding sex with a woman who has aborted or miscarried. Other suggested preventive measures included strengthening the individual and family; sexual abstinence if the client is sick; avoiding sex with menstruating or infected women; avoiding sex with widows; and avoiding breaking taboos such as those against adultery (Green et al. 1995).

Traditional medicine also employs personalistic and supernatural explanations for disease, such as those that blame witchcraft or sorcery. For example, when traditional healers learn through divination that a (locally recognized and classified) STI came from outside marriage, witchcraft or sorcery is often suspected. Women involved in non-sanctioned sex such as adultery might not exhibit symptoms, but the male seducer is believed to become sick from the medicine or spell from the husband of the unfaithful woman. Variants of this theory of STI can be found in other parts of Africa such as Ghana (Warren 1979), Zimbabwe (Gelfand et al. 1985), Botswana (Ingstad 1990:34), Liberia (Green 1992a), and Swaziland, Mozambique, and South Africa (Green 1994, 1999a). Common to these societies is the belief that transgression of social norms, as in adultery or violation of other sexual taboos, provokes mystical punishment either by means of sorcery or retribution from ancestor spirits (Green 1994:61–68, 77, 182, 191).

DANGEROUS SEX

Eminent AIDS researcher Caraël observes of Africa, "Sexuality is the domain *par excellence* of rules and regulations, the prime area where nature and nurture are linked. It belongs to the world of impurity and filth. It is dangerous, an inexhaustible source of individual and social problems" (2006:100). The pioneering work on African pollution beliefs by anthropologist Mary Douglas showed that pollution beliefs tend to involve wrongdoing. Her work among the Lele of present-day Democratic Republic of Congo showed that rules of pollution arise when "a forbidden contact" has taken place, meaning when social norms and rules governing sex are transgressed (1992 [1966]:155). She further notes: "Sex is likely to be pollution-free in a society where sexual roles are enforced directly."

AIDS is not the first disease linked to the breakdown of culture in an African context. African historian Benedict Carton writes of similarities between AIDS and the great rinderpest cattle disease epidemic that led to catastrophic death and starvation in southern Africa in the 1890s:

> Both outbreaks evolved from epi- to pan-phenomena, prompting the urgent attention of Western medical scientists. They also highlighted the unremitting pressures on African families and restlessness of their youths. The epizootic, which originally leaped from Europe into Africa in the late nineteenth century, eradicated a prized source of exchange upholding customs regulating fertility. In the absence of bridewealth cattle that sealed

nuptial negotiations sanctioning reproduction, Zulu-speaking youths at the turn of the twentieth century increasingly engaged in premarital intercourse. (Carton 2006:98)[5]

Such transgressions alarmed the elders who tried to safeguard sexual norms. Carton observes that in the AIDS era, "forbidden sex, a source of hazardous bodily pollution" began to coincide with strong *umnyama,* a more epidemic disease that annihilates people on the scale of the great rinderpest epidemic. A Zulu-speaking informant of Carton in Pietermaritzburg in the early 2000s observed that "promiscuity and *ukufa*" ("bad or calamitous death") are rife because "no one marries anymore." In her opinion, "if a couple could afford to formalize its relationship, fidelity would be more important." Another informant attributed "bad death" among young people to "taboo breaking and the curse of death via HIV/AIDS (Carton 2006:110–11)." (See Chapter 9 for a more detailed discussion about HIV risk and marriage.)

Most if not all African cultures associate sexual intercourse with some degree of danger, as it involves the co-mingling of potent sexual fluids between males and females and has the potential to threaten family, clan, and lineage relations. Sex is also a serious matter because one's social identity is determined by membership in family, lineage, and clan. Intercourse leads to pregnancy, and when this occurs out of wedlock, one's social status can be indeterminate. Full adult social identity is also achieved only with reproduction, especially for women. Social controls around sex are sustained by indigenous beliefs about not offending ancestral spirits. To the extent that ancestor veneration prevails in most of sub-Saharan Africa (despite the powerful influence of Christianity and Islam), one's connection to ancestral spirits of the appropriate partrilineage or matrilineage is part of a person's spiritual health and well-being as well as part of one's social and cultural identity. In much of Africa, traditional mechanisms of social control have been augmented in recent years by the growing popularity of Christianity (especially Pentecostal and Charismatic) (Gifford 2004; Meyer 2004). These churches have contributed to the spread in Africa of an ideology that equates personal respectability and success with adherence to a moral code that prohibits premarital sex, extramarital sex, and polygyny.

Thus, traditionally at least, sexual intercourse in many African cultures is heavily regulated, and there are felt to be dangers inherent in the act itself, even apart from the social and legal consequences of children born out of wedlock. These ideas might seem quaint and even unfamiliar to urban, educated Africans but they are ingrained in African culture and alive and well in more rural traditional areas. The view that there should be no considerations when it comes to sexuality other than fun seems to

be in conflict with African culture and traditions—to go by the accumulated body of ethnographic findings.

In more traditional cultures, existing beliefs and norms about sexual
restraint and rule adherence could provide a foundation for AIDS
prevention strategies. For example, and according to archival materials
from KwaZulu Natal, "until fairly recently, [unmarried Zulu] men were
typically discouraged from engaging in penetrative sexual intercourse. . . .
The practice of non-penetrative thigh sex, *ukuhlobonga* or *ukusoma*, was
central to the control of sexuality and prevention of illicit pregnancies"
(Hunter 2002:105; see also Krige 1936). In a survey of traditional
healers representing the major (black) ethnic groups of South Africa,
Green and colleagues asked whether thigh sex was still common among
the Zulu. Only 13 of the traditional healers (19%) said yes, usually with
the qualification that the practice has become increasingly rare. In some
urban areas such as Cape Town, healers commented that the practice
is "unknown" among younger people (Green et al. 1995). So, sexual
behavior has changed in South Africa, and to varying degrees throughout
the continent.

Working with Culture

Rather than working parallel to or in opposition to indigenous theories
of disease, HIV prevention programs should find ways to work within
these systems, such as recognizing and building on common beliefs about
the cause of disease. To quote Kenyan anthropologist Elizabeth Onjoro
(2003):

> Recognizing the validity of these local [health] beliefs . . . opens room for
> the existence of diverse systems. This also demands greater flexibility in
> prevention and treatment planning and action, [and] allows for acknowl-
> edging other models of folk knowledge as expert systems authoritative
> within their own cultural contexts. . . . Studies in the past two decades
> show that development, including health prevention, projects continue to
> fail for the same reasons they did in the past: the neglect of integrating
> indigenous perspectives as part of development discourse.

Like culture itself, traditional leaders have often been circumvented
in health and development programs, whether funded by local governments or foreign donors. It is uncommon to find examples of efforts
of AIDS programs that *build on the indigenous sector* or its leadership. Yet traditional leaders and healers are often eager to collaborate
in such efforts, as in the case study of research with traditional leaders
in southern Africa that follows. Part of the reason for this motivation
is that involvement in externally funded programs legitimizes the role

of traditional leaders, who are struggling with marginalization vis-à-vis national governments. It makes sense to involve traditional leaders in setting up HIV prevention program that are locally driven and culturally competent, thereby creating a sense of local ownership and minimizing the discord that exists between traditional leaders, government, and donors. It also opens the door to a horizontal (community-based or person-to-person) rather than a top-down model of communication. Such an approach is particularly appropriate for rural populations for whom traditional structures and leadership remain important and who are often hardest to reach through mass media and other standard outreach campaigns.

There are many "entry points" in African cultures that AIDS programs might build on. For example, many ethnolinguistic groups place value on premarital virginity for girls and often for boys as well. Customary law in many African cultures ideally forbids premarital sex, and in southern Africa a cow was often the fine imposed on a man for deflowerment. If pregnancy followed, the fine might have become five cows. Fear of this fine kept young people practicing nonpenetrative thigh sex. Virginity testing was used to gather the evidence to levy the fine, and thus played an integral function in discouraging premarital sex. Some groups still use rites of passage to teach life skills that include responsible behavior, abstinence or moderation, and/or nonpenetrative sex or thigh sex. Social controls could also apply to adults. In a study of 15 African countries, Bingenheimer observes: "Considerable evidence suggests that at least some men in present-day sub-Saharan Africa are subject to a set of rigid social controls that prohibit and severely sanction premarital and extramarital sex and, in many cases, polygyny" (2010:3). All of these are cultural practices that are protective in the context of HIV/AIDS and can be built on to reduce HIV infections.

Virginity testing provides an instructive case study of the conflict that often erupts between a Western paradigm of AIDS prevention and African values and traditions. Virginity testing is understood by some anthropologists and many Africans as an indigenous attempt to protect girls from HIV infection, to control premarital sex, and to bring negative sanctions on men who seduce, coerce, or rape girls, thereby acting as a deterrent to these behaviors (George 2007; Leclerc-Madlala 2001; Ubuntu Planning Meeting 2008).

In July 2000, teenage girls and middle-age virginity testers marched through the main streets of Natal (provincial capital of KwaZulu Natal), waving placards to demonstrate their support for the revival of virginity testing. In a letter to the *The Natal Witness* before the march, supporters of virginity testing wrote:

We are the organization which does virginity testing of girls from six years old up to marriage status. Initially we started from 12 years old but by doing so we found that half of the girls tested had already lost their virginity. The reason? Because most of them have been abused by their relatives— brothers, fathers, uncles and also cousins. . . . We Africans must work together to prevent sexually transmitted diseases and AIDS. I don't believe in Western civilization and culture as they say we must use condoms and contraceptives, which promotes [sic] adultery. (Leclerc-Madlala 2001:533)

Leclerc-Madlala, in quoting this letter, notes that South Africa has "among the world's highest statistics for rape." Our own research suggests that virginity testing also helps build a support network for girls, because the girls come to look out for one another and report sexual abuse through channels made available in the indigenous sector (Green et al. 2009). Yet in the AIDS literature, in the press, and at public forums, virginity testing is typically not seen as an indigenous solution to the threat of HIV/AIDS but as an outdated and destructive practice. Many critics of virginity testing view it through the lens of Western individual-centered human rights and deem it a source of shaming, marginalizing, or humiliating girls rather than as protecting them or building their self-esteem and social support systems. In 2005, South Africa passed the Children's Act, which allows voluntary virginity testing only for girls 16 and older. We are not arguing for or against virginity testing, only presenting it as an example of an indigenous, endogenous response to the threat of AIDS. Westerners ought to attempt to understand it in those terms before judging it by Western standards of women's rights and condemning or dismissing it out of hand.

In her critique of the U.S.-funded, massive South African loveLife campaign, Leclerc-Madlala offers another example of the mismatch between Western and African values and priorities in AIDS prevention. She notes that this slick, loveLife campaign that had found its way into nearly every South African home has little relevance for black South Africans. Leclerc-Madlala writes, "The youth are portrayed as middle class, sophisticated, and seem likely to spend their weekends enjoying multi-racial camaraderie in suburban rave clubs. Wittingly or unwittingly, the thrust of our national HIV/AIDS prevention effort speaks primarily to a narrow band of privileged youth" (2002:19). She points out that South Africa should be looking not to Beverly Hills for answers to AIDS, but to Uganda, where people changed their behavior—and not for the most part by using condoms. She concludes, "As unlikely as it may sound, Uganda's experiences suggest that the promotion of abstinence before marriage and mutual faithfulness in relationships may be the keys to halting the spread of AIDS in Africa" (2002:19).

Unfortunately, Leclerc-Madlala is more the exception than the rule, at least among those of us involved in AIDS. The majority of anthropologists involved in AIDS seem more likely to take a social and political activist position that often requires suspension of the normal rules and conventions of our discipline. At the least, anthropologists should avoid perpetuating stereotypic thinking that views African culture as the problem in the context of AIDS, rather than as part of the solution. African culture is, after all, what we have to work with in changing behaviors that lead to HIV infection, including solving the puzzle of how to discourage multiple and concurrent partnerships and increase rates of male circumcision.

Anthropologists should be identifying entry points for behavior change efforts and bringing change agents such as implementers of AIDS programs together with local and indigenous leaders to explore what kinds of solutions might work. Indigenous leaders such as chiefs and healers are more open to such collaboration than many assume. For example, at a 1992 workshop for traditional healers in South Africa, the president of a healer organization observed: "When tradition and the health of our people are in conflict, it is traditions we must sacrifice (Green 2000)."

Anthropologists might also point out more forcefully that peer education can be seen as being at odds with the tradition of younger people learning from elders. Peer education is especially effective at reaching the type of high-risk groups where most HIV infections are found in the West—gay men, IDUs, sex workers—but this is not necessarily the optimal approach in African general populations. Daniel Halperin relates hearing a young man in Mozambique comment that, "In our communities, everyone thinks those 'peer-to-peer' [HIV] prevention programs are a joke. Sending youth to talk to older people is so disrespectful, and even the youth themselves want to hear from elders, not other youth."[6] One of the many lessons from Uganda is that whole populations can be mobilized once key opinion leaders are on board—including chiefs, religious leaders, traditional healers, women's group leaders, and local government officials.

Anthropologists could also show the missing "other side" of what is extant in culture that can be built on to fight AIDS. If politics and ideology were stripped from AIDS and our only aim was to limit HIV infections, an anthropological approach to prevention could begin by identifying those existing aspects of culture that lead to restraint and caution in sexual behavior, and then reinforcing and building on these. But AIDS involves something anthropologists feel very strongly about—sexual behavior. We seem to be less capable of objectivity and cultural relativism in this domain than in virtually all others. In fact, we seem to project our own wish for sexual liberation on Africans, who are widely believed to be less rule bound and less restrained than Westerners.

The (perhaps unintended) meta-message in the Western approaches to AIDS is that *sex is fun and there should be no worries or inhibitions, as long as a condom is used.* For example, a recent AIDS prevention campaign in Swaziland not only avoided warning about risky sexual behavior, but actually adopted the campaign slogan, "Fun and sex are part of my life. So is HIV" and "Condoms . . . where the fun is at."[7] (Note the American syntax; Swazis don't say "Where it's at.") This campaign was aimed at young people and it certainly did nothing to strengthen existing traditional prohibitions against premarital sex. In fact, it seems not so different from promoting the message that smoking is fun in the same less developed countries where Big Tobacco is building new markets.

Similarly, an ad was developed by Population Services International (PSI) in Botswana in which a teenage girl smiles and says "I am going out with an older man who adds flavour to my life and one thing I do is have protected sex using Lovers Plus condoms every time" (Motlogelwa 2007). This ad provoked local outrage and was pulled after only one appearance in a newspaper, under instructions from PSI headquarters in Washington, DC, which expressed regret for the ad. Yet the view expressed—that sex with a sugar daddy is all right as long as condoms are used—remains deeply disturbing. In fairness, PSI is currently involved in cutting-edge partner reduction campaigns in Botswana, following a new trend among many international donors in that country toward such behavior change programs after heavy investment in condom-centered prevention campaigns has not paid off (Allen and Heald 2004).

Those of us who work on the intervention side need to be certain whether we are teaching that sex is fun and should be enjoyed as much as possible as long as condoms are used or whether sex is potentially dangerous. We really can't have it both ways. Although so-called fear appeals are often claimed to be useless or counterproductive, Uganda's early program shows that the deliberate and apparently successful use of such appeals did succeed in changing hard-to-change behaviors and "cutting through the denial" surrounding AIDS, at least at that time (Green and Witte 2006). In fact, four meta-analyses of the role of fear appeals in motivating change of hard-to-change behaviors, such as smoking and sexual behavior, all reached the same conclusion: The stronger the fear appeal, the greater the changes in attitude, intention, and behavior change.[8] These seem to work in concert with "self-efficacy," when people believe there is a way to avoid a dreaded outcome and they themselves can do something to avoid it. We see the failure to use fear appeals combined with self-efficacy as another example of a disconnect between what is known empirically and what is widely held to be true in the field of AIDS prevention.

CASE STUDY: ENGAGING TRADITIONAL HEALERS
IN HIV PREVENTION

In 1990, the Mozambican government asked Green to help develop AIDS prevention approaches that would build on indigenous knowledge and traditional healers. Mozambique, one of the last African countries to gain independence from a colonial power, had been ruled by the Marxist FRELIMO (Frente de Libertação de Moçambique) government since Mozambique gained independence from Portugal in 1975.

In FRELIMO's attempt to create a modern, nontribal, nonracial, equitable nation, it embarked on a radical program to transform the country's economy and society as quickly as possible. The traditionalism of the various ethnolinguistic groups seemed to stand in the way of "scientific socialism," so there was an attempt to abolish traditional authorities such as chiefs (formerly known as *regulos* or *chefes de zonas*) as well as practices such as bride-price (*lobola*), polygamy, initiation rites (which sometimes included male circumcision), land tenure, and traditional healing and healers. The rural masses were obliged to regroup into communal villages to engage in new forms of collective agriculture. FRELIMO attempted to achieve full equality of women (in societies that were for the most part strongly patriarchal) through legislation. In 1978, People's Tribunals were set up and headed by judges chosen on the basis of having "good sense." This was an assault on traditional adjudicative systems, including the traditional authorities who convened and presided over adjudicative councils.

With FRELIMO'S "marginalization" or suppression of traditional political authorities, many went underground or simply continued to exercise power informally and behind the backs of FRELIMO officials. Traditional healers, spirit mediums, and cult figures were discouraged, and sometimes oppressed, as purveyors of superstition (*obscurantismo*). With the alienation of traditional and ritual leaders and healers, as well as many among the rural masses, FRELIMO lost political control of most of the geographic area of Mozambique. One reason for this loss was its assault on African culture and social structure, which is not easily transformed by fiat. As this period proved, governments cannot easily and quickly transform societies or reinvent culture simply because they deem it in the best interests of the masses.

Beginning in the mid-1980s, there was a growing awareness within the ranks of the FRELIMO government that traditional systems might, in fact, be well suited and responsive to the social, psychological, and other needs of participants in these systems; that they provided security and continuity in an unpredictable, changing world; and that they might be a great source of comfort to Mozambicans suffering the stress of rapid culture change and the prolonged trauma of an unusually vicious civil war (with the rival party RENAMO) that had directly affected the civilian population since independence. By the 5th FRELIMO Party Congress (1989), the government formally recognized the mistakes it had made in its zeal to create a new, equitable, and unified national society. In an April 1992 national workshop held in Mozambique, a presenter noted that FRELIMO's attempt at radically transforming society

> was extremely altruistic, but the way it was implemented entered into direct confrontation with the cultural system hitherto existing in the countryside, which was ignored or set aside to make way for the new, modern progressive and urban culture. A phenomenon which in Europe had taken centuries to evolve was attempted here from one day to the next, and in general the results were not good. There was resistance, difficulties, and failures which might not have occurred if there had been an attempt to conciliate the culture of the peasants and the new forms being proposed, in order to achieve a more gradual and less confrontational transition. A situation of contradictory norms emanating from the traditional authorities and the central government generated disrespect for norms of any kind.[9]

In 1990, the Mozambique Ministry of Health asked Green for advice about its policy on indigenous healers, following the model of a collaboration with healers for health promotion in Swaziland that Green had set up in the 1980s. Despite the new thinking about traditional culture, there was uncertainty, suspicion, and fear regarding collaboration on the part of the government and traditional healers.

It is estimated that between 80% and 85% of Africans consult traditional healers, at least some of the time for at least some conditions (UNAIDS 2006). In Mozambique, the proportion relying on traditional healers was even higher because of poverty, inaccessibility of biomedical health services, and years of attacks against the government's rural health personnel and infrastructure during the country's long civil war. Preliminary census studies by the Department of Traditional Medicine (Gabinete de Estudos de Medicina Tradicional, or GEMT) of the Mozambique Ministry of Health suggested a ratio of roughly one traditional healer to every 200 people. This estimate is comparable to estimates made elsewhere in sub-Saharan Africa (Green 1994). Thus, with a population of about 17 million (in 1990), Mozambique was estimated to have approximately 85,000 healers. In contrast, the physician-to-population ratio in Mozambique was about 1:50,000, with some 52% of doctors concentrated in the capital city.

One might wonder why a country that did not recognize or permit indigenous healing or healers (remember the official resistance to *obscurantismo*) even had a department like the GEMT. In fact, it was established to discover useful phytomedicines (medicines of botanical origin) by finding, classifying, and cataloging those in use, in the hope that foreign chemists or better yet, pharmaceutical companies, would study the medicinal properties and perhaps some royalties or other benefit sharing from the discovery of new drugs would follow. Green argued that "traditional healers" (the term preferred by healers themselves) were needed as well as their medicines, as they were the de facto primary health care workers. If the government had a chance of realizing its public health goals, it was hardly possible without developing some role for, or collaboration with, Mozambique's ubiquitous traditional healers.

The GEMT and Green proposed a three-year project to establish a foundation for public health collaboration between traditional healers and the National Health Service (Green et al. 1991). They designed and implemented preliminary ethnomedical research in Manica Province in a pilot program focusing on STIs, including AIDS. (Childhood diarrheal disease was the other focus.) Green trained the staff of the GEMT in the "take culture seriously" approach and in basic qualitative research methods. The GEMT project produced a model for collaborating with traditional healers, and before long other donors began to undertake similar initiatives. The project also conducted rapid research in three provinces (Nampula, Manica, and Inhambane, covering the northern, central, and southern areas of the country), followed by workshops that brought healers and Ministry of Health staff together. The Ministry of Health was gearing up to address what was then expected to be an explosion of HIV infections. In fact, UNAIDS and other organizations were expecting explosions in many countries, most of which have never materialized.[10] UNAIDS estimates that Mozambique's current HIV prevalence is 12.5% (UNAIDS 2008a), making it one of the highest HIV prevalent countries; the prevalence is still rising at a time when it has stabilized or declined in surrounding countries.

At the time of this project, there was surprisingly little recognition of the role of having multiple sexual partners in HIV transmission. The thinking then was that the condom is the best weapon we have in the war against AIDS. Mass or syndromic treatment of STIs was considered a possible intervention for reducing HIV incidence, especially after hopeful results from the Mwanza study in Tanzania. (As will be discussed in Chapter 6, the results of the Mwanza trial were never replicated, so mass treatment of STIs is no longer considered an evidence-based intervention for reducing HIV infection rates.) There was some recognition that male circumcision might decrease risk of HIV infection, but the AIDS community was far from the point where this might be considered an intervention worthy of promotion. Green (Green et al. 1995) raised the possibility of male circumcision for HIV prevention, noting that some traditional healers in South Africa were promoting it as a way to prevent STIs and HIV (Green et al. 1993). For the most part, the AIDS community was unaware of the landmark article by John Bongaarts, Priscilla Reining, and others (Bongaarts 2006), which, based on data from the Human Relational Area Files, showed a seemingly strong connection between HIV prevalence rates in Africa and ethnolinguistic groups that do not circumcise. Yet some traditional healers in the region claimed to have noticed that it tended to be clients from noncircumcising ethnic groups who kept showing up with STIs. So they put two and two together and began to advise men to consider circumcision as a way to decrease chances of getting both STIs and AIDS. One Xhosa healer organization even published a brochure to this effect, dated 1992, more than a decade ahead of medical researchers (Green et al. 1995).

There was an internal evaluation of workshop impact in Inhambane Province. Twenty healers who participated in a workshop in June 1994 were reinterviewed October–November 1995. Eight patients who were being treated by these healers for STIs were also located and interviewed. Patient interviews provided a means of verifying healers' self-reported behavior and yielded valuable insights into the healing process and the reinterpretation and dissemination of information and advice presented at the workshop.

Among the most important findings were that 85% of healers had learned that AIDS is caused or transmitted by sexual contact with a person with the illness and that use of condoms or fidelity to one (uninfected) partner can prevent AIDS. The role of blood, or contaminated blood, in AIDS transmission was well understood. Virtually all healers said they now used only one clean razor per patient, or boiled or sterilized a razor if they had to reuse it. Most (81%) claimed that they had promoted condom use with their STI patients. However, most of the condoms distributed by healers were those supplied by the GEMT in the 1994 Inhambane workshop; most healers had never been resupplied nor had they taken their own initiative to find condoms. Among other weaknesses encountered, there was still confusion about transmission of AIDS through superficial contact, such as using the same toilet, eating food touched by a sick person, using clothes of a person with AIDS, or kissing a sick person. There was also poor understanding about the role of STIs in increasing vulnerability to AIDS (Green 1999b).

Green developed collaborative programs of this sort in Nigeria, Zambia, Swaziland, and South Africa, focused on family planning, AIDS prevention, and diarrheal disease. Green and colleagues realized that holding a workshop for a limited number of healers had a limited impact, so in South Africa they developed a different model based on "training of trainers." In November 1992, a program using this approach to train traditional healers in AIDS prevention was initiated jointly by the AIDS Control and Prevention (AIDSCAP) project, funded by USAID and administered by Family Health International.

An initial generation of 28 healers was trained in preventing AIDS and STIs, and these healers, in turn, trained a total of 630 additional healers (the second generation) in formal, week-long workshops. By the end of 10 months, 1,510 healers had been trained, and it was estimated that over 200,000 patients and clients may have benefited from AIDS education as a result of the training. AIDSCAP supported the later workshops or sessions financially, but the training was left to healers who had been previously trained. It was recognized that peer education would be somewhat different from training that came from U.S. advisors or trained South African medical staff, and there was great interest in comparing the impact of training done in the usual manner (first generation) versus through peer education (second and third generations).

An internal evaluation was conducted as part of the ongoing program. Perhaps surprisingly, the second generation appeared to be as well trained as the first, going by measures such as reporting correctly how HIV is transmitted and different ways HIV transmission can be prevented. Healers also reported advising their patients to use condoms, and demonstrating methods of correct condom use (Green et al. 1995). Green and colleagues wanted this program to continue and undergo an external evaluation in which clients of trained healers were interviewed. That might have happened but for the vagaries of funding for nonmainstream programs like this.

Whatever national-level impact this program might have had, the South African government was not doing a very good job of gearing up for the impending HIV explosion. (This is one country where the UNAIDS prediction of an AIDS explosion did come to pass.) President Nelson Mandela, like U.S. President Ronald Reagan, never mentioned the word AIDS in any speech while in office, and his successor President Thabo Mbeki famously denied that HIV was causally related to the disease AIDS.

NOTES

1. See Epstein (2007) for a discussion of how this myth originated in the reporting of a small group of Western journalists. After a nationally publicized trial in South Africa in which a nine-month old baby was raped as a crime of revenge having nothing to do with HIV, news reports began to claim that some African men believed that raping a virgin (even a baby) could cure them of AIDS. Epstein

writes, "The idea that virgin-rape myths are a significant cause of either child abuse or the spread of AIDS in Africa is itself a myth, perpetuated by stigmatizing attitudes toward people with HIV and racist fears of black sexuality" (p. 229). Epstein reports that surveys have shown that belief in the virgin-rape myth is now common among South Africans, although the number of such rapes appears to be tiny. Epstein also notes that such a belief was at one time attached to eastern European immigrants in the United States, who were reported to be raping virgins to cure themselves of syphilis.

2. Whatever the risk of HIV transmission from reused razor blades, the risk of Hepatitis B and C is clear, as these viruses can survive longer outside the body and are thus more infectious. HIV/AIDS programs that collaborate with healers typically warn them of the dangers of using the same razor with more than one client or provide them with razor blades (see, e.g., Peltzer et al. 2006).

3. See Green 1999. "Biomedicine" refers to Western-style, cosmopolitan medicine, including its branch of public health, and it is distinguished from African "traditional" (although dynamic, adaptive, and changing) systems of "indigenous medicine." "Contagious" disease usually refers to disease transmission that is direct, by contact, whereas with "infectious" disease, transmission is indirect, through water, air, or contaminated articles (Pelling 1993:309).

4. Participants were Xhosa (12), Zulu (7), South Sotho (3), Tsonga (3), Swazi (2), North Sotho (1), and Pedi (1).

5. On sex pollution, see also Carton 2003.

6. Halperin, personal communication. Halperin heard this comment during an August 2009 visit to rural Mozambique.

7. The campaign was sponsored by PSI Swaziland, the Health Ministry of Swaziland, and the United Nations Population Fund (UNFPA). See "Have responsible fun this festive," *Times of Swaziland*, December 12, 2008. http://www.times.co.sz/index.php?news = 3849 (accessed September 30, 2009) and R. Poglitsh, "Advert is not the answer," *Times of Swaziland*, December 28, 2008. http://www.times.co.sz/index.php?news = 4171 (accessed September 30, 2009).

8. These meta-analyses were done by four different investigators utilizing different statistical methods, namely Boster and Mongeau 1984, Mongeau 1998, Sutton 1982, and Witte and Allen 2000, cited by Witte in Green and Witte (2006:249).

9. Workshop on Strengthening Civil Society and Community Development in Southern Africa, Maputo, April 1992.

10. See Chin (2007) for a discussion of how UNAIDS has overblown its estimates, particularly in Asia, and see Pisani (2008) for an insider's view of the same process at UNAIDS.

Chapter 3

HOW THE GLOBAL AIDS RESPONSE WENT WRONG

Anthropologists have been called on to use their expertise to contribute to the global response to AIDS since the beginning of the epidemic. But anthropologists have not been the only ones responding to AIDS, and in this chapter we discuss other actors and their contributions as well as ways in which the global response went wrong. As we have noted, much of global AIDS prevention continues to be dominated by the values and priorities of the West, particularly certain groups in the West. This has its roots in a certain history of how AIDS (and the first responses to AIDS) unfolded in the United States and West and later in the rest of the world. Thus, it is important to consider this history. We believe that America's first response to AIDS might have made sense for high-risk subgroups in America, but that it was not suited to the generalized or population-wide epidemics of Africa or other epidemics that had little in common with the largely MSM- and IDU-driven epidemics of the West.

A SHORT HISTORY OF THE GLOBAL AIDS RESPONSE

The earliest medical response to AIDS—at least the first that was sympathetic and empathetic—came in the early 1980s, from doctors and health personnel who were themselves gay-identified. It is impossible to discuss the history of AIDS and the global response without going into the history of gay men in America, as they were among the first to be widely affected by AIDS (for a short time, AIDS was known as Gay-Related Infectious Disease, or GRID) and were the first to mount a response to the newly identified disease (Shilts 1987). It should be possible to discuss the history of gay men and AIDS (both their successes and mistakes) objectively without fear of accusation of homophobia. We are not criticizing the gay men who led this first response, or minimizing the tremendous contribution that gay men have made to the field of AIDS, but simply noting how this particular part of the history of the

AIDS pandemic unfolded. Any group that responded to such a complex and poorly understood disease would doubtless have made mistakes but if we can learn from the mistakes that have been made, we can avoid repeating them.

In the early years of the AIDS pandemic, few non-gay men or women felt they had a stake in this new disease or that it threatened them, so not many people were interested in working in the emerging field of AIDS *except* gay men. From the very beginning, the strong identification of AIDS as a "gay problem" in the West shaped Western responses to global AIDS. To the extent that anyone could be considered an expert in the early years of the crisis, many of the first AIDS experts sent by the United States and Europe to Africa were gay men. One of the unintended consequences of this first wave of technical expertise was that Africans could dismiss AIDS as not being a threat to them.

Many Africans, when seeing openly gay men for the first time, and simultaneously learning from AIDS experts about the "gay plague" and anal sex in America, reasoned that they themselves could not get the disease. Caraël has observed this about Africa in the early years of the pandemic:

> The refusal to recognize the existence and the extent of the epidemic was demonstrated by both the authorities and the African elites including the great majority of the medical fraternity. AIDS became a political and cultural stake before being a health problem. Reactions of nationalistic pride were exacerbated by the debate on the African origin of the virus or on "African sexual promiscuity." The African elites denounced AIDS as a foreign disease spread on the continent by white homosexuals, as an attempt to bring down the birth rate by imposing the use of condoms, as an attack associated with the puritanism of Christian sects in the face of African traditions such as polygamy. (2006:27)

In former Zaire, the French acronym for AIDS, SIDA, was said to stand for Syndrome Imaginaire pour Décourager les Amoureux (an imaginary syndrome to discourage lovers) (Echenberg 2006). Neighboring Uganda, which launched a tremendously successful response to AIDS, had to take very deliberate steps to "cut though the denial"[1] that Ugandans were at risk of this new disease, which was seen as an American plot to spoil fun and force condom use.

Both within anthropology and the United States as a whole (soon to be followed by Western Europe and the rest of the world), the norms, values, and perspective of gay men predominated in the AIDS world. The outspoken, in-your-face so-called fast track gay men (Rotello 1997)[2] who belonged to organizations such as ACT-UP became the face of the gay response to AIDS and were extremely effective in determining the content and parameters of AIDS prevention. They were also highly instrumental in shaming governments into directing ever larger amounts of money to AIDS prevention, which, by the early 2000s, came to also include public funds for expensive ARV drugs, not only in the United States but around the world. It is possible that if AIDS had not impacted so many gay men in the United States and Europe (creating a natural and effective lobby for global AIDS spending), AIDS never would have become the most highly funded disease in history. Further, it is also possible that the risk-reduction approach that came to dominate global AIDS prevention, which had its origin in the MSM epidemics of the West, might then not have become the standard model of prevention everywhere.

In fact, billions of dollars were directed toward HIV/AIDS, first as a trickle and then as a tsunami, at first only for prevention but then for relatively expensive treatment as well. This departure from a prevention-focused public health approach and shift to the free offering of expensive treatment is part of AIDS exceptionalism (treating AIDS as exceptional and different from all other diseases). AIDS has also been treated differently in the high degree of confidentiality conferred to tests and diagnoses; the practice of not reporting the names of individuals carrying a deadly communicable departs radically from standard public health practice in the United States and many other parts of the world.

But gay activists were not the only ones shaping global approaches to mobilizing resources to fight AIDS. They were strongly supported by and allied with the feminist movement, from whom gay activists learned political tactics (Parker and Easton 1998; Rotello 1997). The developing lesbian, gay, bisexual, transgendered, and queer (LGBTQ) coalition would also be guided by sexology, social constructionist or sexual liberation anthropology, reproductive health, and family planning, all drawing strength and inspiration from one another and pursuing many of the same progressive social and health goals. Some of these constituent groups had always been on the periphery of power prior to AIDS, and they began to exercise real power for the first time in global AIDS. Suddenly, *they* were in charge; they were the Establishment. They also found themselves allied with the pharmaceutical industry; an ethos of sexual freedom and "rights" came with a demand for drugs and medical devices that would make possible sex without risk of disease or harm.

Family planning groups were also key players in the early response to AIDS. Among the first non-governmental organizations (NGOs) to become involved in global AIDS prevention were those which were already working in family planning (Greeley 1988), and the first prominent idea about AIDS prevention in America and most of the world was to promote the condom for the dual purpose of avoiding unwanted pregnancy as well as sexually transmitted infections, including HIV. This is one of several ways that AIDS prevention developed as a condom-centered enterprise. The U.S. government believed—and would often claim—that it had a comparative advantage in condom social marketing because social marketing originated in the United States and it had up-and-running contraceptive social marketing programs. Because of the early influence of U.S. family planning advocates, virtually all the donors also emphasized condoms above all other approaches without looking at the different patterns of HIV transmission in different countries and populations and without evidence that condoms were effective in any of these diverse situations.

Mistaken Priorities

Thus, the first experts in AIDS prevention, mostly gay men and members of the family planning community, agreed about the priorities and guiding values of AIDS prevention. Relying on the triumvirate of condoms, HIV testing, and drugs (for treatment of STIs and later HIV) avoided awkward, thorny issues of changing (or restricting) sexual behavior. If harmful consequences of sexual behavior could be mitigated or prevented through medical and technological solutions, there was no reason to address sexual behavior itself. A risk-reduction approach had seemed to work among Western MSM, although how well it worked is now in question (Stoneburner and Low-Beer 2003), and indeed HIV infections among U.S. MSM are today on the increase. But a risk-reduction approach already had the allegiance of the U.S. MSM who were working in AIDS prevention and was also logical to and popular among family planning experts and health professionals, who tended to trust medical rather than behavioral approaches and solutions. Condoms in particular were favored as they were cheap and easy to distribute and count (thus making AIDS prevention activities easy to quantify and monitor), and they were, after all, the quintessential symbol of sexual freedom, its essential technology.

This risk reduction approach has been embraced by the majority of international development professionals and by all major foundations (Gates, Soros, Clinton, Ford, Hewlett and Packard), major international development organizations (UN, the World Bank, the Global Fund to Fight AIDS, Malaria, and Tuberculosis), and bilateral agencies (USAID, DFID [U.K.], CDC, GTZ [Germany], CIDA [Canada], and SIDA [Sweden]). These organizations together form and control the powerful global AIDS industry, and their priorities (rather than the priorities of the communities and countries affected by AIDS) have determined the global AIDS response. As we will discuss later, the standard approach to AIDS prevention has recently begun to shift somewhat, and solutions other than condoms, drugs, and testing are being considered and funded. But for much of the AIDS epidemic there has been one standard approach to AIDS, and deviations have generally not been supported or tolerated.

To many, this alliance of gay activists, family planning advocates, and big donors sounds ideal. What could be wrong with using condoms, testing, and drugs as a strategy to control an HIV epidemic? The short answer (discussed in greater detail in Chapter 6) is that none of these measures have been shown to decrease HIV prevalence in African population-wide epidemics, and the jury is still out about MSM epidemics. HIV infection rates are rising among U.S. MSM, who have more access than virtually anyone else in the world to both condoms and life-saving ARV drugs. Risk reduction measures have also not been an unmitigated success in IDU-transmitted HIV epidemics, as we will discuss in Chapter 5.

Some critics of standard AIDS prevention have spoken critically of the condom code, as noted in Chapter 1. Robin Gorna observes that condoms fail to address women's inequality and oppression and that the contexts within which sexual behavior occur "are sufficiently diverse and complicated that it would be logical to expect *a range of technologies* to reduce the risk of HIV transmission. Not so." (Gorna 1996:296, emphasis added). Since Gorna's writing, female condoms have been introduced, but no other female-controlled HIV prevention method is yet available, and female condoms remain quite unpopular (and infrequently used) among women worldwide. This reduction of HIV prevention options to condoms alone is very strange when compared to the range of contraceptive technologies available for women (Farmer 2003).

We wonder if anthropologists would have seen more clearly to support simple behavior change, as opposed to a "techno-fix," if sexual behavior had not been central to the new disease of AIDS and had gays not faced intense stigma. Had AIDS not crossed paths with deeply cherished notions about sexuality, would anthropologists still have sided with the condom industry over simple solutions such as reducing number of sexual partners? Would anthropologists have been more willing to at least question a prevention approach that requires the constant export of commodities from the north to the south, at the price of endless dependency on the largesse of wealthier countries?

More recently, an emphasis on using anthropological tools and methods to understand sexual behaviors and other proximate determinants of HIV transmission has largely been overtaken both in and outside the anthropological community by a focus on other political and social causes and on drugs and devices. At the August 2008 International AIDS Conference (Mexico City), for example, and at many similar meetings, much greater attention was given to sexual and gay liberation, women's emancipation, gender equality, poverty eradication, and rights for sex workers than to basic questions of how to reduce risky sexual behaviors. Many of these causes are laudable and critical to human well-being, but they divert attention from a more effective, straightforward public health approach to preventing new HIV infections.

Progressive social and political causes are compatible with the values and beliefs of the great majority of anthropologists, as well as nearly all Westerners who work in the AIDS industry and allied fields such as reproductive health and family planning. It is understandable that anthropologists and health experts feel passionately about these issues. Yet identification with these causes has resulted in a lack of attention to the culturally imbedded *behaviors* that spread HIV and it has kept anthropologists from a much-needed critique of what the AIDS industry has become: a giant medical, technological, multinational behemoth.

For all it undertakes in the name of public health, the AIDS industry has repeatedly failed to adequately address the very *behaviors* that drive the pandemic: sexual intercourse with multiple and concurrent partners, injecting drug use, and commercial sex. AIDS has been treated as an "exceptional" disease and therefore not subject to the usual rules of public health, which might be defined as beginning with primary prevention and then promoting the maximum health benefits for the greatest number of people, at the lowest cost, in the most sustainable manner. AIDS has provided a smokescreen for diverting massive spending towards programs to promote human rights and a number of political causes, not to mention toward AIDS prevention interventions that lack an evidence base.

These social and political causes are no less important—maybe even more so—than that of HIV prevention. However, achieving them will not necessarily achieve an end to the AIDS pandemic, or even a reduction in infection rates, and they have been distractions from focusing on the real drivers of HIV infections. Furthermore, the challenges of bringing about human rights and bringing about fewer AIDS infections diverge in some important ways. As will be discussed, in the world's worst epidemics in eastern and southern Africa, the wealthier and more educated are often more likely to be HIV infected, and, as women become more empowered and achieve equality with men, this does not necessarily put them at lesser risk of HIV infection.

It has been difficult for anthropologists and others not to assume *a priori* causal links between reducing inequalities and oppression and reducing rates of disease, especially one such as AIDS for which stigmatization of the infected and their behaviors is so prominent. It's hard not to think primarily (or only) of *victims* of AIDS, rather than people who may bear responsibility for becoming infected. For example, Paul Farmer responded to a 2003 essay of Green's about the success of HIV prevention in Uganda by agreeing that risky sexual behaviors must be addressed and that AIDS prevention had been "by and large a failure." But Farmer asked why Green didn't "go further":

> Why is HIV concentrated so heavily in the poorest parts of the world? Why do social inequalities, including gender inequality and racism, seem to fuel the AIDS pandemic whether in Africa or in the cities of the US? Why do economic policies foisted on poor countries tend to heighten HIV risk? (Farmer 2003)

Like Green, Farmer acknowledged that condom promotion and social marketing are not "the" solution to the problem, instead arguing that "risk for HIV goes hand in hand with not having. The have-nots constitute the global risk group . . . current AIDS prevention tools work least well precisely where individual agency is most constrained, usually by poverty and gender inequality, because what the have-nots lack is agency." In response to Green's claim that AIDS is a "behavioral problem with behavioral solutions," Farmer responded, "Perhaps. But AIDS is also, surely, a social problem with social solutions."

In *The Anthropology of AIDS: A Global Perspective*, anthropologist Patricia Whelehan (2009) also argues that HIV infections are a product of vulnerabilities including poverty, stigma, discrimination, and homophobia. Whelehan does not hide her bias against "views about sexuality and gender carried over from our puritan ancestors" (p. 123) and sees AIDS as driven by poverty as well as "erotophobia, homophobia, and sexism" (p. 149). Conquer these, Whelehan seems to argue, and AIDS will take care of itself. Whelehan fails to acknowledge the ways in which Africa does not fit her assumptions—for instance, that poverty is often inversely associated with HIV infection within a population (Mishra 2007a) or that HIV infections are rising in some of the places in the world (such as San Francisco) where economically and politically empowered gay men face less stigma and discrimination than perhaps anywhere in the world.

Whelehan is particularly concerned that nonheterosexual and non-monogamous expressions of sexuality be accepted as normative (she labels them "sex-positive"), and, without evidence, implicates "sex-negative" views such as those deriving from Anglo European Christian traditions in the spread of HIV. Her defense of sexual freedom extends to labeling condom campaigns "authoritarian" and defending non-use of condoms, even in extremely risky behaviors such as anal sex, as long as it is "an informed choice" that involves "responsibility for the behavior" (p. 139).

Susan Hunter is another anthropologist who has written widely about AIDS in Africa (*Black Death: AIDS in Africa*, 2004) and other continents. Her books have picked up back cover endorsements and glowing reviews from the likes of former UN Special Envoy for AIDS Stephen

Lewis and business magnate Donald Trump. Unfortunately, *Black Death* exhibits common Western biases, such as presenting African and other cultures as hyper-sexualized. For example, she accepts Kinsey's now discredited data on hyper-sexuality and prevalence of MSM experience in the United States,[3] and writes that extramarital sex is found in "73% of cultures worldwide." No doubt extramarital sex occurs in virtually 100% of cultures worldwide among *some* percentage of the population, but Hunter's implication seems to be that extramarital sex is normative. The best behavioral data we have suggest that extramarital sex, particularly among women, is far from normative. In much of the world, the vast majority of women report only one *lifetime* partner.[4] Even in the highest HIV prevalence countries in Africa, the great majority of women do not report more than one sexual partner in the past year. We acknowledge that there may be significant underreporting by women, but these data should not be entirely ignored.

Hunter calls for ever greater funding levels for AIDS, which she erroneously says is "still in its infancy." Although AIDS may arguably be the most devastating disease in human history, when these words were written, HIV incidence was already in decline globally and had been for some time. HIV prevalence stabilized globally in about 2000, and since then has declined somewhat in Africa (UNAIDS 2008b:35). Incidence, the rate of new infections, must have stabilized and begun to decline even earlier than this.

VALUES CLASH

The AIDS epidemic has taken place within the context of an increasingly "sex positive" culture in the countries of the West. Messages appealing to fear or stressing the risks of sexual behavior have been labeled as anti-pleasure and sex-negative and deemed ineffective. Communication campaigns have been crafted on the assumptions that messages that were more comfortable to see and hear (i.e., erotic, humorous messages) must work better in influencing behavior. In a post-1960s, postsexual revolution generation, the ethos in the West has become that people's sexual practices and preferences should not be denied or discouraged in any manner that might interfere with their freedom of choice and ability to do what feels good. Of course, what feels good and seems personally gratifying can also lead to harm to both oneself and others. This is especially true in the case of tobacco, drug, and alcohol use and some sexual practices.

This approach is drastically out of sync with the values of much of the developing world, which is largely rural, conservative, and religious. Religious communities (especially more conservative branches) often draw ire for their values-based approach to AIDS and have been treated as less than full partners by much of the AIDS establishment. Faith-based organizations (FBOs) own and operate many of the schools, hospitals, and clinics in Africa, yet FBO involvement in AIDS is often dismissed with comments about how religion contributes to stigma, and the important contributions of faith-based communities to AIDS are overlooked (Green 2003a; Green and Ruark 2008a). Worse, religious communities are blamed for exacerbating the spread of AIDS. In *AIDS in America*, Susan Hunter writes, "I interviewed far too many innocent Americans who have HIV because of the ignorance and greed of our conservative, right-wing 'Christian' government" (2006:ix). One might ask if Americans' choices to engage in risky behavior, and a culture that encourages those choices, are not at least as much to blame as the government, which after all does not give anyone AIDS.

Many African religious leaders believe that the West is forcing homosexuality and other liberal sexual practices and values on Africans. When asked in an interview if there was a Western campaign to corrupt African values, the archbishop of Ghana's Catholic Church Charles Palmer-Buckle replied, "We don't only suspect that there is a campaign, we think it's deliberate" (Okyne 2009). In a 2008 op-ed in *The Washington Post*, the architect of the (Anglican) Church of Uganda's first AIDS program similarly protested Western interference:

> Because we knew what to do in our country, we succeeded . . . the proportion of Ugandans infected with HIV plunged. . . . But international AIDS experts who came to Uganda said we were wrong to try to limit people's sexual freedom. Worse, they had the financial power to force their casual-sex agendas on us. . . . We, the poor of Africa, remain silenced in the global dialogue. Our wisdom about our own culture is ignored. (Ruteikara 2008)

In early 2010, an international furor exploded over proposed anti-gay legislation in Uganda, which has grabbed world attention because of the severity of the proposed penalties for gays (life imprisonment or death). Western heads of states and major newspapers condemned the law, while Ugandan lawmakers seemed to grow more entrenched in their support of the legislation, which they saw as defending traditional African values. We raise this issue not to condone the Uganda reaction (we strongly condemn a law that would kill or terrorize people based on their sexual behavior or orientation), but to highlight the extreme clash of values about sexuality that it represents. Might the proposal of such a law be a backlash to the myriad ways in which Western organizations have imposed their values and agendas regarding sexuality on Africans, especially in a country such as Uganda that has been flooded with donor AIDS funds?

One of the unspoken assumptions of many AIDS programs and AIDS professionals is that more traditional cultures are still in the dark ages when it comes to sexual norms and values but will gradually become more enlightened and more like "us" with increased contact with the West. Sexually liberated Western AIDS activists sometimes seem to expect to see a sexual revolution and the overthrow of patriarchal systems during the life of a five-year AIDS project. Anthropologists should know better and remember that anthropology's values-neutral understanding of cultural difference should also extend to sexuality. Why should we assume that non-Western societies will have their own Western-style sexual revolutions, or that they should?

Of course, cultures everywhere do change and evolve, and many have their own unique "culture wars" over sexuality. Unfortunately, when it comes to AIDS prevention, we in the West have exported our own culture wars, on such issues as abstinence education for youth and in debates over the place of religion in AIDS prevention. The "ABC" approach to AIDS prevention (Abstain, Be faithful, use Condoms) has been extremely controversial in the West, despite its wide acceptance in the generalized epidemics of Africa. In 2003, a heated discussion over the ABC approach arose on the AARG listserv. Talking about Uganda's ABC approach (Abstain, Be faithful, or use Condoms), Feldman commented,

> Trying to impose a sex-negative morality across all African cultures will not only fail to reduce HIV seroprevalence, but it will only bolster the rapidly growing danger of fundamentalist religion on the continent, and take Africa on a downward spiral into sexual repression and hostility. (AARG 2003)

Kenyan anthropologist Elizabeth Onjoro strenuously objected to Feldman's statements, protesting:

> I guess our friend Douglas is taking the stand that he knows more about Africans' sex life and behavior than Africans themselves. Better yet, that sexual behavior must be understood by the standards set by his own culture. Or mirrors his own culture. . . . As an anthropologist, I am perturbed to see that many in our profession still evaluate and narrowly interpret culture through their own ethnocentric ideals. . . . His school of thought is driven by lack of understanding of the TRUE African (or let me limit it to Kenyan since that is where most of my experience lies) sexual behavior and culture. Africans are not the crazed sexual animals we have been portrayed. . . . It may appear that way on the surface but underneath, that sex life is very well organized. . . . I grew up in Africa and as (an) anthropologist, I have a totally different belief of what Africans sexual behaviors are. Abstinence is built into many African cultures as part of various rituals.

The term or practice did not come to Africa from the conservative Christian wing as it seems to be the case here in America. (AARG 2003)

In a later post, Onjoro argued that although A, B, and C should be presented as options, a condom-focused strategy owed more to ideology than evidence. She noted that even in the United States, where knowledge and availability of condoms were high, new HIV infections were on the increase. She suggested that Western AIDS organizations may have been unable to absorb the success of Uganda's ABC strategy because they had not invented it, and that "ABC is an African-owned response, an indigenous and . . . integrated approach to HIV prevention." Onjoro posed a number of challenging questions:

> What if the CDC and USAID had promoted ABC in equal strengths in Africa? What if field officers did not impose their ideological beliefs about prevention on the African continent? . . . Do you know how many lives have been lost because the US had to uphold their ideological ideal of prevention? . . . What happened to giving Africans a chance to come up with their own ideology and models that work for them? (AARG 2003)

American anthropologist Brooke Schoepf entered the debate to express strong doubts about an approach centered on faithfulness and abstinence:

> I find myself heartily agreeing with Doug Feldman that sex-positive and anti-fundamentalist approaches have more to recommend them than abstinence/fidelity backed by moralist preachments AND the stigma that falls on those who do/can not comply. . . . We already know several ways to bring African men to use condoms, even at home. Is anybody listening? (AARG 2003)

In a special issue of the *AARG Bulletin*, Schoepf elaborated further: "Uganda's good news is remarkable. Nevertheless, 5 percent national adult HIV prevalence means that more and better condom promotion is needed. . . . In my view, more not less money needs to be allocated to condoms" (2003:13).

Anthropology should provide tools to better understand HIV risk behaviors and their sociocultural, economic, and other determinants. It should also serve as a corrective to Western medical approaches to AIDS prevention that are culturally inappropriate or simply ineffective. The standard approach to AIDS prevention has *not* put emphasis on behavior change beyond adoption of certain risk-reduction technologies, such as condoms. Reducing people to potential consumers of a marketed product and HIV prevention to little more than distribution of products does not invite the kind of in-depth research of behavior embedded in a particular culture that anthropologists are known for. If donors, governments, program implementers, and researchers *were* to focus on the key behavioral drivers of AIDS, and the sociocultural context of these behaviors, then anthropology would be in the best position of all disciplines to tease out the determinants of these behaviors, along with the context and conditions associated with them.

CASE STUDY: THEY DID IT THEIR WAY

In 2004, Green evaluated a small, low-cost program implemented by Africare in three southern African countries and funded by the Bill & Melinda Gates Foundation and known as the YES! Program. These programs were so low cost that they fell under the radar screen and were pretty much left to fend for themselves. By default, then, they actually resembled what they were supposed to be: locally designed and community-run AIDS prevention programs. They had an income-generation component so they could be self-sufficient, and they operated largely without direction from the Gates Foundation. The project was so low cost that none of the youth groups were even trained in AIDS prevention, so they fell back on common sense and carried out AIDS prevention in a way they knew would be locally acceptable. This is an example of how less direction from foreign donors led to better outcomes.

These programs targeted youth with messages about delaying sexual debut and not having multiple partners. Although programs like PSI and loveLife which commanded comparatively vast financial resources, were promoting condoms, testing, and STI treatment to high-risk youth, the YES! Program targeted youth who were not engaging in casual or multi-partner sex and were, in fact, the majority of the youth population. There were two reasons youth groups in South Africa, Zambia, and Malawi did not focus prevention primarily on condoms. First, they were operating in remote rural areas, where a steady supply of condoms could not be assured. Second, many parents in these rural areas would not have let their daughters participate in these programs if condom distribution were the main activity, and Africare policy called for gender balance in its projects. In fact, it was hard to enlist teenage and young women early in the project, until program "trustees" (local community supporters) explained that the goals of the program were actually promoting delay of sexual debut and not having multiple partners (Green 2004b). Green concluded:

> The single most important finding from this evaluation was that there is a viable model of AIDS prevention that seems replicable elsewhere in Africa and beyond. The model is low-cost, low-tech, culturally appropriate, sustainable, and to a great extent non-dependent on outside technical

assistance or commodities, except for condom supply (and condom use is not the only behavior promoted) (p. 2).

NOTES

1. Discussed at a workshop as an early accomplishment, Kampala, Uganda, AIDS Education and Control Project, April 21, 1993.
2. Gabriel Rotello's name for American gay men who exchanged partners often and frequented bars and gay bathhouses (see Rotello 1997).
3. As discussed in Jones (1997), Kinsey's data was skewed by a lack of random sampling and oversampling of men in prisons.
4. For example, India's 2005–2006 *National Family Health Survey* found that the average number of sexual partners among women who had ever had sex was only 1.02 (International Institute for Population Sciences [IIPS] and Macro International, 2007, National Family Health Survey [NFHS-3], 2005–06: India: Volume I. Mumbai, India: International Institute for Population).

Chapter 4

REFOCUSING HIV PREVENTION ON PRIMARY PREVENTION

A lthough we believe that there is a place for reducing the harm or risk of inherently harmful or risky activities (such as through wearing a condom or using a clean needle), we believe that fundamentally the goal of AIDS prevention should be to prevent harm and risk through primary prevention (such as through avoiding risky sex or not using drugs). We believe it is fallacious to begin with the premise that the underlying risk behaviors cannot—or *should* not—be influenced. We don't know these behaviors cannot be changed until we try. Otherwise, the belief that these behaviors can't change becomes a self-fulfilling prophecy. Besides, there are countless examples of people who have changed both sexual and addictive drug behaviors.

By primary prevention, we mean a focus on changing fundamental risk behaviors, such as risky sex or drug use. If these high-risk behaviors are eliminated, we have achieved not just risk reduction, but risk *avoidance*. We are not against risk or harm reduction measures, which may help individuals to reduce the risk of HIV infection. But these harm-reduction measures have had a poor record of halting the spread of HIV in many contexts, and we believe that they fundamentally do not go far enough toward protecting the health of those involved in high-risk activities. (Health, of course, encompasses more than just avoiding HIV infection, and there is ample evidence that activities such as sex work and drug use bring a host of other health risks besides that of HIV.) Sound public health means limiting disease and promoting health as much as possible, and, according to such an approach, activities that promote the spread of HIV should be discouraged as much as possible.

Unfortunately, risk or harm reduction has been not only the preferred but often the only approach used in prevention programs aimed at both sexually transmitted and IDU-transmitted HIV infection. There has been little or no *primary prevention* in HIV/AIDS, in spite of public and private sectors pouring more money and resources into this single disease than any other in history. Harm-reduction programs favor technology and medical solutions (drugs, condoms, syringes, methadone, or other substitute drugs) rather than any interventions that could be construed as interfering with sexual or drug use behavior. This assumes that harm-reduction strategies can sufficiently mitigate the HIV risk incurred by high-risk activities such as IV drug use, sex work, and sex with multiple partners. Proponents of harm reduction favor and defend people's "rights" to engage in a variety of high-risk behaviors, in the belief that they are helping people, but may not adequately consider the impact of these "rights" on the health of high-risk individuals, their partners and family members, and society at large. In our view, harm reduction takes a defeatist view of human capacity for change and treats symptoms rather than underlying problems.

Understanding the role of harm-reduction measures requires understanding how such measures are adopted by different populations in different epidemics. There are two primary types of HIV epidemics—generalized and concentrated—and they require very different prevention strategies. Yet AIDS prevention experts have often failed to recognize crucial differences between epidemics and have therefore targeted populations with inappropriate prevention interventions or targeted the wrong population altogether. To borrow the definition of David Wilson, Global HIV/AIDS Program Director at the World Bank (2005):

> Epidemics are concentrated if transmission occurs mostly among vulnerable groups and if protecting vulnerable groups would protect wider society. Conversely, epidemics are generalized if transmission occurs mainly outside vulnerable groups and would continue despite effective vulnerable group interventions. (2005)

Most HIV epidemics are concentrated, although generalized epidemics, mostly in Africa, account for the majority of the world's HIV infections. In concentrated epidemics, most infections occur among most at risk population (MARPs) and their sexual partners, more men than women are typically infected, and vaginal intercourse may not be the predominant mode of transmission. MARPs include sex workers (usually female) and their clients (usually male), injecting drug users, and MSM. Interventions for these populations are an essential part of AIDS prevention. Harm reduction would potentially yield far greater health benefits for these populations—and might even become risk avoidance—if it would promote far safer forms of drug taking and altered MSM sexual behaviors, behaviors that may have been the norm historically.

In generalized epidemics, most infections are found not among MARPs but among seemingly low-risk, sexually active people. The predominant mode of transmission is heterosexual vaginal intercourse, there are more women infected than men, and perinatal transmission is relatively common. One fundamental problem with prevention strategies in generalized epidemics has been that they have not been calibrated for where the HIV infections are primarily found—in general populations. For example, condom promotion has been a successful strategy among high-risk populations such as sex workers and their clients, and this can have national-level impact on HIV prevalence in epidemics driven by these populations. But condom promotion has utterly failed to increase usage rates enough to impact these epidemics in the generalized epidemics of Africa (Hearst and Chen 2004; Potts et al. 2008).

For those who continue to have multiple sexual partners or inject drugs despite being fully informed of the risks, the only preventive options may be risk reduction. However, we should not decide at the outset that no one has any control over his or her behavior, thereby eliminating primary prevention. Much of the problem with prevention stems from the global AIDS industry's insistence that solutions for high-risk groups are also appropriate for everyone, for general populations, for people who could make informed choices if we only informed them. We have learned too little from the mistake of misapplying the risk-reduction approach, especially in the generalized epidemics of Africa.

Decreases in risky behaviors (e.g., fewer multiple partners) and increases in risk-avoidance strategies (e.g., abstinence and faithfulness) have been linked to reduced HIV infection rates in generalized epidemics, although it is difficult to link this to specific AIDS prevention *interventions*, outside of Uganda in the period between the mid-1980s and the mid-1990s. Recently, many AIDS organizations and some major donors have become interested in finding ways to address multiple and concurrent partnerships, which involves influencing sexual behavior. Prior to this, there was little interest among most donors (with the notable exception of PEPFAR) in trying to change sexual behaviors, and few resources have been allocated to such approaches. Similarly, in IDU-driven HIV epidemics, there has been far less interest in trying to change injecting behavior in fundamental ways, than in distributing sterile needles, methadone, bleach, or other commodities or drugs. As we will discuss in Chapter 5, the success of such harm-reduction programs has been mixed.

Why do we persist in spending billions of dollars for programs with little or no impact? There are many possible reasons, including financial self-interest and inertia. It is difficult to scale down a multi-billion dollar per year industry. There are also subtler reasons related to ideologies and biases held by the West. To reform AIDS prevention, we who comprise the Western AIDS industry must not be blind to our own ideological biases, especially as we are making decisions about billions of dollars (most of it public funds) that lead to life or death for millions of people. To most in the AIDS industry, speaking of ideology in the context of AIDS conjures up images of George W. Bush, abstinence-only programs, and the religious right wing. But for most of the epidemic, the multi-billion dollar per year enterprise has actually been in the hands of those who label themselves progressives and liberals. Given that, we must ask: Why have we ignored primary prevention? Why have we failed to warn people about the risk behaviors that drive the pandemic, to the point that in a national survey South Africans were found to believe they had a greater risk of getting infected through blood transfusions than through having multiple partners (Shisana et al. 2005)?

Adding Risk Avoidance to Risk Reduction

To answer these questions, it is necessary to understand a bit of the history, politics, and ideology behind the AIDS prevention risk-reduction model that developed in the West and was exported to the rest of the world. Risk reduction seems to have grown out of (or alongside of) harm reduction, which developed in the field of substance abuse. Harm reduction starts with the premise that all addicts will engage in the most dangerous mode of drug ingestion, intravenous injection, just as risk reduction assumed that all MSM will engage in the most dangerous form of sexual behavior, anal intercourse. When we promote condoms or treat STIs but do not discourage sexual risk behaviors themselves, we call it risk reduction. When we provide syringes or bleach to reduce the risks of self-injection, we call it harm reduction. Harm and risk reduction do not focus on or even consider the full *range* of behaviors available to the addict (or person engaging in risky sex) or try to promote less risky alternative behaviors. In neither case are the risk behaviors themselves targeted for change.

Whether we speak of reducing risk or harm, the underlying thinking is the same. We can adopt the Open Society Institute definition of harm reduction:

> Harm reduction is a pragmatic and humanistic approach to diminishing the individual and social harms associated with drug use, especially the risk of HIV infection. It seeks to lessen the problems associated with drug use through methodologies that safeguard the dignity, humanity and human rights of people who use drugs. (Open Society Institute 2001)

Harm reduction sees itself as a pragmatic and a progressive alternative to the prohibition of certain lifestyle choices (Winstanley 2008). The Harm Reduction Coalition "believes in every individual's right to health and well-being, and believes they are competent to protect and help themselves, their loved ones, and their communities" (Harm Reduction Coalition n.d.). Unfortunately, people engaging in risk behaviors do not always have accurate information about the failure rates of harm reduction approaches. For example, correct and consistent condom use reduces HIV risk by only 80% (Weller and Davis 2002). Further, people addicted to drugs may *not* be competent to protect themselves and their loved ones from the consequences of their addiction, and being under the influence of drugs or alcohol increases the risk of violent, commercial, anonymous, unprotected, or otherwise risky sex.

Yet within the AIDS community, risk reduction continues to be synonymous with effective or standard AIDS prevention. According to a press release of the Global HIV Prevention Working Group during the 2008 International AIDS Conference in Mexico City, "successful HIV behavior-change programs deliver a combination of scientifically proven risk-reduction strategies" (Global HIV Prevention Working Group 2008b). Risk-avoidance strategies such as mutual fidelity and abstinence are not mentioned, although in the final report released by the Prevention Working Group, prevention is defined more broadly (Global HIV Prevention Working Group 2008a). When the United States, alone among major donor organizations, added risk-avoidance strategies (promotion of mutual fidelity and abstinence) to its mix of risk-reduction interventions, there was a strong negative reaction among HIV/AIDS activists and health professionals. This was probably inevitable, but with the policy coming from the unpopular George W. Bush administration, and with the initial program emphasis placed on abstinence (rather than faithfulness), the rejection of risk avoidance (or genuine primary prevention) by the vast majority of Western AIDS professionals became categorical and nearly complete.

When dealing with a disease that can be so easily prevented, it is tragic that greater efforts have not gone toward encouraging people to give up risky activities such as sex with multiple partners, or injecting drug use. Serious efforts to change high-risk behaviors themselves have been conspicuously absent from AIDS prevention. Solutions such as drug users abstaining from drugs, young people abstaining from sex, or sexually active individuals being faithful to their partners have been treated as being profoundly unrealistic. An Institute of Medicine report on preventing HIV transmission among IDUs stated: "The most effective way to reduce the risks of HIV transmission among injecting drug users is to stop drug use. However, not all drug users are ready or able to take this step" (Committee 2006:3). Programs aimed at helping addicts to stop drug use are relatively rare. But it's a false argument to assume or assert that *everyone* has to be ready to take the step of stopping before *anyone* can be helped out of active addiction.

Similarly, many HIV prevention programs have treated everyone as if they were sexually active and already engaging in risk behaviors that were unlikely to change. Consider the statements of Stephen Lewis, former UNAIDS special envoy for AIDS in Africa, when interviewed in March 2008 on a national news program (Rather 2008). Lewis explained why we need a condom approach for youth in Africa, saying: "In the United States, more than 50% of teenagers are sexually active by the age of 18. Why should it be different in other countries?" Actually, a large majority of Africans ages 15–19 report that they are not sexually active unless they are married. (African girls marry early, often before the age of 19, in a number of countries.) See Table 7.1 in Chapter 7 for data on premarital sex among African youth.

One wonders why U.S. taxpayers spend millions of dollars on detailed studies of sexual behavior of Africans, such as the Demographic and Health Surveys, if such data are not understood and used by so-called experts on AIDS in Africa. Lewis continued, "Hormones are churning in Africa! So why the devil would you insist upon abstinence when you know people are sexually active! If you want to protect them, you gotta use a condom" (Rather 2008). Lewis then blamed rising HIV rates in Uganda on an overemphasis on abstinence, stating: "There are so many problems with abstinence, that one hardly knows where to start!"

Besides the fact that such statements as "hormones are churning" are little more than racial stereotyping, Lewis seems to be unaware of, or unwilling to provide, clear evidence that HIV infections have been increasing in Uganda while condom usage rates have increased. Although the number of young people abstaining has been steady and may even have increased slightly, the most likely explanation for recent increases in infections is increasing numbers of partners among adults (see discussion of current trends in Uganda later in this chapter). As will be discussed in Chapter 6, higher condom usage rates are often associated with higher rates of casual sex, and more (not less) risk of HIV infection. Yet Lewis is apparently so intent on creating a false dichotomy between abstinence-only and evidence-based programs that he never mentions the intervention and behavior most associated with HIV decline in Uganda and elsewhere: fidelity or reduction in numbers of sex partners.

Comprehensive HIV prevention should offer risk reduction as well as risk avoidance and options for those at various levels of risk. A broader approach will surely have greater impact than a narrower one, given the variability of human behavior and circumstances. A single preventive approach to influencing something as complex as human sexual behavior will never appeal to all people, let alone influence

Table 4.1 Risk avoidance versus risk (or harm) reduction in sexually and IDU-transmitted epidemics.

	Sexually transmitted epidemics	IDU-transmitted epidemics

Risk avoidance	Sexual abstinence
	Mutual fidelity/monogamy
	  with an uninfected partner[†]
		Not injecting, stopping IDU
		Substituting oral (opioid)
		  drugs[*]

Risk (or harm) reduction	Partner reduction[•]
	Correct and consistent
	  condom use
	STI treatment
	Knowing one's HIV status
	Male circumcision
		Syringe provision or exchange
		Bleach for needle
		  sterilization
		Reduction in number of
		  needle-sharing partners

[†] Or mutual fidelity within a polygamous relationship.
[*] This avoids risk of HIV transmission through infected needles but addiction continues.
[•] This term implies something less stringent than mutually faithful monogamy or polygamy.

their behavior. For those who continue to have multiple sexual partners or who are otherwise at risk, the only preventive options may be those classifiable as risk reduction, namely condom use, male circumcision, and appropriate treatment of STIs (see Table 4.1). But we should be realistic about the risks that continued high-risk behaviors incur (even when harm-reduction measures are taken), and seek to promote the best possible health outcome, which is avoidance of high-risk activities.

A RIGHT TO HARM?

AIDS advocates and activists see themselves as the protectors and defenders of the poor, the downtrodden, and the socially marginalized, and as such protest anything they believe would restrict and further marginalize these groups. Supporting "human rights" in the context of AIDS has come to mean supporting the legal rights to engage in risk behaviors, whether they be injecting drugs or sex work. Support of any other position is seen as tantamount to committing the worst transgression in the AIDS world: making moral judgments. Yet, in what we might call our rush to *non*-judgment, we fail to make a sober, objective assessment of the pros and cons of legitimizing and legalizing sex work, heroin, crack cocaine, and methamphetamines. We don't ask whether social acceptance and legal protection of sex workers and addicts also leads to the social acceptance and legal protection of drug dealers, pimps, traffickers and brothel owners (Farley 2006). We fail to ask what is ultimately best for sex workers and drug addicts themselves—nor do we really ask these individuals themselves. We instead rely largely on self-selected activists who claim they speak for all people in their situation.

At the 2008 International AIDS Conference, there was a clear agenda among the organizers and many represented organizations toward not only legalizing and legitimizing sex work, but denying any risk associated with it. The first sex worker ever to be a plenary speaker was greeted with a frenzy of applause and cheering when she said that sex workers were not part of the problem but part of the solution and when she defended her right to continue to "work" even though she was HIV positive. But there were no speakers who had been trafficked into sex work as young women and held against their will, or women who would gladly do anything else to feed their children, given the opportunity. The reality of women who are forced into and traumatized by sex work was not even presented. Based on what was said at the conference, one would have thought that the "happy hooker" was the global norm.

At a satellite session organized by the International Planned Parenthood Foundation and moderated by Mary Robinson, former president of Ireland and former United Nations high commissioner for human rights, the pipe dream of high-risk behavior without risk of HIV was on full display. One of the speakers, a sex worker, declared, "We want pleasurable and risk-free sexuality." Another speaker, also a sex worker, added, "You can't expect us to practice A, B, or C [abstinence, be faithful, or use a condom] all the time." No one in the room seemed perturbed at the implication that sex workers should not be expected to use condoms consistently. Robinson added, "Repression of sexuality is life threatening," as if the real threat to life was not HIV and the real possibility that sex work will exacerbate its spread, but rather not freely expressing one's sexuality, in whatever form one chose. In response to this discussion, a member of the audience protested, "I question whether we have a common agenda here. I'm a woman living with HIV and I don't agree that a 'risk-free agenda' actually works. Sexuality is not risk free for me."[1]

In recent years, a happy hooker parallel has emerged from the injecting drug world: the happy and responsible drug addict. There seems to be a growing constituency within the harm-reduction movement to promote a "pleasure maximization," or "drug positive" philosophy, parallel to the "sex positive" philosophy that guides AIDS prevention. The International HIV/AIDS Alliance reported on the 2009 International Harm Reduction Conference by saying,

In much the same way safe sex programs have switched from a disease approach to a sex positive approach, harm reduction programs in the context of drug use need to be more drug positive in order to reflect the true nature of using drugs. . . . "Pleasure maximization and harm reduction" are integrally linked, and it is important for us to . . . acknowledge that there are positive aspects to drug-taking, and incorporate this concept into our work. (Chamberlain 2009)

The International Network of People who Use Drugs (INPUD) was established to represent on the world stage the interests of people who use drugs recreationally and to seek money from donors for such advocacy activities. At a 2009 harm-reduction donors meeting in Amsterdam, INPUD claims to have "demonstrate[d] that people who use drugs can indeed self-represent and donors should be funding groups of people who use drugs directly" (Gray and Page 2009).

The agenda of accepting drug use, as positive and "maximizing pleasure" is drastically out of sync with the experience of many drug users who find their lives dominated and ruined by drug use and certainly runs counter to the goals of public health. *If* our aim is to minimize sickness and death from injecting drugs use—and we must question if some working in AIDS prevention really have this as their primary aim—then anything that supports or encourages injecting drug use will work against this goal. Furthermore, the cost of addiction in terms of addicts' emotional and psychological health should be considered, as well as the impact on the family (including children), friends, and coworkers of the addict, and on society as a whole. The current treatment paradigm in the United States treats drug addiction as a "family disease," given the impact on spouses, children, and others close to the addict, and it is almost uniformly based on the 12-step Alcoholics Anonymous model, which requires abstinence from alcohol (and mood-altering drugs) as an immediate goal. Finally, let us not forget that many addicts are desperate to break their addiction.

We submit that human rights should *not* be interpreted to mean an individual's right to do whatever he or she chooses regardless of the personal cost or cost to society. Public health *cannot* pursue a policy of individual rights at any cost, or it ceases to be *public* health. Consider the logic of a Thai drug addict in calling for the legalization of drug use, in a statement made at the 2004 International AIDS Conference in Thailand:

In Thailand, injecting drug users or "IDUs" are the only group whose 50% HIV prevalence has not changed in fifteen years. One third of all new HIV infections are IDU-related, and this number is increasing. Yet there has been no effective response from the government. . . . Even

though the Thai government says its current policy is to treat drug users as "patients," not "criminals," it is still illegal to be a drug user. We
continue to be arrested and offered the choice of prison or military-run
rehabilitation centers. . . . We often do not enjoy even the most basic human rights. (Suwannawong 2004)

This addict seems to suggest that the only alternative to being
arrested and sent to prison or a military rehabilitation center is legalization of drug use. A similar argument was made at the opening plenary
of the 2008 International AIDS Conference by a speaker who protested
the "harmful consequences" of anti-trafficking laws in Cambodia. She
claimed that such laws led to violation of the rights of sex workers,
transgender people, MSM, drug users, and beggars, including wrongful
arrest and physical and sexual abuse (Pen 2008). In the addict's call for
legalizing drug use and in the Cambodian activist's call for ending anti-
trafficking laws, a false choice was presented: Legalize high-risk behavior, or violation of human rights will occur.

But there is a third option: *not* legally sanctioning activities that are
inherently risky to individuals and society yet also *not* arresting, harass-
ing, or allowing violence to be perpetrated against drug users, sex workers, and others engaging in high-risk activities. As an example, Sweden
has adopted a model in which *buying* sex is illegal and those who do
so are prosecuted, but those who sell sex are not criminalized or pun-
ished. A policy of treating drug users as patients and not criminals would
also achieve the goal of decreasing drug use, without criminalizing drug
users.

Similar to the "pleasure maximization" promoted by some drug users,
in recent years there has been an increasing resistance within the MSM
community to anything that is perceived to reduce pleasure, including
not only partner reduction but also condom use. (A notable exception to
this is the Netherlands, which we will discuss.) This is in spite of rising
HIV infection rates. Randy Shilts, in his highly informative and influential book *And the Band Played On* (1987), describes how this attitude
originated among gay men in the very beginnings of the AIDS epidemic
in the United States:

> The politically correct line, emerging from a handful of "AIDS activists,"
> maintained that talking about the gay community's prodigious promiscu-
> ity was part of a "blame-the-victim mentality." Michael Callen [a well-
> known early gay AIDS activist] saw a fine line between blaming the victim
> and taking responsibility, and he thought it was time for some straight
> talk about the disease if gay men were to survive. Merely moderating
> sexual behavior, as most gay doctors and health officials counseled, was
> not enough, he and Berkowitz wrote in the *The New York Native*. Strong

measures needed to be taken; it was time to think about closing the bath-houses, they wrote. "If going to the baths is really a game of Russian roulette, then the advice must be to throw the gun away, not merely to play less often." (1987:209)

Callen and Berkowitz were quickly denounced and angry rebuttal letters were fired off to the *Native* editor.

Shilts continues:

Writer Charles Jurrist responded with his own *Native* piece, "In Defense of Promiscuity," which highlighted the popular party line that a gay man was more likely to be killed in a car accident than by AIDS. An infectious agent might be hypothesized, Jurrist wrote, "but that's all it is—a theory. It is far from scientifically demonstrated. It therefore seems a little pre-mature to be calling for an end to sexual freedom in the name of physical health." (1987:210)

By the time incontrovertible evidence had accumulated that the new disease was viral and that promiscuity was indeed the primary risk factor for both homosexuals and heterosexuals, the "don't judge" and "hands off sexual behavior" ideologies were already entrenched. According to these ideologies, the problem was not found in behavior but in the reac-tions of narrow-minded people to certain behaviors, leading to stigma and discrimination.

HIV first arose in the United States among groups that were—and still to a large extent remain—marginalized and which suffered discrimi-nation and rejection by the wider society. Gays and gay activists were certainly victims of stigma and discrimination, and they died in droves at a time when the governments of the United States and other coun-tries seemed to care little about the new disease that primarily infected gay men. Gay men were also victims of discrimination, hate, stigma, and other things that come under the rubric of homophobia. There was much blaming of the victim, and some even said publicly that "These people are getting what they deserve" (Marcus 2001).

We can only guess at the anger and resentment—even paranoia—this treatment provoked among gays. But this should not cause gay men to turn on themselves and on those who have advocated taking stock of and changing high-risk behaviors. Larry Kramer and Gabriel Rotello are two gay men who have called for a modicum of restraint and been subsequently pilloried by other gays. Mark Schoofs, in a criti-cal comment on Rotello's explosive book *Sexual Ecology* (1997), asks with a note of sarcasm, "Should prevention workers print posters say-ing, 'Reduce your number of partners'?" (Schoofs 1997). Green wrote in 2003:

Rotello's (1997) book provoked great controversy within the gay community. Judging by the reviews I have read, the controversy was not over Rotello's analysis of condom use but rather over his suggestion that gay men—at least highly sexually active, fast-lane urban gays—developed values and behavioral patterns that led to self-harm, as well as built-in mechanisms that resisted critical self-examination and more fundamental change in sexual behavior, such as having far fewer sexual partners. Rotello refers to this as the multipartnerist ethic of the gay sexual revolution. (p. 119)

In a 2004 speech at Cooper Union College, Larry Kramer suggested that gay men should take responsibility for their behavior: "I wish we could understand and take some responsibility for the fact that for some 30 years we have been murdering each other with great facility and that down deep inside of us, we knew what we were doing." Kramer was accused of sex negativity, gay homophobia, and anti-eroticism.

Some members of the gay community have suggested that biological survival is less important than sexual freedom. Gay activist and psychologist Walt Odets, quoted earlier, has argued that avoiding HIV infection should be "secondary to the primary goal of continuing unrestrained gay sexual practices." Odets writes:

> If some gay men feel that the fullest, richest possible life demands behaviors that may also expose them to HIV, who are educators to tell them that they are wrong. It is homophobia that motivates these authoritarians—many of them gay men—to dictate to the rest of us. It is homophobia that drives us into retreat from intimacy and sexuality that once gave our lives meaning. . . . Also homophobic is the expectation that gay men ought to feel shame and guilt for not liking condoms and, often, not using them. (1994:1)

Surely a word like homophobe loses its power when used manipulatively and punitively against someone with whom one disagrees. Gay men are not being told what the real dangers are and are lulled into thinking that if they use a condom they have adequately managed their risk. But they have a right to the truth, even when the truth (such as the fact that partner reduction is a crucial component of HIV prevention at an individual and population level) could be deemed "sex negative."

A HUMAN RIGHTS AGENDA OR DISEASE PREVENTION AGENDA?

The rhetoric of human rights and social justice now permeates AIDS conferences, literature, and press releases, and HIV prevention, treatment, and care are increasingly seen through the lens of a struggle for human rights. Within the AIDS community, a "rights-based approach" has become normative; a human rights agenda is assumed to be synonymous with the goals of preventing AIDS and mitigating its impact. The struggle of people living with HIV (PLHIV), MSM, and other marginalized individuals for access to treatment and services, protection under the law, and against stigma and discrimination is certainly a struggle for human rights.

We are not denying the intersection of human rights with issues of AIDS prevention, treatment, and care. But it is unusual (and possibly unique) for the political agenda of human rights to be elevated to a major theme for disease prevention, as it has been for HIV/AIDS. For example, "Access to Services and Human Rights" was named the theme of the 2009 World AIDS Day. Yet never has there been a theme along the lines of "Stick to One Partner," the clear call to behavior change used when Uganda mounted the most effective AIDS prevention response the world has ever seen.

According to the logic of most of the international AIDS community, effective HIV prevention primarily requires two things, both of which fall under the rubric of human rights: access to services and decreasing the vulnerability of those at risk of HIV infection. The right to services is often invoked as a fundamental right and has been the theme of National Strategic Frameworks for HIV/AIDS of countries throughout the world. We certainly support the provision of biomedical services such as testing and treatment of HIV and other STIs and acknowledge that such services may be of great use to individuals. Yet, as we will discuss in Chapter 6, there is strong evidence that nothing that is found in a hospital or clinic will succeed in curbing generalized epidemics if there are not also fundamental changes in sexual behavior. We should not think that we are doing all we can to prevent HIV if we are not also addressing the behaviors that spread the virus.

Botswana provides a telling example of this reality. Probably no country in Africa will ever be able to invest as much money per capita as Botswana has invested in AIDS-related medical services, but this has had little or no apparent impact in national HIV prevalence. Botswana is stable, democratic, offers free education through university level, and is wealthier than virtually any other country in Africa. HIV infections are found in all parts of the population, and education and wealth do not seem to significantly decrease risk of being HIV infected.

What does it mean in a situation like this to concentrate HIV prevention efforts on achieving human rights? Researchers Tim Allen and Suzanne Heald, in their article "What Has Worked in Uganda and What Has Failed in Botswana?" state: "It seems to us that human rights activism linked to HIV/AIDS in Botswana has hindered public health measures" (2004:1152). Allen and Heald believe that focus on condoms and human rights diverted attention and resources from trying to change sexual behavior. They further note: "In this region of the world the pandemic has been allowed to become a public health disaster. It urgently demands appropriately tough responses to bring it under control" (2004:1152).

As evidence has accumulated that decades of condom promotion have not paid off in terms of lowered HIV rates in the world's hyperepidemics (and treating STIs has been shown by multiple research trials not to be an effective HIV prevention approach), major donors have responded not by questioning an "access to services" approach, but rather by investing in another medical service: HIV counseling and testing. Voluntary counseling and testing (VCT) is certainly one of the more expensive ways to go about AIDS prevention. A comparative study of the different costs per case of HIV prevented found that VCT was the most expensive nondrug method, at around $400–500 per infection averted (Creese et al. 2002). And as we will see in Chapter 6, VCT may not always result in lower HIV risk, and some studies show that testing negative may result in more risky behaviors.

A group of HIV prevention experts argued in a 2008 article in *Science* (Potts et al. 2008) that "the largest donor investments are being made in interventions for which evidence of large-scale impact is increasingly weak" (namely condom promotion and distribution, VCT, and STI treatment). They protested that "much lower priority is given to interventions for which the evidence of potential impact is greatest" (p. 750), specifically male circumcision and reducing multiple sexual partnerships. UNAIDS' response was to defend its HIV prevention spending priorities (DeLay 2008), and there is little evidence that the international community will abandon massive investments in the "three 'established' pillars of HIV prevention" (Potts et al. 2008) anytime soon.

Toward the end of his tenure as executive director of UNAIDS (which ended in 2008), Peter Piot was known to urge that rather than being evidence-based, AIDS prevention should be evidence-*informed* (Piot 2006), which seems to suggest a much less rigorous use of the evidence than one might expect from the world's most prominent AIDS organization. In fact, UNAIDS has always been primarily an *advocacy* organization (Chin 2007), which perhaps explains its priorities and at times selective use of evidence when it comes to HIV prevention.

In the last few years, epidemiologists Elizabeth Pisani and James Chin have both published insider exposés about UNAIDS' selective use of data to make HIV epidemics seem even worse than they were, for the purposes of raising global concern and ever-expanding levels of funding (see Chin 2007; Pisani 2008). But not everyone consults insider accounts. The official viewpoint of ever-increasing HIV incidence prevailed at least as late as the 2007 Institute of Medicine assessment of the PEPFAR program. It states: "The epidemiologic facts are clear . . . the rate of new HIV infections continues to grow" (p. ix). It is now widely acknowledged that global HIV incidence peaked more than a decade ago.

Addressing vulnerability to HIV is the other HIV prevention approach that is championed by the AIDS community. In this view, stigma and discrimination, social marginalization, poverty, lack of education, women's lack of empowerment, gender-based violence, homophobia, and other violations of human rights are seen as the causes of HIV transmission. According to Pedro Cahn, then head of the International AIDS Society, we must "fight the gender inequality, homophobia and poverty, which continue to drive this epidemic." In the same speech at the 2008 International AIDS Conference, he called for programs "grounded in both human rights principles and sound public health that meet the needs of men who have sex with men, injection drug users and sex workers" and said nothing about non-MARP populations, which account for most infections worldwide (see Cahn 2008).

In a like manner, the resolution adopted by the UN General Assembly Special Session on HIV/AIDS (UNGASS) in 2001 states: "The full realization of human rights and fundamental freedoms for all is an essential element in a global response to the HIV/AIDS pandemic, including in the areas of prevention, care, support and treatment, [and] reduces vulnerability to HIV/AIDS and prevents stigma against people living with or at risk of HIV/AIDS" (General Assembly 2001:point 16). This resolution further states that "poverty, underdevelopment and illiteracy are among the principal contributing factors to the spread of HIV/AIDS," that "stigma, silence, discrimination and denial, as well as a lack of confidentiality, undermine prevention," and that "gender equality and the empowerment of women are fundamental elements in the reduction of the vulnerability of women and girls to HIV/AIDS" (General Assembly 2001:points 11, 13, 14).

In such a view, HIV infection is seen as primarily being a result of vulnerability to HIV caused by underlying societal or structural factors, rather than a result of individual choices and behaviors, or cultural factors that may lead to those behaviors.[2] The key to HIV prevention thus becomes reducing vulnerability and ensuring basic human rights, such as through reducing poverty and empowering women. The *Operational Guide on Gender and HIV/AIDS: A Rights-Based Approach*, published by UNAIDS, captures the opinion of many in AIDS prevention when it says:

> Addressing gender equality is possibly the most effective strategy in reducing vulnerability to HIV infection. . . . When the human rights of women and girls are truly respected and when women and girls are able

to engage their male counterparts as equal partners in the household, the community, the workplace, at school and in politics, the epidemic will cease to spread so rapidly and will no longer cause such devastation. (Mukhopadhyay et al. 2005:4)

In concentrated epidemics, those who are at high risk of HIV infection (primarily IDUs, MSM, and sex workers) are also marginalized within society. Working with such marginalized, high-risk groups in any meaningful way involves gaining access to such people, gaining their trust, and developing some level of sympathy for their plight. These groups are often looked down upon, even despised, perhaps more openly in more tradition-bound and religious societies. In the not-so-distant past in the United States, for example, gays were considered by some to be "plague carriers" who threatened to contaminate mainstream America (Fumento 1990). Those working to prevent AIDS in high-risk groups naturally find themselves becoming involved with the human rights of these marginalized groups. The danger is that the cause of human rights may be used to justify investing significant prevention resources in programs that have little or no *prevention* impact. Surely the right to accurate information on how *not* to become sick and die ought to be high on the list of human rights we defend and promote. To fail to provide this information is to take the position that "we" know what is best for those at real risk of a fatal disease. It is very disempowering to start with the premise that people are merely passive victims in their own lives, with no agency to change or improve their situation. A further disempowering corollary is that *individual* behavior change is of little of no consequence.

We wholeheartedly support causes of human rights, including empowering women, reducing poverty, and increasing access to HIV treatment and any services that might help an individual avoid HIV infection. As a global community, we should not need the impetus of AIDS to make protecting human rights a matter of prime importance and urgency. But we would question if the AIDS community's focus on human rights has not been an impediment to effective HIV prevention, in that it has distracted us from a more direct approach to HIV prevention that focuses on risk behaviors and proximal causal factors of infection. Which is the primary agenda of the AIDS community, that of promoting human rights or preventing HIV infections?

AIDS is not, after all, *caused* by poverty or discrimination or any other number of supposed culprits; it is caused by a virus, which can be spread in a relatively small number of ways. Preventing HIV transmission requires addressing the proximal factors of HIV transmission: sex with an infected individual, or exposure to infected blood, or transmission from a mother to child. Vulnerabilities such as poverty or lack of empowerment may increase the risk of exposure to the virus, or they may not. Even when more distal factors (such as socioeconomic factors or gender-based violence) are associated with higher HIV risk, influencing them will only reduce HIV transmission if in doing so the proximal factors themselves (exposure to HIV through blood or body fluids) are addressed. If raising a person's economic status simply results in new risk behaviors (which may occur, for instance, when a person becomes wealthier and has greater mobility and access to more sexual partners), addressing economic vulnerability will not result in effective HIV prevention.

The question we need always ask—but seldom do—is what impact, if any, would achieving greater human rights have on reducing HIV infections? If the true answer is little or none, then using AIDS prevention funds to promote social and political ends—no matter how worthy those ends—is hard to justify. The most recent South African National Strategic Plan lists as its first three HIV prevention strategies reducing poverty, empowering women and educating men and women on human rights (and women's rights in particular), and addressing gender-based violence (*HIV and AIDS and STI Strategic Plan for South Africa 2007–2011*, 2007:10). Prevention strategies such as strengthening behavior change programs and specific interventions for youth, in workplaces, and for MARPs are mentioned further down the list.

In its 2008 global report, UNAIDS claims that "sufficient evidence exists to guide national initiatives that aim to minimize the societal sources of HIV risk and vulnerability" (p. 65). We challenge the view that there is "sufficient evidence" for many of the structural interventions promoted by UNAIDS (and others) for HIV prevention. As UNAIDS notes in the same report, relatively few studies have examined such interventions and the ones that have done so have thus far failed to show any impact on HIV transmission. Some of these failures will be discussed in Chapter 8.

Another aspect of a human rights approach to AIDS prevention that deserves consideration is that within this paradigm, expanding access to human rights—and therefore reducing AIDS—is seen as primarily being the role of government. In the words of Gruskin and colleagues, when discussing the link between health and human rights:

> Governments are therefore responsible for enabling their populations to achieve better health through respecting, protecting, and fulfilling rights (i.e., not violating rights, preventing rights violations, and creating policies, structures, and resources that promote and enforce rights). This responsibility extends beyond the provision of essential health services to tackling the determinants of health such as, provision of adequate

education, housing, food, and favourable working conditions. These items are both human rights themselves and are necessary for health. (2007:450)

Governments should do what they can to protect their citizens from HIV infection, including instituting laws that protect girls and women from sexual coercion and rape, providing HIV testing and prevention of mother to child transmission (PMTCT) services, and investing in communication campaigns to inform people about the risks of AIDS and attempt to change social norms. But even the most beneficent government policies will not solve the key problems of AIDS prevention if communities are not mobilized and if risky behaviors do not change. We would also ask whether this focus on *government* action is not somewhat misplaced: Is HIV prevention primarily the responsibility of individuals and communities, or governments? Is it individuals, communities, and social norms that must change, or governments that must change? The answer may be that change is needed on all sides, but we would certainly argue against a view that sees governments, and not communities, as being the key to effective AIDS prevention.

Balancing Rights

Promoting human rights can promote HIV prevention (e.g., by increasing access to PMTCT services), but there may also be tension between the two agendas. There is clearly tension between the "right" of an HIV-positive sex worker to work and the goal of reducing HIV infections among clients of sex workers. How does the "right" of a sex worker to have clients relate to the "right" to health of the wife or regular partner of that client? Which "right" is more important? An HIV-positive sex worker might argue, as one did in a plenary session at the 2008 International AIDS Conference, that she has the right to work "because that's what condoms are for."[3] But condoms do have a failure rate. How many women would support the "right" of their husbands or partners to have sex with an HIV-infected sex worker as long as a condom was used, no matter how small the possibility of condom failure?

To take another example, former Botswanan President Festus Mogae defended Botswana's decision to pursue "opt-out" HIV testing (in which HIV testing became part of routine procedure at health facilities, although people had the option to opt-out) at the opening session of the 2008 International AIDS Conference:

We must not be afraid to take controversial steps so long as we are careful and caring of people's needs and rights. One of the examples is the heated debate a few years ago over Botswana's decision to adopt provider initiated opt-out HIV testing. The evidence now supports the decision. We must distinguish human rights which are absolutely sacrosanct from civil rights which are contextual. What do I mean by contextual? I will give an example. Eighteen months ago, there was a new outbreak of measles in Southern Africa, in Botswana and Namibia. And in both countries, there were communities who absolutely refused for their children to be vaccinated. We could not afford for that to happen, so we vaccinated the children against the will of their parents. I think we may be guilty of having violated their civil rights, but certainly not their human rights. But this is not only about individual efforts, but also about collective responsibility to our families, to our friends, to our communities, our countries and continents, and to our global village. (Mogae 2008)

The "rights" of people not to know or not to disclose their HIV status are in tension with the public health good of having people be tested for HIV as routinely as possible, just as the "rights" of parents to not have their children be vaccinated are in tension with the imperative of preventing a measles outbreak. In such cases, "rights" may indeed be contextual, as Mogae suggests.

We believe that it is important for the public health community to acknowledge ways in which a human rights agenda and the mandate of decreasing HIV infections might diverge and to discuss ways in which the two agendas can be reconciled. This tension between public health and individual rights is not unique to HIV prevention. When the state requires vaccinations for school-age children or forbids smoking in public places, it has decided (often with the support of the public health community) that the public's health is more important than an individual's right to practice harmful behavior. It may be that HIV/AIDS also requires that certain individual rights yield to the priority of protecting the public's health.

If our objective is to bring down HIV rates rather than pursue social, economic, or political goals, responses need to be in line with public health priorities, rather than with primarily economic or political goals. Many activists and groups with various social agendas have sought and found opportunity to promote various worthy causes, using both the financial resources and the intense interest the world has shown in AIDS. As the world's most politicized disease, opportunities abound for attaching a political cause to the coattails of AIDS. One downside of this is that it has complicated and compromised a public health response to AIDS.

An individual rights-based approach is also limited in that it doesn't help us make tough decisions about resource allocation, decisions that are at the heart of public health. Proponents of the human rights approach to AIDS admit this limitation and correctly note that "no single analytical framework—whether grounded in economics, social sciences, ethics, or human rights—can determine to everyone's satisfaction who should benefit from services first, second, or last" (Gruskin and Tarantola 2008:S124). Gruskin and Tarantola assert that a human rights framework helps ensure that "the processes of setting agendas and priorities, as well as the expected outcomes, are based on justice, dignity and fairness and that a level of accountability is built into decision-making processes" (Gruskin and Tarantola 2008:S124). Gruskin and Daniels (2008) suggest an approach which they call "accountability for reasonableness," in which "'fair-minded' people, who seek mutually justifiable terms of cooperation . . . agree on and justify, even when resources are constrained, the reasons for the priorities they determine necessary to meet health needs fairly" (p. 1576).

Fairness, reasonableness, dialog, and accountability are all vital when it comes to setting priorities, even if they may not provide much clear direction on how resources should be allocated. The challenge of deciding how to distribute scarce resources among multiple claimants is not unique to AIDS, and the human rights approach is not alone in struggling to provide clear guidelines on how to do so. In practice, however, the claim of "rights" often becomes a trump card that squelches further dialog. Experience suggests that global resources go to the activists who call most stridently for their rights, rather than to where it would promote the maximum health benefits for the greatest number of people. And when one group successfully invokes its "right" to claim resources, this may in fact shut down the crucial process of deciding how to distribute scarce resources *equitably* among a number of claimants with equally urgent needs and equally valid "rights."

AIDS activists—in partnership with not a few anthropologists—have been extraordinarily effective in defining services such as antiretroviral therapy (ART) in terms of rights, with the result that huge sums of money have been mustered for treatment. Millions of people worldwide are alive as a result. But the problem with defining treatment as a "right" is that it precludes any difficult yet necessary conversations about what our priorities should be in global AIDS spending. At a time of decreasing global resources, and when the cost of treatment for all those who need it is increasing exponentially, we cannot pretend that there will be enough money in the global AIDS pot for everyone who needs treatment. Further, increasing resistance to first-line drugs in poor regions of the world will force difficult decisions about whether and when more expensive treatment options should be offered and about whether offering more expensive treatment for some is justified when many have not even been able to access first-line treatment.

As of early 2010, major donors such as the U.S. government have decided to essentially flatline HIV treatment budgets, meaning that the number of new patients who can be enrolled will be extremely limited. After several years of both the rhetoric of AIDS treatment as a basic human right and the reality of rapidly expanding access to free ARV drugs, many HIV-affected populations around the world have come to expect access to treatment, but it seems inevitable that we will soon reenter an era in which, for many HIV-infected people, the hope of treatment will seem dim. Conflict may arise among the HIV infected, between the treatment haves and have-nots or between those in need of life-prolonging treatment and the governments and programs that provide it. How will governments and treatment programs make decisions about allocating treatment, should funds become scarcer? Should the teachers and health care workers be given priority, or the young, or those with children?

If we widen the view from HIV, the funding dilemmas become even more severe. The world has poured forth an unprecedented amount of money for AIDS, while other health interventions that could save lives at pennies to the dollar compared to HIV/AIDS remain severely underfunded. As AIDS expert Daniel Halperin wrote in a 2008 *New York Times* op-ed, the fact that the United States spent almost $3 billion on AIDS programs in Africa in 2007 and only $30 million on safe-water projects on the continent is "disastrously inequitable," and "many millions of African children and adults die of malnutrition, pneumonia, motor vehicle accidents and other largely preventable, if not headline-grabbing, conditions" (p. A9).

We are not arguing that PLHIV not be given state-of-the-art HIV treatment, even if such treatment is extremely expensive. Nor are we saying that PLHIV should automatically be given such treatment as a "right." There is no easy answer to the question of an equitable distribution of health resources and who should get what in a world of finite resources (and in which global health likely will never attract more than a tiny fraction of the world's resources). Yet in such a discussion an uncompromising rhetoric of "rights," which refuses to make compromises or acknowledge competing priorities, is not helpful. Statements such as "it should never, ever be a question of either or" may draw applause at an AIDS conference. (Pedro Cahn was, in fact, applauded for this statement, when he fought back at the criticism that AIDS was taking money away from other vital health services in his speech at the opening plenary of the 2008 International AIDS Conference.) But if we truly care about the best health for *all*, there are hard choices to be made.

CASE STUDY: THE RISE (AND FALL?) OF THE WORLD'S MOST
EFFECTIVE AIDS RESPONSE

In recent years, Uganda has become something of a Rorschach test for
AIDS prevention, with interpretations of "what really happened in
Uganda" being used to support all manner of foregone conclusions about
what really works in AIDS prevention. It is undeniable that Uganda
experienced the most dramatic turnaround of an AIDS epidemic the
world has ever seen, with HIV prevalence declining by approximately
two-thirds, from 18% in 1992 to 6% in 2002 (Wabwire-Mangen et al.
2009). In our view, Uganda's success against AIDS is a remarkable example of the success of a primary prevention approach. In the late 1980s
and early 1990s, Ugandans developed a response to AIDS that was culturally grounded, innovative, low tech, low cost (and therefore sustainable), and more effective than any other AIDS prevention program that
has ever been implemented anywhere before or since. Unfortunately, the
recent history of AIDS in Uganda is a much sadder tale, as AIDS prevention there has come to resemble AIDS prevention elsewhere, and the
number of new infections has again begun to creep up.

Some background: President Museveni of Uganda received a phone
call from Fidel Castro soon after taking power in Uganda in 1986;
Castro told him that 18 of the 60 Ugandan officers training in Cuba
were infected with HIV (Allen 2002:14). Museveni then called his top
medical advisers to develop a strategy for combating AIDS.[4] There was
an urgency about the matter comparable to the task of ridding Uganda
of its previous dictators, Idi Amin and Milton Obote. Museveni was the
first African head of state to declare war on AIDS.

The news from these medical advisers was at first alarming. One advisor was Vinand Nantulya, who had been working for African Medical
and Research Foundation in Nairobi, and he well remembers his first
meeting with Museveni about AIDS. Nantulya told the president that the
bad news was that this new disease was progressive, incurable, and fatal.
Yet Museveni also quickly understood a feature of AIDS that is often
forgotten: HIV is actually quite difficult to spread. As he once said,

> (AIDS) is a good disease. We know the few ways it is transmitted and it *is*
> *in our control.* You have a choice! You can decide *not* to get it. How can
> you stop it? You can abstain from sex. Or you can stay with one partner.
> Be faithful to survive. You can decide not to get it. You have to agree with
> me, what a good disease! (Uganda AIDS Commission 2003)

Five months after Museveni came to power, his newly appointed minister of health, Dr. Rukahana Rugunda, shocked delegates to the World
Health Assembly in Geneva with a simple, frank admission: "Fellow

delegates, I have to inform you that we have a problem with AIDS in Uganda, and we would like the support of the international community in dealing with it" (Kaleeba et al. 2000:9). The rest of the African continent remained in denial that AIDS was a problem in Africa for years to come.

The government did not promote condoms at first. For example, in the first booklet on AIDS prevention put out by the Ugandan government, there was no mention of condoms until page 32.[5] On this page, the original draft of the booklet showed a doctor talking to a patient. The patient asks the doctor if a condom can prevent AIDS. The doctor says no, and then explains the various shortcomings of condoms. This page concludes: "The government does not recommend using condoms as a way to fight AIDS." However, the booklet was paid for by UNICEF, and because it controlled final publication, UNICEF literally pasted over a new, more pro-condom page before releasing the booklet. The pasted over version deleted the statement that had been on page 32 as well as part of the dialog with the doctor. But the doctor still tells the patient that he could get AIDS even if he uses a condom, a statement unlikely to be seen in a donor-funded message anywhere else.

We are not anti-condom, but we want to underscore the fact that Uganda, almost alone in the world, crafted its own response to AIDS rather than following the advice being offered by international experts. There has been much revision of the history of Uganda's response to AIDS. By 2003, when USAID/Washington decided to do a comprehensive study of "What Happened in Uganda," Americans who had worked in Uganda for years were saying that Museveni had promoted condoms from the start. Yet Green's former colleagues at The Futures Group, which brought the first condom social marketing program to Uganda, told him what an ordeal it was to get the Ugandan president to agree to this program.

As early as 1991, there was a sense that Uganda was being mobilized to address AIDS in ways unlike any other country in Africa.[6] Accordingly, President Museveni was invited to give a speech at the International AIDS Conference in Florence, Italy, that year. He made it clear that Uganda was going its own way and did not accept the "magic bullet" approach (as he called it) that the West offered in the form of the condom. He commented:

In Africa sexually transmitted diseases such as gonorrhea and syphilis were a big health hazard before the advent of modern Western medicine. To discourage the spread of these in society, Africans had evolved cultural taboos against premarital sex and strict sanctions had been established against premarital sex or sex out of wedlock. I have been emphasizing a return to our time tested cultural practices which emphasized fidelity and condemnation of pre-marital or extra-marital sex. (Museveni 1991)

President Museveni was clear that the best response to the threat posed by AIDS and other sexually transmitted diseases was to be found in behaviors or values such as "reverence and respect and responsibility," which in Africa are often polite code words to refer to fidelity between spouses or sexual partners. This was a powerful statement: AIDS is an STI (at a time when much of Africa was in denial that AIDS existed, or considered it only a new form of witchcraft) yet it can be controlled simply by adhering to certain familiar behaviors already embedded in the culture by the wise ancestors. But this was not what the Western AIDS establishment wanted to hear, and Museveni was not invited to speak at another International AIDS conference until 2004, when his speech was similar in tone and again upset Western activists.

Jesse Kagimba, Museveni's presidential adviser on HIV/AIDS, recalled to Green in 2003 that there was little mass media available in the early years of HIV in Uganda, but government radio and TV (one station each) carried messages about AIDS awareness and prevention. According to Kagimba, President Museveni set the tone and the approach. Museveni's message was that AIDS is caused by a virus and is a heterosexual disease, not just something gay men get in America. AIDS has no cure and it kills you. But he also said, "It is preventable, we can control it. As a matter of fact, it's not very infectious. It's not born by the air, nor carried by insects. Behavior alone can control epidemic disease."[7] In an earlier conversation in 2001, Kagimba had stated that there were three steps to Museveni's approach: Realize how severe the problem is; convey that fact every person is at risk (Museveni used to say AIDS is spread by "promiscuity"); and then clearly show that *you don't have to get it*. Museveni would say, "There's something *simple that you yourself can do to avoid it*."[8] This concept is known as self-efficacy.

Another distinctive feature of Uganda's approach was the deliberate use of fear appeals. Museveni used political rallies and public broadcasts to educate people about AIDS. He has stated, "When I had a chance, I would shout at them: 'You are going to die if you don't stop this [risky sex]. You are going to die'" (Zeelie 2002). Clearly, Museveni was not soft-peddling the message that AIDS is a fatal disease. Jesse Kagimba reflected in a personal interview with Green: "We were told that we shouldn't use fear in our messages. But I am not sure that is right. I still believe fear helped us achieve our goals." He said fear "cut through the denial" that AIDS was an American disease that didn't affect Africans, a theory popular in Africa in the early years, and made people open to the message of what they needed to do to not get this dread disease. In fact, research has shown that fear messages, when combined with high self-efficacy (also part of AIDS messages in Uganda, as discussed), can be very effective (Green and Witte 2006).

Uganda's earliest AIDS posters used imagery of human skulls, coffins, and the grim reaper. There were somber radio messages accompanied by the slow beating of a drum and a stern, raspy voice of an old man talking about AIDS in the manner of announcing funerals. The AIDS Support Organization (TASO), the first organization of its kind in Africa to support people living with AIDS, sent people living with HIV/AIDS to conduct AIDS education in local communities, including schools. Ugandan informants have reported that this strategy increased personal perception of threat, arousing responses such as "I, too, can get this new disease," and "There but for the grace of God go I," which motivated behavioral change (Green and Witte 2006). The high level of fear, paired with the knowledge that Ugandans could *do something* to avert infection (self-efficacy), created optimal conditions for behavior change (Green and Witte 2006; Witte 1992, 1998).

In sum, Ugandans were made to fear AIDS, to feel personally at risk of infection and to believe that their very lives depended on their actions. There was also an appeal to national unity and national defense ("We will fight this enemy together"), and it came from the then very popular president who had ended brutal years under the bloody regimes of two dictators. This sense of vulnerability was especially true of the period 1986–1991, when HIV incidence (the number of new infections) is calculated to have peaked and when behavioral studies show there was fundamental behavior change: reduction in partners and delay of sexual debut. According to a national survey carried out by the Global Programme on AIDS in 1989, 9% of Ugandans reported that they had already changed their behavior (or intended to do so) by practicing abstinence, faithfulness, or reducing number of sexual partners, and 1% of Ugandans reported that they had changed their behavior (or intended to do so) by using condoms (Kirby 2008). Any incidence or prevalence decline attributable to condoms would have come later, as condom social marketing only began to distribute condoms in significant quantities after this early period, and Uganda did not produce its own condoms during the 1990s (Green et al. 2006; Kirby 2008). A good description of Uganda's approach from a Ugandan perspective can be found in the book *Open Secret* (Kaleeba et al. 2000) and in a 2005 article coauthored by the former director of Uganda's National AIDS Control Programme (Okware et al. 2005).

Thus, we see an African approach to AIDS prevention that was different from the way the rest of the world was gearing up to combat

AIDS. The Ugandan approach took a clear aim at sexual behavior. It was behavior based, and the key behaviors emphasized were fidelity, "zero grazing" (which originally meant fidelity within a polygamous relationship), and delay of the age of first sex. Okware and colleagues (2005) recount some of this early history, noting that at the establishment of the National AIDS Control Programme in 1986, condom promotion messages were limited to the dissemination of "technical information" and that availability and use were very low. In 1991, the government adopted a policy of "quiet promotion and responsible use of condoms with appropriate education." Condom procurement rose (from 10 million in 1994 to 120 million in 2003), as did usage. Yet Okware and colleagues note:

> It is clear, however, that national HIV prevalence began to fall in the late 1980s and early 1990s, several years before condoms were available in large numbers; and this means that much of the credit for turning the tide must go to the "home grown," community derived solutions to the problem: A [abstinence] and B [being faithful]. (p. 627)

Researchers Tim Allen and Suzette Heald (2004) have asked: What was it that worked in Uganda and failed in Botswana, a country which has achieved the world's second-highest HIV prevalence? They proposed that "the promotion of condoms at an early stage proved to be counter-productive in Botswana, whereas the *lack of condom promotion* during the 1980s and early 1990s contributed to the relative success of behavior change strategies in Uganda" (p. 1141, emphasis added). Green argued in a report to the World Bank in 1998 that behavior change (this meant faithfulness and abstinence in Uganda at that time) and not condom use was the key to HIV decline, and authored a USAID report in 2003 with similar conclusions. From 2004 onward, most peer-reviewed articles about what happened in Uganda, and why, concur that it was primarily behavior change, in particular partner reduction, that account for Uganda's AIDS success (Genuis and Genuis 2005; Green et al. 2006; Kirby 2008; Shelton et al. 2004; Stoneburner and Low-Beer 2004).

HIV prevalence decline in Uganda sputtered out in about 2004, and a national sero-behavioral survey in 2004–05 showed prevalence was 6.7% (Uganda HIV/AIDS Sero-behavioural Survey 2004–05), higher than previously estimated. Other data also suggest an increase in new infections. An ongoing study of HIV incidence in Rakai District, Uganda, found that an uptick in incidence began in 2003 (Arroyo et al. 2006). Data from 203,000 VCT clients tested between 1993 and 2003 (the data were national but overrepresented urban residents) found an increase in annual HIV incidence per 100 uninfected persons from 0.9 in 1993 to 2.3 in 2003 (Baryarama et al. 2007). HIV prevalence was declining during this period even though the rate of new infections appeared to be rising (Bessinger et al. 2003).

The important question is why HIV infections began to rise again in the world's greatest AIDS success story. The answer has immense implications for how we spend billions of dollars on HIV prevention worldwide. In the absence of clear empirical evidence a number of explanations emerged; two of the most prominent were not enough condoms and too much abstinence forced on Ugandans by the George W. Bush administration. For example, Human Rights Watch released a rapid assessment report in March 2005 which alleged that Uganda was discontinuing condoms in favor of an abstinence-only strategy (Cohen 2005b). A version of this report was also published the next year in *The Lancet* (Cohen et al. 2005). Uganda's purported change in strategy was even discussed in Congress and in the Institute of Medicine's 2007 overall evaluation of PEPFAR (Sepulveda et al. 2007).

Many Western observers have alleged that abstinence was not an indigenous Ugandan response but was a strategy imposed by the U.S. religious right through the policies of the Bush administration. This view is contradicted by statements made by some of the architects of Uganda's HIV prevention response (see quotes by Museveni and Okware), and by data (which will be discussed in Chapter 7) showing that fewer Ugandan youth were having sex long before the advent of PEPFAR. Ugandan researcher Busulwa found in his survey of abstinence among Uganda's various ethnolinguistic groups that although they vary somewhat in their sexual practices "the avoidance of pre-marital pregnancy appears to have been a key factor in the shunning of pre-marital sex" (Busulwa 1995). (He also found that there was typically a double standard between the sexes.) Ruark conducted a series of focus groups with Ugandan youth in 2003 that found that Ugandan youth saw many risks to premarital sex. They were highly aware of how HIV infection or (more likely) a premature pregnancy could cut short their educations and have devastating consequences for themselves and their families, and they saw abstinence as a strategy to avoid risk and achieve "bright futures."[9] However abstinence was understood and practiced historically, in the era of AIDS a great many Ugandan youth see abstinence as a positive and pragmatic choice.

In 2006, the Uganda AIDS Commission issued a report in which the Ugandan authors synthesized a number of peer-reviewed articles and other data sources and gave their perspective on Uganda's purported increase in new infections (Wabwire et al. 2006). This report gave no recommendations about needing more condoms and no warnings about Uganda abandoning evidence-based prevention for an excessive focus on abstinence. The report did note that "[t]here has been a shift of focus towards service access messages as opposed to behavior change messages [and] reliance on mass media with limited individual and community contact/dialogue" (p. 37). A section on youth again mentioned "more focus on service access messages as opposed to behaviour change messages" (p. 24). According to this report, the problem in Uganda did not seem to be a dearth of condoms, but rather an overemphasis on service access messages (for such services as counseling and testing) and a lack of behavior change messages.

For those who had ideological differences with the Bush administration, it might be tempting to pin the blame on that administration's policies. However, evidence gleaned from behavioral surveys, a review of government policies, and qualitative research, points elsewhere. As noted, it has been the consensus in the research community that monogamy, fidelity, and partner reduction were the behaviors most responsible for prevalence decline in Uganda (Green et al. 2006; Shelton et al. 2004; Stoneburner and Low-Beer 2004). (This epidemiological evidence will be discussed in more detail in Chapter 7.) Yet from 1995 to 2006, the proportion of men and women reporting high-risk sex (sex with a non-marital, noncohabiting partner) has increased somewhat—from 11% to 16% of women, and from 31% to 35% for men (Uganda Demographic and Health Surveys 2000–01, 2006).

Second, if one looks at recent AIDS strategy documents in Uganda,[10] it is clear that condoms and testing have been increasingly emphasized at the expense of sexual behavior change. "Zero grazing" and partner fidelity are seldom mentioned in recent documents, nor are abstinence or delay of sexual debut. Initial drafts of the *2007/8–2011/12 National HIV & AIDS Strategic Plan* (subtitled *Moving Towards Universal Access*) did not include any impact indicators for abstinence and faithfulness, despite the protests of members of the prevention committee about the document. Rev. Sam Ruteikara, one of the co-chairs of the prevention committee, said about the process:

> Repeatedly, our 25-member prevention committee put faithfulness and abstinence into the National Strategic Plan that guides how PEPFAR money for our country will be spent. Repeatedly, foreign advisers erased our recommendations. When the document draft was published, fidelity and abstinence were missing. . . . When Washington insiders were alerted to these scandals, the words "abstain" and "be faithful" were quietly re-inserted into the plan—on paper. But that doesn't guarantee these methods will be implemented or promoted. (2008)

The "Washington insiders" to which Ruteikara refers were officials at PEPFAR, a funder of the document and an ostensible promoter of abstinence and faithfulness as part of a comprehensive prevention approach. As an apparent result of pressure brought to bear on PEPFAR officials, an Annex was added to the document, supplying language about behavior change. Such a cautionary tale causes us to wonder who pulls the strings with other national prevention documents and strategies in Uganda and elsewhere.

Recent qualitative research conducted by Green in collaboration with researchers at Uganda's Makerere University and at University of California, San Francisco (UCSF) also points to shifts in Uganda's prevention priorities that may explain Uganda's slipping gains against HIV. Interviews and focus groups conducted in 2009 in peri-urban and rural areas near the capital of Kampala discovered evidence of major changes in prevention messages. The peri-urban location was the same area where Norman Hearst of UCSF and Phoebe Kajubi and Moses Kamya of Makerere University conducted an earlier study, which showed that increased condom use led to greater HIV risk (Kajubi et al. 2005).

The purpose of the 2009 research was to gain a better understanding of the changes that have occurred in AIDS prevention in recent years. As this book goes to press, some preliminary findings provide a disturbing picture. When asked to rank the effectiveness of different methods of prevention, both men and women ranked HIV testing first, followed by condoms. Significantly down the scale of responses came fidelity, with abstinence ranked last. Respondents were then asked, "Over the last 6 months what is the main AIDS message you have heard or seen?" Three-quarters of men and women answered HIV testing or condoms.

Preliminary findings from the focus groups were similar. In transcripts of these discussions, "test" or "testing" appeared 267 times; "condom(s)" appeared 194 times; "faithful" or "faithfulness" appeared 57 times; and "abstain" or "abstinence" appeared only 33 times. The terms "zero grazing" and "love faithfully" were not mentioned. In contrast, a USAID survey in 1991 had found that these were the two most remembered AIDS prevention slogans (Moodie et al. 1991). These results show a clear shift in emphasis from promotion of fidelity and partner reduction (the behaviors most emphasized in Uganda's successful HIV response and most critical to declining HIV rates), to testing and condoms.

Additional factors may also be implicated in the reversal of Uganda's AIDS fortunes. The recent Uganda research found ample evidence that AIDS has come to be seen as a treatable, chronic disease like malaria. Because of the availability of ARVs, and because Ugandans no longer see PLHIV wasting away before their eyes, AIDS is no longer as feared. Focus group respondents made comments such as, "Ever since people began getting ARVs, it has caused them to have irresponsible sex. They don't fear each other any more, [or fear] that they might infect each other with the AIDS virus" (Green et al. 2010).

We are certainly not arguing that people should not be given ARVs, but rather acknowledging that wider availability of treatment may have unfortunate effects on risky sexual behaviors and on HIV transmission. Prevention fatigue was also probably inevitable, regardless of the availability of treatment. A country cannot stay on high alert forever, and the widespread feelings of personal vulnerability and cautious behavior that were evident in the late 1980s were probably bound to decline. But Uganda's adoption of the global standard approach of treatment, testing, and condoms (and its turn away from emphasizing behavior change) has almost certainly hastened the process. And infection rates seem to be rising in Uganda at a time when they are declining elsewhere in Africa.

NOTES

1. Ruark, personal notes, August 5, 2008.
2. According to the last UNAIDS global report,

   Risk is defined as the probability or likelihood that a person may become infected with HIV. Certain behaviors create, increase, and perpetuate risk. . . . Vulnerability results from a range of factors outside the control of the individual that reduce the ability of individuals and communities to avoid HIV risk. These factors may include: (1) lack of knowledge and skills required to protect oneself and others; (2) factors pertaining to the quality and coverage of services (e.g. inaccessibility of service due to distance, cost or other factors); and (3) societal factors such as human rights violations, or social and cultural norms. (UNAIDS 2008a:65)

3. Ruark, personal notes, August 3, 2008.
4. Nantulya, personal communication, October 15, 2003. Also see Allen 2002:14–15.
5. *Guidelines for Resistance Committees on the Control of AIDS: Action for Survival*. Prepared by UNICEF Kampala with the approval of Directorate of Information and Mass Mobilisation, NRM Secretariat and the Health Education Division, Ministry of Health, Republic of Uganda n.d. Green was given a copy of this book in 2004 by Filippo Ciantia, an Italian medical doctor, who had worked in Uganda even before Museveni came to power and dated the booklet to 1988 or 1989 (there is no date on the booklet itself). Those who produced the first edition of this booklet didn't bother to change the condom page; they just pasted over the toned-down comments on a new page. It was possible to peel back the paste-on and read the original version.
6. Senegal and Gambia developed programs around this time that had some similarities with Uganda. Their success was largely hidden by the high rate of male

circumcision and preexisting low prevalence of partner exchange for females. It takes multiple partner sex from women as well as men, as well as lack of male circumcision and other factors, to develop and sustain a hyper-epidemic (Green n.d.).

7. This statement summarizes two of three widespread African indigenous theories of contagious disease discussed earlier: Diseases are believed to be caused by contact between people, tiny insects or worms, and by wind or air that carry disease.

8. Kagimba, personal communication, November 5, 2003.

9. These comments are based on research Ruark conducted with 13–16-year-old in-school Ugandan youth and 13–21-year-old out-of-school Ugandan youth in Soroti and Masaka Districts in 2003.

10. Such documents include The Revised National Strategic Framework for HIV/AIDS Activities in Uganda: 2003/04–2005/06 (July 2004), The National Monitoring and Evaluation Framework for HIV/AIDS in Uganda (July 2004), and the Uganda Ministry of Health's National Condom Policy and Strategy (June 2004).

Chapter 5

Primary Prevention in Concentrated Epidemics

A s we noted at the beginning of this book, basic principles of public health teach that avoiding an infectious disease is better than reducing the risk of infection. Risk avoidance is often dismissed as being unrealistic for most at-risk populations, the populations most in need of HIV prevention interventions in concentrated epidemics. But it is unjustified to dismiss risk avoidance before investigating and determining the evidence for the effectiveness or ineffectiveness of both risk reduction and risk avoidance, with most-at-risk populations (MARPs). Let us consider these questions with the three main categories of MARPs: sex workers, IDUs, and MSM.[1]

Sex Workers

One reason for the near-exclusive emphasis on risk reduction, when considering prevention experience in concentrated epidemics, is that *some* of the strategies developed for MARPs have worked for *some* of those groups. Condoms seem to have had significant impact on the HIV epidemic in countries like Thailand and Cambodia, where it was possible to enforce condom-use policies in certain environments, notably in brothels. Thailand in particular has been repeatedly cited as justification for a primary focus on condom promotion, regardless of the part of the world or type of HIV epidemic.

It may be possible to enforce a "100% condom" policy in an *accessible* population and in a situation that is to some extent controllable, such as among sex workers and their clients in brothels. But outside of settings such as brothels, condom use is not enforceable, and consistent condom use is achieved by only a small number of people in *general populations*, where people cannot be "bribed or blackmailed" (in the words of epidemiologist Elizabeth Pisani) into condom use (Pisani 2008). Furthermore, a less-often mentioned aspect of the prevention success in both Thailand and Cambodia is that the proportion of men reporting contact with sex workers also declined significantly. It is difficult to know how much prevalence decline can be attributed to condom use and how much to less contact with sex workers and fewer men reporting any type of extramarital sex (Phoolcharoen 1998).

Moreover, the impact of condoms may not be sustainable. For one thing, in many countries sex work has drifted out of brothels into locations where it is difficult or impossible to enforce condom policies or rules. And some data challenge the belief that when reported condom use reaches high levels among sex workers, HIV prevalence will decline significantly for sex workers and their clients. For example, 99% of sex workers in Uganda report ever use of condoms (although usage is inconsistent), but HIV prevalence among sex workers nevertheless rose from 28.2% in 2001 to 47.2% by 2003 (Wabwire et al. 2006).

In Thailand, HIV prevalence among brothel-based sex workers fell by about half in the late 1990s, but according to a 2004 United Nations Development Programme (UNDP) report, prevalence remained "high" at 7% to 12%, partially due to the increasing numbers of non-brothel-based sex workers who operated in settings that were less easily regulated or reached (UNDP 2004). This report also noted that the 100% condom policy was less rigorously enforced than a decade previously and that sex workers' use of condoms had dropped, with one 2003 study of major cities showing only one-fourth of Thai clients were likely to use a condom (Buckingham and Meister 2003, cited in UNDP 2004:53). By 2005, reports from Thailand showed that the rate of HIV infection among gay and bisexual men in Bangkok had risen more than 50% in two years (from 17.3% to 28.3% between 2003 and 2005). This caused Mechai Viravaidya, the architect of Thailand's 100% Condom Use Policy, to declare: "For 12 years Thailand has been winning the war against AIDS, but now the champion has been knocked out . . . I'm going to let the world know that Thailand is no longer a model for AIDS prevention" (MacIsaac n. d.).

Likewise, a study of sex workers in Cambodia found that, "Despite the implementation of a nationwide 100% condom use policy, the prevalence of STIs among female sex workers in 2005 was comparable to 2001" (Sopheab 2008:167). There is substantial evidence that condoms work much better at protecting male clients than at protecting the female sex workers themselves, probably because the men have far fewer exposures.

There is a risk avoidance versus reduction debate concerning sex work: Should AIDS prevention be limited to providing condoms and treating the curable STIs of sex workers (risk reduction), or does such a policy ignore the health of sex workers (physical, psychological, and emotional) as well as social and criminal problems associated with sex work? Might risk reduction actually work *against* protecting women and girls who are trafficked and prostituted because provision of risk reduction requires some sort of working relationship with those who control prostituted women and the business of prostitution, as well as "looking the other way" with criminal activities related to prostitution? (Farley 2006; Farley and Seo 2006).

Green had a crisis of conscience in which this dilemma was indelibly imprinted in his mind. One night in Georgetown, Guyana, in 1999, he was interviewing sex workers and brothel owners as part of design activities for that country's first USAID-funded AIDS program. He interviewed one girl in a brothel who was no more than 15 years old. She was clearly terrified of her pimp and brothel owner, who insisted on sitting close enough to hear all her answers. It was understood by prearrangement that Green could ask her questions only about oral-anal-vaginal practices and use or nonuse of condoms. He could not ask how she might have been trafficked by the menacing-looking man seated nearby.

Green was reminded that evening that he was part of a risk reduction-only industry. He could not ask this girl if she wanted to be where she was, doing what she was doing, or whether it was at all involuntary. Raising questions about the ethics of a 15-year-old girl working in prostitution would have been judged interfering or moralizing or "imposing his own values." It would have threatened the cozy, collegial relationship that had grown up between the brothel owner, his "girls," and the local donor-financed, AIDS prevention industry of NGOs and the government. Green was struck with how this relationship makes brothel owners and pimps, often known to be violent, seem semi-respectable partners and stakeholders in internationally funded programs, much as any NGO. Feminist activist Melissa Farley has long made just this argument.[2]

Imagine how this cozy relationship between AIDS prevention NGOs and brothel owners would look to a girl who had been kidnapped, trafficked to a distant city, had her documents confiscated to prevent escape, and locked in her room until some man wanted sex—sometimes violent sex—with her. The AIDS industry typically views "sex workers" (the preferred term in public health and one that makes prostitution seems like any other job) quite shallowly, as vectors for disease, as condom recipients, and as people who occasionally need antibiotics. Ideally, they can be turned into peer educators and spread information and condoms to other sex workers.

But there appears to be little consideration of the whole person, sympathy over the coercion and violence sex workers often suffer, or referrals to legal aid or counseling—nothing that interferes with the business of prostitution. That would be judgmental, it is argued, and would drive prostitution underground. The health worker, the AIDS prevention specialist, and the anthropologist are asked to check their brains and their ethics at the brothel door, so to speak.

There are two divergent views of sex work, and each is invoked to support political positions. One view is of a 12-year-old girl who is kidnapped, sold into slavery, and chained to a bed in a brothel. The other archetype is the happy hooker (think Julia Roberts in the movie *Pretty Woman*). From our own experience in Africa, Asia, the Caribbean, and elsewhere, both types are found, as are all types in between. Yet even where women (and less often, prostituted boys and men) appear to have made a choice, it is not that simple. As Farley summarizes, a number of prostitutes have described this vocation as:

> *"volunteer slavery"* and as *"the choice made by those who have no choice."* If you're a woman or girl, global forces that *choose you* for prostitution are sex discrimination, race discrimination, poverty, abandonment, debilitating sexual and verbal abuse, poor education or no education, and a job that does not pay a living wage. All drive girls and women into the commercial sex industry. Defined as whores when they were young, women who appear to choose prostitution have been sexually abused as children at much higher rates than other women. One way that women end up "choosing" prostitution is that they are paid for the abuse that they have already grown up with. They assume that's all they are good for. (2006:103)

What are the risk avoidance options? Conventional thought tells us that sex work is "ineradicable," that prostitution is the world's "oldest profession." But women do leave prostitution, and in some countries we have seen significant drop-offs in clients visiting sex workers.

We can encourage men not to participate in commercial sex, using health and perhaps even moral arguments from culturally appropriate sources. We can prosecute men if they engage the services of sex workers. This protects not only the men and their non-sex worker partners, but also sex workers by reducing the demand for their services and ultimately reducing the number of sex workers. Sweden has undertaken to charge and prosecute *clients* and *not* sex workers, which can be seen as a structural or "ecological" intervention (Farley 2004).

Another ecological intervention that may have accounted for fewer visits to sex workers in Thailand and Cambodia is the "100% condom policy" that forced men to use condoms in brothels—a policy that could be enforced by telling the brothel owners that their businesses would be shut down if they didn't cooperate. Cambodia's National HIV/AIDS Center survey showed:

The percentage of soldiers who said they had visited a prostitute in the previous month dropped from 47% in 1999 to 20% in 2001. The proportion of police officers who reported visiting a prostitute within the previous month dropped from 37% in 1999 to 18.5% in 2001, while the proportion of motorbike taxi drivers who visited a prostitute dropped from 34.5% to 8.5% within the same time period. (Kaiser Daily HIV/AIDS Report, 2001, cited in Green 2003b:114)

There are also programs that help rescue girls and women from being trafficked and then provide shelter and job training for the victims. All of these alternatives get at the underlying problem of prostitution and go beyond putting a band-aid on the problem, so to speak. This does not mean that we should not also be providing condoms and STI treatment for sex workers while working on more lasting solutions.

MSM

Considering prevention for MSM, there are two behaviors that put them at high risk of HIV infection: having multiple and concurrent partners, and anal intercourse. Early in the U.S. epidemic, as the theory evolved that the new disease was caused by a sexually transmitted virus, health officials soon realized that not all gay men were getting the disease, but rather it was those who reported a great many concurrent sexual partners (see Chapter 3). For the first time, non-gay health officials were gaining some understanding of how far the gay sexual revolution had progressed in some cities and in some bathhouses. Gay activists had fought long and hard for the right to practice sex as they wished, without fear of arrest, public shame, beatings, or worse.

A culture of extreme sexual freedom developed in the years after gay men flexed their political muscles and stood up to police in Stonewall in New York (June 1969), and this carried over into the beginning of the AIDS era. Gay doctors and gay leaders like Larry Kramer who counseled against having many partners, strictly from a public health or survivalist perspective, were derisively labeled "monogamists" with "sex negative" attitudes (Shilts 1987:245).

We have already noted great resistance to changing sexual behaviors, at least among some of those who choose to speak for the gay community. Gay anthropologist Ralph Bolton cautioned that calls for a reduction in the number of sexual partners could be viewed as a criticism of gay culture, as well as that "calling for a reduction in the number of sexual partners implied a radical restructuring of all gay social life" (1992:168). Still, there was some fear-driven, mostly spontaneous reduction in partners among U.S. MSM, that seemed to reduce the rate of new infections.

Psychological anthropologist Robert Edgerton holds that although some cultural traits are positively adaptive to their environments, others may be neutral, inefficient, or unambiguously harmful by any objective measure, such as human health and well-being. Inspired by Edgerton and ecological anthropology, Green has observed: "Health beliefs may arise and persist because they serve a useful function, because they are useful in some way, because they are adaptive to a particular environment, or, in the context of our discussion, because that are adaptive to conditions in an environment that threaten health" (1999a:249). Traits can also be maladaptive. But for the availability of ART, natural selection would select for those individuals and those elements of culture that favor some degree of sexual caution and restraint, which guards against fatal sexually transmitted disease.

Rotello, in his 1997 book *Sexual Ecology* (and personal communication), presented an extended argument for fundamental behavior change among his fellow gay men. He challenged the popular view that gay men are biologically wired for promiscuity, that:

> Human males are inherently promiscuous, and a sexual society consisting only of men must, by an implacable law of nature, lead to the kind of promiscuity we experienced in the seventies. If this is true, gay men can do little for themselves but hope for an early and complete cure for AIDS. . . . However, if this concept is not true, it is vital to say so, because the very belief that it is may make change impossible. (p. 222)

Is it really the case that gay men, once liberated from artificial social controls, must "tend toward biological self-destruction unless continually rescued by modern science" in the form of improved condoms or anal microbicides (Rotello 1997:222)? Rotello rejects this, and points out that men have always lived in societies that control sexual behavior:

> Throughout history the voluntary control of sexuality has been a major preoccupation of all religions, all cultures, all peoples. Every society on record has attempted to channel sexual drive in ways that promote stability, usually by enacting explicit rules about whom you can and cannot have sex with, and then backing up those rules with powerful rewards and penalties, social customs, religious beliefs, laws, and taboos. (p. 223)

All men, gay or not, can and do control their sexual behavior provided they live in a culture (or subculture) that provides them sufficient incentives to do so. For that to be the case, there have to be things in men's lives that are more valuable than complete sexual freedom. As Rotello put it: Fellow gay men must accept the fact that "the unlimited, unstructured pursuit of absolute sexual freedom [is] biologically disastrous for gay men" (1997:290–91). On the other hand, replacing maladaptive behaviors and norms with new norms of partner reduction and monogamy (including serial monogamy) could radically curb new infections among MSM.

From the beginning of the AIDS pandemic, anal sex has always been assumed by the AIDS establishment to be a "given," a universal and immutable behavior of gay men. If challenged, the response would be that anal sex is an essential part of a gay man's identity and that anal sex for a gay man is as natural and unavoidable as vaginal sex is for heterosexual men. Yet there are whole traditions of male homosexuality that allegedly did not involve anal sex, starting with the ancient Greeks (Dover 1978) and continuing today in some countries. In the Netherlands and some countries of Asia, the practice is still relatively unknown and is practiced by a minority of MSM (Hospers and Blom 1998; Hong Kong Community Planning Process on HIV/AIDS MSM Working Group 2002).[3] A 2006 meta-analysis of studies of MSM in Asia found that the prevalence of "ever had sex with a man, in lifetime" is typically several times higher than lifetime prevalence of "anal sex with another man" (Cáceres et al. 2006:82). Research of non-anal alternatives for MSM is limited by the fact that surveys of MSM practices—including the most recent survey done by the U.S. Centers for Disease Control (CDC)—conflate oral and anal sex, meaning prevalence of anal sex alone is not available. Other studies limit the definition of MSM to "those who admitted engaging in anal sex since a year prior to the studies," meaning they leave out what might well be, in some countries, a majority of MSM (Lesbian and Gay Legislative Advocacy 2006).

There was some small effort in the U.S.-government funded AIDSCOM project to promote alternatives to anal sex, such as through developing a "hierarchy of risk" pyramid, with the most dangerous behaviors listed at the top and the least dangerous ones at the bottom. Receptive anal sex was at the highest level. Yet tools like this, showing levels of relative risk, were rarely used in AIDS preventive education, then or since.

Anal sex is by far the major mode of HIV transmission among MSM (Buchbinder et al. 1996). Furthermore, a study of gay men in California showed little difference in risk between anal sex with a condom or without a condom. The authors note:

> Many studies have demonstrated that receptive anal sex is most strongly associated with prevalent and incident HIV infection in MSM and carries the highest per-contact risk of acquiring HIV. This study found that URA [unprotected receptive anal] sex with either HIV-positive or unknown serostatus partners explained one quarter of new infections in this cohort. Surprisingly, we also found an independent increase in the risk of HIV seroconversion among men reporting PRA [protected receptive anal] with an HIV-positive partner. (Buchbinder et al. 1996:954)

One explanation for this might be that condom effectiveness is lower in anal than in vaginal sex (Halperin 1999). Moreover, there is little evidence that consistent condom use is the norm, even among American gay men, who must be among the most AIDS-educated and condom-accessible group in the world (Rotello 1997). After remaining constant in recent years, HIV prevalence among U.S. and especially African American MSM rose from 2001 to 2006 (CDC 2008), and U.S. syphilis rates have risen every year since 2001, with 63% of cases among MSM (CDC 2009). Largely missing from prevention programs for MSM are any risk-avoidance interventions that seek to change basic patterns of high-risk sexual behavior, such as discouraging anal sex itself or discouraging multiple partners.

There is at least one well-documented risk-avoidance program, targeting Dutch MSM, which discouraged anal sex. After being presented with facts about the risk, a large proportion of Dutch men discontinued anal intercourse (which had only a relatively recent history in the Dutch gay community) and went back to sexual practices which had risk of HIV infection several orders of magnitude lower (Hospers and Blom 1998; Van Griensven et al. 1987). Thus, in the early Dutch response to AIDS, men were encouraged to give up anal sex completely, and many apparently did. Cohort studies of Dutch gay men reported that the practice of anal sex declined dramatically from 1984 to 1985. Since the level of HIV prevalence in these cohorts remained lower than in most American cities—the rate of new infections actually reached zero in one cohort in 1987—this advice may have been quite effective (King 1997, cited by Rotello 1997).

An evaluation of this program concluded:

> The decline in transmission of HIV in the AIDS cohort from 1985 onwards was probably a result of the decrease in sexual activity in the studied population and more specifically the decrease in the number of partners with whom anogenital intercourse was performed. The alternative explanation, that the decline in transmission of HIV was a result of a so called saturation effect, is unlikely given that 60% of the participants were still not infected. (King 1997, cited by Rotello 1997:222)

This important example of a successful risk-avoidance approach for MSM does not seem to be widely known or discussed within the AIDS field. By the 1990s, Dutch AIDS prevention was under increasing pressure to promote condoms (risk reduction) as an "equally valuable" AIDS prevention option for Dutch MSM, according to Dutch scientists Hospers and Blom (1998). That condom use is equivalent to not practicing anal sex is, of course, not true, but it is in keeping with the so-called condom code. According to this code:

> Gay sex is fine as long as a condom is worn. Not wearing a condom violates obligations to other gay men as well as obligations to the larger gay

community. A consistent condom user is under no obligation to be tested for HIV or to inform prospective sex partners of his HIV status even when he knows himself to be infected. (Chambers 1994:353)

In a powerful essay published by The Gay Men's Health Crisis in 1997, Richard Elovich wrote:

What is so seductive about reducing HIV prevention to what is now called the "condom code" is that it papers over some of these painful distinctions: it allows us a way to feel that HIV status doesn't make a difference; to pretend we are all the same; to act as if having a fatal virus doesn't even make a difference in our sex lives; that we don't have to deal with disclosure; and most painful of all, we don't have to deal with the meanings of the differences between being positive and negative. (1998)

Equating condom use with safe sex has had a disastrous effect on the gay community, even without factoring in organized promotion of bareback sex among a minority of gay men (Scarce 1999). As with generalized heterosexually transmitted HIV epidemics, condom use does not seem to be containing the epidemic, and different kinds of behavior change (partner reduction or fidelity, and shifts away from anal sex) may be needed to significantly impact infection rates.

IDU

The great political and ideological battle in the IDU arena is about harm reduction. The argument, in our view, is not about the inclusion of harm reduction as *a strategy* for those who cannot or will not refrain from injecting various mood-altering drugs (which we support), but whether this approach as the *only* realistic or legitimate way to prevent HIV infection. The efficacy of drug substitution (such as methadone) and needle exchange programs is unquestioned within the HIV prevention community. The Global HIV Prevention Working Group recently stated "Multiple studies conducted in resource-limited settings have confirmed the public health benefits of harm reduction programs" (Global HIV Prevention Working Group 2008a:14). A 2004 WHO report states, "In the absence of an effective and widely deployed vaccine against HIV, measures to improve access to sterile needles and syringes will remain the most effective tool available to reduce the spread of this virus among (and from) IDUs" (p. 5).

How has harm reduction fared among IDUs? The evidence has been quite mixed. The most sophisticated studies yet to assess the impact of needle exchange programs on new HIV infections (incidence) among IDUs found that greater attendance at needle exchange programs

(NEPs) was actually associated with significantly *increased* risk of HIV acquisition among IDUs in Montreal (Bruneau et al. 1997). In discussing this research, a Gates Foundation–supported study of the Institute of Medicine (2006) reminds us that IDUs who attend needle exchange programs may be higher risk IDUs and that the availability of clean needles in pharmacies confounds the results of NEPs. These are valid points but don't negate the lack of clear evidence that NEPs provide any proven benefit to higher risk IDUs. Even the Institute of Medicine study, which was highly positive toward the evidence for needle exchange, concluded that evidence regarding the effect of needle exchange on HIV incidence was "limited and inconclusive" (Institute of Medicine 2006).

Even if it does not have a clear HIV prevention benefit, a visit to a needle exchange program or other health center may provide an opportunity to reach addicts and at least theoretically provide them access to an array of comprehensive ancillary services. Yet it has been difficult or impossible to demonstrate through carefully designed studies any positive impact of harm reduction on biological outcomes or actual HIV infection rates (Bruneau et al. 1997; Institute of Medicine 2006; Langendam et al. 1999; Strathdee et al. 1997; Van Den Berg et al. 2007; van Haastrecht et al. 1996). As with MSM and sex worker-related prevention, there are comparatively few risk avoidance programs that provide primary prevention for IDUs. In their case, primary prevention would mean programs to help addicts become free of addiction altogether (Second International Scientific–Practical Conference 2008).

Although the dominant approach of the HIV prevention community is harm reduction, what do addicts themselves want? A few studies have looked at this and found strong support for getting off drugs (i.e., risk avoidance). For example, in a study of addicts in Scotland:

> Our research has identified widespread support for abstinence as a goal of treatment with 56.6% of drug users questioned identifying "abstinence" as the only change they hoped to achieve on the basis of attending the drug treatment agency. By contrast relatively small proportions of drug users questioned identified harm reduction changes in terms of their aspiration from treatment, 7.1% cited "reduced drug use," and 7.4% cited "stabilization" only. Less than 1% of respondents identified "safer drug use." (McKeganey et al. 2004:423)

And still "safer drug use" (provision of needles, and/or bleach for sterilization of equipment) is the predominant goal of most programs provided to IDUs.

A study of addicts in Baltimore (United States) likewise found that most addicts seeking services wanted to achieve abstinence, a goal that the researchers decided was unrealistic. Researchers from Johns Hopkins

University reflected the harm-reduction philosophy of AIDS prevention when they developed a "step" program that suggests abstinence as a goal set for some time in the indefinite future. Instead of building on a desire to "get clean," this program lowered the expectations to "practice and preach safer injection practices." The program also emphasized not feeling hypocritical about being in a recovery program—one that required addicts to outreach the program to other addicts while still using injecting drugs themselves (Peterson et al. 2006).

The most successful approach in the United States and elsewhere to both alcoholism and drug addiction has been the abstinence or risk avoidance 12-step model of Alcoholics Anonymous (AA) and Narcotics Anonymous (NA). This conclusion is based on available research (Emrick et al. 1993; McKellar et al. 2003; Moos and Moos 2004; Tonigan et al. 1996) and the formal adoption of the 12-step model for the great majority of medical and related treatment facilities in the United States and a growing number of other countries. A National Institutes of Health (NIH) study concludes:

> Unlike other countries such as Australia and most of Western Europe, the US has adopted an abstinence-based response to drug dependence, making 12-step recovery an ideal recovery resource and aftercare modality. We note however that even in countries that have adopted a harm minimization paradigm such as Australia, we have found that the majority of individuals with a chronic history of polysubstance use choose total abstinence from all mind altering substance as their personal recovery goal and report 12-step utilization patterns that do not significantly differ from that of their US counterparts. (Luadet 2008)

Both AA and NA are virtually no-cost (and absolutely no cost to the public) mutual support programs, consisting simply of recovering alcoholics and addicts helping one another *achieve and maintain abstinence*. They are called self-help but are really mutual help organizations. This approach *begins* with abstinence from drugs.

The preferred Russian approach to treatment of IDU also sees abstinence from drugs as the goal, and has been criticized by Western drug experts because it emphasizes detoxification of addicts, not harm reduction. For example, a recent editorial in the journal *Harm Reduction* complained that Russian "narcological dispensaries . . . are structured primarily to provide detoxification for opiate users and alcoholics, and most provide few or no harm reduction interventions to reduce HIV and hepatitis among users." The authors characterize this as an "implacable ideological stance" that amounts to a "rejection . . . of the usual obligations of medicine (as expressed in the Hippocratic oath)" (Elovich and Drucker 2008). Imbedded in this statement is the assumption that harm reduction reduces risk of HIV infection.

A recent meta-analysis of evidence from needle exchange programs concluded that such programs have not had an impact on HIV infection rates, but the authors could not get their findings through peer review in Western journals. Knowing that Russian AIDS experts are skeptical of harm reduction, the authors submitted it to a leading Russian AIDS journal, where it was accepted (Judson et al. in press).

Drug addiction, like human sexual behavior, is an extremely complicated issue. It should be emphasized that in the 12-step NA model, abstinence or detoxification is only the first step. Without virtually unlimited and around-the-clock support from peer groups of recovering addicts, most addicts return to drug use. We believe that efforts should be made to encourage growth of these no-cost, sustainable, popular support groups as a harm *elimination* strategy for addicts. Primary prevention and treatment for those who wish to be free of drugs should be prioritized within HIV prevention programs for addicts.

We are not opposed to also offering drug substitution or other harm reduction for those who will not or cannot undergo treatment. But we believe detox programs and relapse prevention should at least be provided as a complement to harm reduction, so that both halves of the circle are provided. We should not leave out the choice that is optimal on a scale of health options and the one many addicts seek for themselves (sadly, often only to encounter harm-reduction options that prolong their addiction and keep them at high risk). If addicts are supported or enabled in their addiction by substitute opioids, they remain at risk in a number of ways, including of overdose and blood-borne diseases, because addicts on methadone sometimes occasionally inject heroin on top of methadone.

Higher Impact Harm Reduction?

For those who do continue practicing risky behaviors, harm-reduction measures are important although suboptimal. The question arises: How could we make harm reduction better and more effective? One possible means of harm reduction is the promotion of other means of drug ingestion that do not involve needles and injections. According to older studies of IV addicts in the United States, it seems that the transition from snorting and smoking heroin to use of needles occurred between 1930 and 1945, by which time injecting became the norm (Ball and Chambers 1970). In many parts of the world, heroin is still often smoked or inhaled in addition to or instead of injecting it. And in some parts of the world, there has been a transition from smoking to injecting, just as HIV began to spread in the population. A review of drug abuse in Asia found that "about 50% of heroin users take to injecting once they get over the initial phase of consumption through smoking or inhalation" (Brown et al. 2007:Foreword).

How common is such a transition from smoking to injecting, and can anything be done to reverse the trend? A study of the diffusion of heroin smoking in the Netherlands found evidence to challenge the conventional view on heroin use that "assumes an (inescapable) sequence to more efficient self-administration rituals [injecting] as a result of the progressive process of addiction" (Grund 1993). In the Netherlands, it seems there was a transition from "chasing the dragon" (smoking) to injecting heroin, and then back to "chasing." Today, chasing heroin and "freebasing" (smoking) rather than injecting cocaine is more common than injecting these drugs. This phenomenon ought to be studied carefully to assess the potential for campaigns designed to at least promote far safer forms of drug ingestion for addicts who cannot or will not stop using drugs altogether. In the Dutch experiment, the researchers believed that the "transition back" to smoking might be partly explained by cultural factors. Immigrants from Suriname were a substantial proportion of the Dutch addict population, and they together with Dutch of Chinese descent were allegedly averse to injecting drugs. The purity of drugs available for inhalation might also have been a contributing factor explaining the trend away from injecting.

In addition to the Netherlands, increases in *non-injecting* drug use have been documented in the United Kingdom, Spain, Switzerland (Maher and Swift 1997), and even the United States (Des Jarlais et al. 1992). Treatment centers in the United States report that heroin has become purer in recent years, making inhalation more feasible (National Institute on Drug Abuse, 2005). The pattern is different in Asia and Africa, though. A review notes:

> South East Asia in particular, appears to be experiencing an explosion of injecting drug use. . . . Although smoking or sniffing opium and increasingly, heroin, remain significant modes of consumption in the Golden Crescent and some neighboring countries, in many parts of Asia there has been a sharp increase in injecting among populations who have traditionally used opiates by other means. (Maher and Swift 1997:33)

The mode of administration also seems to be shifting toward injection in eastern, western, and southern Africa. And, as recently noted by UNAIDS's former director Peter Piot and colleagues, southern and eastern Africa are now the regions with the world's second highest growth in opiate use (2008).

There has been at least one program in Africa aimed at "rehabilitating" addicts by downshifting modes of ingestion, at a center in Malindi, Kenya, known as The Omari Project (TOP). Addicts were taught very clearly about the risk of HIV infection from injecting and sharing needles. By 2004, "most IDUs had switched to smoking the cocktail (a mix of heroin, marijuana and tobacco) again. . . . The fear of HIV was, and remains really great" (*PlusNews* 2007). One wonders why more programmatic emphasis is not given to this type of harm reduction—strongly warning specifically about *injecting* behavior specifically—as success in this area might have far more impact on preventing HIV transmission and death from other causes than needle exchange or home sterilization of needles.

Note that fear appeals worked in this case, as they did in Uganda, to change sexual behavior, contradicting widespread beliefs in global AIDS prevention. In fact, a meta-analysis of fear appeals and hard-to-change-behaviors shows that they can and *do* work, when linked with self-efficacy or knowing what to do to avoid feared outcomes (Green and Witte 2006; Witte and Allen 2000).

We also need to consider the possibility that our prevention programs are inadvertently promoting the very risky behaviors that should be discouraged. When we offer condoms for MSM and clean syringes for drug addicts, while making no mention of *risk avoidance* alternatives, what unintended consequences might this cause? It would not be surprising if the reaction of MSM who *don't* practice anal sex and drug addicts who *don't* inject is perhaps to consider practicing risky behaviors (anal sex and injecting drugs) that they haven't before, especially if they perceive these behaviors to be normative among other MSM or addicts. In other words, they *might* think that maybe they have been doing it wrong all these years, not like their counterparts in the prestigious, stylish West.

Finally, a discussion of IDU would be incomplete without noting the frequent intersection of drugs and risky sex. Drugs were very much part of the lifestyle of fast-track gay men, according to Rotello and others, to the extent that at the beginning of the AIDS epidemic special research on the specific risk factors and needs of gay men who took amyl nitrate ("poppers") and crystal methamphetamine was required. Crystal meth continues to fuel extremely risky sex among gay men, and, in an age of Internet chatrooms, such sex can be arranged nearly instantly and is increasingly anonymous.[4] Apart from sharing syringes, IDU may also engage in risky sexual behavior including trading or selling sex to support their habits, and research has shown that a significant number of HIV infections among IDU are through sexual transmission (Strathdee et al. 1997). The best solution to both modes of HIV transmission is risk avoidance. Failing that, risk/harm reduction should actively discourage the highest risk behaviors, such as injecting drugs and commercial sex, rather than provide tepid interventions that ignore behavior and rely solely on commodities transfer in the form of condoms and needles.

The U.S. Harm Reduction Coalition (HRC) describes certain "principles central to harm reduction practice." According to the HRC, harm reduction:

- Calls for the non-judgmental, non-coercive provision of services and resources to people who use drugs and the communities in which they live in order to assist them in reducing attendant harm.
- Ensures that drug users and those with a history of drug use routinely have a real voice in the creation of programs and policies designed to serve them.
- Affirms drugs users themselves as the primary agents of reducing the harms of their drug use, and seeks to empower users to share information and support each other in strategies which meet their actual conditions of use.
- Recognizes that the realities of poverty, class, racism, social isolation, past trauma, sex-based discrimination, and other social inequalities affect both people's vulnerability to and capacity for effectively dealing with drug-related harm (Harm Reduction Coalition n.d.).

We see from this language that the HRC sees itself as a defender of the human rights of *victims* of poverty, racism, trauma, etc., who, because of heightened vulnerability to socioeconomic evils, have been addicts. The HRC gives a voice to a subpopulation of socially marginalized if not despised people; it advocate for and defends them. If addicts are seen only or even primarily as victims of unfair social and economic systems, then defending their rights can begin to take more importance than reducing the harms of addiction, which are legion.

There are serious social, familial, and individual costs associated with addiction. First, drug addicts lacking family trust funds need to find a way to pay—usually daily—for their drugs. This often leads to various forms of criminal behavior such as larceny as well as prostitution. Family members of addicts also suffer in various ways, including neglect, abuse, violence, sexual infidelity and being forced or manipulated into enabling the behavior—or enhancing the finances—of the addict. At the individual level, addicts risk death from overdose and are at significant risk of blood-borne diseases such as hepatitis (Smyth et al. 2007).

Whatever their personality traits were before becoming addicts, addicts usually became adept at manipulating others in the constant search for drugs. Nonjudgmental health officials intent on staying in favor with the addict to the point of defending their "human right" to use narcotics, when confronted with manipulative addicts, all too often become enablers of the addicts' intrinsically harmful behaviors. ("Enabling" is the term used in alcoholism and addiction circles to describe giving inadvertent assistance to the facilitation and maintenance of inherently dangerous behaviors.)

For harm reductionists, the "traditionalists" (those who argue for abstinence) are depicted as basing their approach on "anecdotal clinical lore" rather than science (Marlatt 1998:14). Harm reductionists depict the choice as abstinence or punishment ("abstain, or be busted and go to jail"), and claim to explode the myth of uniformity—that all addicts are the same. Of course, they are not, but they all are addicted to drugs, which means they tend to share certain adaptive behaviors regardless of their educational or socioeconomic backgrounds. Addicts are driven by drug-seeking urges so powerful that they lead to certain predictable behaviors. This does not mean that addicts are bad people. Drug addiction is a disease of the brain that is characterized by denial, obsessive thoughts, and compulsive behavior. At any 12-step meeting of recovering addicts, they themselves will be the first to say that their judgment was highly impaired, dulled, and twisted by denial and self-deception during their time of active addiction. Addicts will describe doing many of the same self-defeating things before becoming "clean."

A group of American addiction experts, in criticizing the Russian approach to addiction, wrote:

> Consistent evidence from around the world shows that opiate dependence treatments work most effectively when they widen from an exclusive goal of abstinence and seek to foster multiple outcomes—including reduction in use of illicit opiates, reduction in injections and exposures to blood-borne infections such as HIV and hepatitis, reduction in drug overdoses, better management of existing health problems, and improvement of normative social functioning. (Elovich and Drucker 2008:23)

We basically agree with this observation, except that we would turn it on its head and say that IDU programs within the sphere of HIV/AIDS—with all the attendant new funding for addiction programs in the developing world—need to widen from a near-exclusive goal of harm reduction to include the critical components of abstinence-oriented treatment programs and prevention. This is entirely consistent with recognized best practices of dealing with addiction in the United States and elsewhere, and with the principles of promoting public health, protecting human rights, and achieving long-term, sustainable solutions.

NOTES

1. Some of this argument has been published in Green 2009.
2. Full disclosure: Green played in Farley's folk music band, in Berkley, California, in the 1960s.
3. For example, a survey in Hong Kong found that oral sex appears to be the most popular sexual practice among MSM, practiced by about 90% (see Hong Kong Community Planning Process on HIV/AIDS MSM Working Group 2002). (accessed October 9, 2009).
4. See, for example, Michael Specter's (2005) reporting in the *New Yorker* on the convergence of crystal meth and anonymous gay sex arranged through the Internet.

Chapter 6

FACTS AND MYTHS ABOUT HIV PREVENTION IN GENERALIZED EPIDEMICS

UNDERSTANDING BASIC EPIDEMIOLOGY

Although most of the countries and regions of the world are experiencing concentrated epidemics, in which HIV infections occur primarily among people in most-at-risk populations, a substantial proportion of the HIV infections in the world occur in high-prevalence, generalized epidemics. These epidemics are almost exclusively found in Africa. Even in Africa, not all countries and regions follow the pattern of a generalized epidemic. In much of West Africa, for instance, transmission is largely among sex workers and their clients (and partners of the clients) and thus is not really generalized. HIV prevalence in a number of African countries (including Senegal, Gambia, Mali, Niger, Guinea, and Ethiopia) hovers around 1% and is not in any danger of exploding into the kind of very high-prevalence, generalized, hyper-epidemics that we see in southern Africa. The reasons for this will be discussed, but the point remains that even in much of Africa, HIV transmission seems to happen primarily within vulnerable groups and not within the general population. HIV prevention programs should thus be targeted accordingly.

Effective HIV prevention requires an understanding of the basic epidemiology of HIV transmission, a point that seems obvious but is often forgotten or ignored. It is simply not true that everyone is equally at risk of HIV infection, and every person at risk does not need a primary message of condom use any more than every person at risk needs a primary message of abstinence or using a clean needle. Epidemics differ, as do the needs of people in those epidemics. "Knowing your epidemic" is crucial, as is understanding the dynamics of infection. Even basic terms like "incidence" and "prevalence" are often misunderstood (see Box 6.1), leading to confusion about whether HIV prevention measures have been successful (and when), and which populations are more or less at risk.

BOX 6.1: INCIDENCE AND PREVALENCE

Incidence—the number of *new* infections within a population, or the proportion of a population that is newly infected within a time period such as a year—is a better measure of HIV trends than prevalence, the proportion of a population that is infected at a given time. Note that prevalence, although often referred to as a rate, is actually a *proportion*, as it does not involve a time dimension but refers only to the number of persons or percentage of population that is infected at a single point in time.

For example, knowing that 10% of a population is infected (10% prevalence) does not give one any information about whether the trend of that epidemic is toward fewer infections or more infections. Knowing that the incidence of new infections was 1% in the past year compared to 1.25% the year before (1% of the population was newly infected in the past year, compared to 1.25% of the population newly infected the year before), or that there were 64 new infections per 1,000 women attending antenatal clinics (ANC) this year compared to 47 new infections per 1,000 ANC attendees last year, allows one to track the trend of an epidemic.

In an era in which access to antiretroviral therapy (ART) is causing HIV-infected persons to live longer, using HIV incidence rather than prevalence data to track infections is more crucial than ever. Availability of ART can lead to increase in prevalence as people live longer with HIV, but this increase in prevalence does not necessarily mean that incidence is increasing.

Prevalence data are much more routinely collected and are easier to collect than are incidence data. Although there are a number of cohorts in Africa that regularly test an entire population and so can establish how many people were newly infected in a year or other time period, such a means of establishing incidence is not practical in most settings. Several other methods are therefore used.

BED-assays, which test for the presence of HIV, are a more sensitive test than are standard HIV tests, which detect the presence of antibodies to HIV. As it takes the body several months after infection to produce antibodies, there is a so-called window period in which a person newly infected with HIV will test positive with a BED-assay, but negative with a standard HIV test such as an ELISA. BED-assays can therefore be used to determine if someone is newly infected and in this window period, and data about the number of people in this window period can be used to calculate incidence. Although this method is a powerful tool, it is not perfect. A particular challenge is that a small percentage of any population will never test positive with a test that detects antibodies, such as the ELISA, and so will appear to be in the window period long after initial infection. Incidence estimates that rely on BED-assays attempt to estimate this percentage of false-positives and correct for it, but this is an inexact science and the subject of much scientific debate.

Incidence can also be imputed through prevalence data, especially for young populations such as (commonly) 15–19-year-old women. Infections in this population will almost certainly be recent, and prevalence will be relatively unaffected by die-off of HIV-infected persons. Declines in prevalence will always lag a few years behind declines in incidence because prevalence cannot decline until HIV-infected persons die off and are *not* replaced by newly infected people. Peaks in incidence often occur 5–10 years before peaks in prevalence, so a steep decline in prevalence may point to rapidly decreasing new infections at a point in time 5–10 years in the past.

Dynamics of HIV Transmission

With a few possible exceptions (such as Haiti and Papua New Guinea), all the generalized epidemics in the world are found in Africa, and the highest prevalence countries in the world are all in southern Africa. In this handful of countries, HIV prevalence rose very quickly during the 1990s to reach levels of between 15% and 25%, and prevalence remains in this range.[1] In comparison, HIV prevalence is currently between 5% and 10% in eastern Africa (although prevalence in Uganda was once as high as 15%), and prevalence is below 5% in other regions of Africa.[2]

Why are HIV infection rates so high in Africa, especially southern Africa? It has been suggested that the hyper-epidemics of southern Africa, and to a lesser extent in Africa, have resulted from a unique combination of two volatile elements—low rates of male circumcision and high rates of multiple and concurrent sexual partnerships (MCP) (Halperin and Epstein 2004). We will discuss male circumcision in the next section, but it is crucial to understand several epidemiological facts that contribute to the unique dynamics of HIV transmission and lead to the amplifying effect of concurrent (overlapping) sexual partners. First, an obvious but epidemiologically critical fact is that AIDS is a disease with a very long latency period (typically 5–7 years) between infection and the onset of symptoms, during which time the infected person appears healthy and likely does not know that he or she is infected. He or she is quite capable of infecting others during this period of seeming health, and this is one of the factors that makes HIV such a persistent pandemic. This is in contrast to a disease like Ebola, which produces immediate symptoms and quick mortality, meaning that an Ebola epidemic quickly burns itself out.

An HIV-infected person is not equally infective at all points during infection, which leads to other particular dynamics of HIV transmission. An HIV-infected person has a high viral load and is very infectious immediately after infection, a period known as acute infection, lasting from several weeks to several months. Viral load begins to drop as the HIV-infected person's body begins producing antibodies to HIV and will remain low for the next 5–7 years.

Empirical evidence and epidemiologic modeling exercises have shown that the probability of transmission per sex act during acute infection is increased 10-fold (Pilcher et al. 2004) to as much as 43-fold (Pinkerton 2007), compared to the much longer asymptomatic later stage infection period. When viral load again begins to rise, the HIV-infected person will begin to develop full-blown AIDS and will be visibly sick. At this point, he or she may be less likely to engage in sexual intercourse either because of decreased libido or because a potential sexual partner observes signs of ill health. This last stage of HIV infection may therefore account for relatively few onward infections.[3]

But what of the first, asymptomatic but highly infectious stage of acute infection? Not only does an HIV-infected person not feel sick during acute infection, but he or she will not test positive for HIV with a standard test during this time, as antibodies to HIV have not yet been produced. Some researchers estimate that acute infection contributes up to half of all onward infections,[4] depending on the type of epidemic and the characteristics of sexual relationships in that epidemic.

A further epidemiological fact must be mentioned that may be surprising. When transmitted through vaginal intercourse, HIV is a relatively hard virus to transmit and it is far less infectious than many other common sexually transmitted infections. It is estimated that the risk of HIV transmission *per act* of penile-vaginal intercourse, when one partner is infected and the other is not, is in the range of 1/100 to 1/1,000.[5] Many factors, including ulcerative STIs and lack of male circumcision, increase this risk; correct condom use reduces it by 80% to 90% (Hearst and Chen 2004; Weller and Davis 2002). HIV transmission thus usually requires either a great many acts of intercourse or some other factor that greatly increases infectivity, such as sex during acute infection or the presence of an STI.

Concurrent Sexual Partnerships

The great paradox is that sexually transmitted epidemics can reach such devastating levels in certain countries and populations when most people in those populations do not seem to have large numbers of sexual partners or other obvious risk factors. This is most apparent in southern Africa, where men and women have similar numbers of sexual partners, over a lifetime, to people in other regions of the world, yet infection rates are orders of magnitude greater than those of heterosexual populations elsewhere (Halperin and Epstein 2004; Morris 2002). Poverty, lack of women's empowerment, lack of education, and other socioeconomic factors have often been implicated as fueling the spread of AIDS, but, as will be seen in Chapter 8, these broader realities are sometimes related to HIV in exactly the *opposite* way of what we might expect. Lack of male circumcision is certainly a key factor in the much greater transmission of HIV in some regions of Africa, and there may be other biological factors at work as well, such as differences in infectivity between virus subtypes (clades)[6] or a greater biological vulnerability of people of African descent to the virus.[7]

There is increasing evidence, and consensus, that the crucial factor fueling the hyper-epidemics of southern Africa may be widespread patterns of overlapping or concurrent sexual relationships (Halperin and Epstein 2004; Mah and Halperin 2008; Potts et al. 2008; Shelton 2009). In an epidemic in which sexual relationships are of long duration and in which people have only one sexual partner at a time (what we might call serial monogamy), the virus will spread slowly because it will be "trapped" in monogamous relationships for the duration of those relationships. An HIV-infected person with an uninfected partner may infect that partner, but neither partner will infect anyone else for the duration of the partnership.

Unfortunately, a pattern of concurrent partners facilitates HIV transmission far more than serial monogamy because of the high viral load that occurs during the acute stage of infection and because it is much more likely that other sexual partners will be exposed during the period of acute infection. In serial monogamy, an infected person will put at risk all *future* partners, but those partners will likely not be exposed until the infected person is no longer in the acute phase of infection and the risk of onward transmission is reduced. By contrast, in an epidemic with high levels of concurrent sexual partnerships, many people may be connected in a sexual network and exposed during a short period of time, with one acute infection leading to other highly infectious acute infections and so on (Mah and Halperin 2008; Morris and Kretzschmar 1997). When large numbers of people within a population have concurrent partnerships, they form dense sexual networks through which the virus can quickly spread. In the case of primarily heterosexual epidemics, such dense networks require that both men *and* women have concurrent partnerships.

Interest in concurrent partnerships has recently exploded within the HIV prevention community, with a profusion of meetings and conferences about reorienting prevention programs to address MCP[8] in the generalized epidemics of Africa.[9] This is not a new issue. Green argued in 1988 that number of sexual partners was the most important factor to guide prevention in African epidemics,[10] and Morris and Kretzschmar wrote in 1997 that "compared with sequential monogamy, a pattern of concurrent partnerships can dramatically change the early course of an epidemic, increasing the growth rate and the number infected exponentially" (p. 646). Researchers such as Daniel Halperin, Helen Epstein, and James Shelton have also been writing about concurrent partnerships for a number of years. In a 2004 article in *The Lancet*, Halperin and Epstein observed, "African men and women often have more than one—typically two or perhaps three—concurrent partnerships that can overlap for months or years. This pattern differs from that of the serial monogamy more common in the West, or the one-off casual and commercial sexual encounters that occur everywhere" (p. 4).

The evidence for concurrency significantly increasing the size of HIV epidemics is largely derived from modeling studies. We do know that in every case of HIV prevalence decline in Africa, the proportion of men and women who report more than one sexual partner in the past year has declined (as shown in the case studies in Chapter 7). This refers to partners of any sort. To date, few major surveys of sexual behavior have measured concurrency, and most of the data we have about number of partners per year do not distinguish between types of sexual partners (such as casual or one-time partners versus enduring, long-term partners). Recent Demographic and Health Surveys (DHS) have provided some data about patterns of concurrency, although these surveys have been challenged by the task of capturing complex patterns of sexual relationships using a standard interviewer-driven survey. One analysis of DHS data from four African countries found, not surprisingly, that couples who were married or cohabiting and reported an additional (concurrent) sexual partner were more likely to be HIV infected. Perhaps more surprisingly, this analysis also found that having concurrent partners was more likely among urban, more educated, and wealthier men and women (Mishra et al. 2009b). Until we have more data about the particular risk of concurrency, the implications for prevention are to discourage multiple sex partnerships of *any* sort.

Anthropologists and others have used qualitative data to explore patterns of concurrent sexual partnerships. For instance, Soul City, a major health communication initiative in southern Africa, carried out a 10-country study of multiple and concurrent partners in southern Africa that focused on qualitative findings about the motivators and sociocultural context of these behaviors (Jana et al. 2008). The South Africa-based Ubuntu Institute conducted a four-country study which used in-depth interviews and focus groups with indigenous leaders to explore ways to address multiple and concurrent partners (this research will be discussed in Chapter 10). According to the findings of Soul City, the Ubuntu Institute, and others, such concurrent partnerships are often long term and are viewed not as casual sex but as regular and trusted relationships. Within such trusted relationships, condom use tends to be low. It is perhaps ironic that a relationship based on a degree of commitment and responsibility may be considerably more dangerous than casual, commercial, or one-night-stand sex, liaisons that typically do not involving commitment or responsibility (but are more likely to involve condom use).

In our view, the relatively recent realization of the importance of targeting multiple and concurrent partnerships has brought more attention and acceptance to the notion that changing sexual behavior is fundamental to HIV prevention. We would add that rather than focusing on concurrent partners narrowly, the focus should continue to be on discouraging risky sexual behavior of all kinds, including multiple (but nonconcurrent) sexual partnerships. Data have repeatedly shown a strong correlation between number of sexual partners and HIV risk, at an individual level and at a population level. Demographic and Health Surveys from all regions of the world consistently show a higher HIV prevalence among those reporting greater numbers of sexual partners, for both men and women. An analysis of data from the large UNAIDS Multicentre Study (conducted in the 1990s) found that among four African cities, when male circumcision was controlled for, average number of lifetime sexual partners was itself an important determining factor in the spread of HIV (Auvert 2002). Rates of condom usage were not predictive. We have long known about this risk factor, yet global AIDS organizations have been reluctant to address sexual behavior directly and are only now starting to think of ways to discourage sex with multiple and concurrent partners.

Male Circumcision

Understanding the role of male circumcision in reducing HIV transmission within populations is also critical to understanding the dynamics of the HIV epidemic within Africa. An association between male circumcision and lower HIV infection rates was first noted around 1989

(Bongaarts et al. 1989). Since then, over 40 epidemiological studies, several meta-analyses, and randomized trials in South Africa, Kenya, and Uganda have investigated this association (Weiss et al. 2008). The UNAIDS Multicentre study of four African cities found that prevalence of male circumcision was one of the most significant factors explaining levels of HIV infection, with cities where there were high rates of male circumcision having lower HIV prevalence even when behavioral risk factors were similar (Auvert et al. 2001). The first randomized trial of male circumcision, held in South Africa, found that it has the potential to reduce HIV infection rates 60%–70% (Auvert et al. 2005). Subsequent randomized trials in Kenya and Uganda found that male circumcision reduced HIV infection rates by 53% and 48%, respectively (Bailey et al. 2007; Gray et al. 2007).

On the basis of these findings, voluntary male circumcision programs are being rolled out in many countries in Africa. It may be of anthropological interest that as early as 1992, traditional (indigenous) healers in South Africa recognized this risk factor and recommended that men from noncircumcising societies become circumcised to decrease their chances of contracting HIV and other STIs (Green et al. 1993).

Anthropologists have been prominent among those studying male circumcision long before the three randomized, controlled trials changed—or initiated—the prevention policy focused on it. Priscilla Reining and Francis Conant were among four coauthors of a landmark 1989 article that used data from the Human Relations Area Files to show a strong association between lack of male circumcision and higher HIV infection rates (Bongaarts et al. 1989). Anthropologist Robert Bailey conducted one of the three definitive randomized controlled trials (Bailey et al. 2007). Anthropologists have contributed in other ways as well, such as studying local beliefs and perceptions about male circumcision in African societies that do and do not have the practice and the relationship to religion and cultural practices (Bailey et al. 2001; Drain et al. 2006; Halperin et al. 2005).

LIMITED EFFECTIVENESS OF STANDARD HIV PREVENTION MEASURES

Sexual behavior, particularly the number and overlap of sexual partnerships, is the critical factor in sexually transmitted epidemics. Such a point seems obvious: If a sexually transmitted epidemic is going to be contained, sexual behavior must change (or existing protective behaviors must be maintained), toward lower numbers of partners and less concurrency in partnerships. Yet standard HIV prevention programs have typically done everything *but* address sexual behavior in a straightforward way, out of the assumption that sexual behaviors would not change no matter what the approach or that they *should* not be changed because such an approach is repressive or sex-negative. The HIV prevention approaches that have received the vast majority of prevention resources since the beginning of the epidemic are interventions that attempt to reduce risk of HIV transmission without fundamentally changing risky sexual behaviors. Condom use or treatment of ulcerative STIs such as herpes (which increase risk of HIV transmission) have been promoted to reduce per-act risk of HIV transmission. (Condom use is a type of behavior change, but it can be adopted without changing the sexual risk behaviors themselves.) HIV testing has been promoted with the expectation that knowing one's status (whether positive or negative) would lead to changes in behavior, specifically greater condom use.

Such outcomes seem logical, but an abundance of research has shown that these three prevention approaches—condom promotion, STI treatment, and HIV testing—have failed to reduce HIV in generalized epidemics. Although much of the HIV prevention community still defends them as "best practice" (and they continue to account for the lion's share of HIV prevention spending), others acknowledge the lack of evidence of effectiveness. As discussed in Chapter 4 a group of HIV prevention experts recently noted this lack of evidence in an article in *Science* and called for a reallocation of global prevention resources toward male circumcision and reducing MCP, two interventions which receive only a small fraction of global HIV prevention resources (Potts et al. 2008). UNAIDS, clearly a target of this critique, responded that the proposed focus on partner reduction and male circumcision in hyper-epidemics was too narrow. In his speech at the opening plenary of the International AIDS Conference later the same year, then UNAIDS Executive Director Peter Piot criticized "those who claim that we just need one or two things to prevent HIV," and called "combination prevention" the "only feasible option" (2008).

"Combination prevention," taking its cue from combination treatment (the use of several drugs together to treat HIV), is increasingly invoked as the solution to HIV prevention. The term is rarely defined, beyond the usual statements that the prevention response should be tailored to the local reality and that no prevention approaches should be excluded. (As an example, after calling for combination prevention, Piot gave no real clues about the specifics of such an approach, beyond stating, "No more stigma around HIV, no more homophobia, no more ostracism of sex workers, no more gender-based violence," and briefly mentioning harm reduction for drug users.) Piot's successor as UNAIDS director, Michel Sidibé, characterized combination prevention in a recent *Lancet* editorial as "programmes [which] deploy a blend of biomedical, behavioural, and structural approaches tailored to address the particular and unique realities of those most vulnerable to HIV infection." He added: "Human rights must remain at the core of prevention. Women, young people, migrants, people who inject drugs, sex workers and their clients, and sexual minorities continue to face societal barriers to protecting themselves from HIV. Prevention must include efforts to promote dignity, justice, and equality" (Sidibé and Buse 2010:534).

Using the full arsenal of prevention strategies sounds fine, and no one will argue with the fact that a prevention response should be tailored to the reality of the local epidemic. But in reality, a combination prevention mindset may keep a country or program from identifying prevention priorities, focusing on what epidemiologically speaking is most crucial and effective, and using scarce resources in the most effective way. At the least, the prevention community should deal objectively with the evidence and stop sinking a majority of prevention resources into interventions that have not been shown to be effective.

HIV Counseling and Testing

HIV testing is one of the main components of the universal access paradigm that has become the dominant prevention approach within global AIDS. Knowing one's status is assumed essential to keeping one from spreading HIV to others, if HIV positive, and to help one stay uninfected, if HIV negative. Advocates of testing point out that in parts of the world, a majority of HIV-infected individuals do not know their status; in sub-Saharan Africa, it is four in five, and even more do not know their partner's status (Bunnell and Cherutich 2008). In some of the most AIDS-affected countries in the world, universal testing has been a linchpin of the government's HIV prevention strategy. Lesotho launched a "Know Your Status" campaign in 2006 that included door-to-door testing and mobile services, and, by the end of 2007, 169,000 people (out of a population of 2 million) had been tested under the campaign (Motlalepula et al. 2009). In early 2010, South Africa launched a campaign similarly aimed at universal testing, with a target of testing 15 million South Africans and featuring public testing by high-profile South Africans, including President Zuma (Sapa 2010).

We certainly support full access to testing and the right of all people to know their HIV status so they can stop onward infections to sexual partners, manage their infection, and seek treatment, care, and support. But the evidence simply does not support a significant prevention role for testing, either in terms of primary prevention (preventing those who test negative from becoming infected), or secondary prevention (preventing those who test positive from infecting others).

Numerous studies have examined HIV testing as a prevention strategy and have nearly universally found that although there may be positive behavioral changes among those who test positive (including among those in discordant partnerships), there are few if any behavioral gains among those who test negative (the majority even in the world's highest prevalence epidemics).[11] Most studies have shown that being tested does not cause people to reduce their number of sexual partners, and evidence of increased condom use is limited. Even more crucially, several trials have shown that expanding access to VCT in a population does not result in fewer HIV infections (Corbett et al. 2007; Matovu et al. 2003).

There is even some evidence that testing negative may lead to *riskier* sexual behavior, a phenomenon known as risk compensation or behavioral disinhibition. A study in rural Zimbabwe found that those who were tested did *not* engage in less risky behavior or have fewer HIV infections during follow up compared those who were not tested (Sherr et al. 2007). Women who tested positive were more likely to report consistent condom use in their regular partnerships, and men and women who tested positive reported fewer partners subsequently. However, men and women who tested negative (as most did) were *more* likely to adopt risky behaviors such as greater numbers of partners and concurrent partners. Lifetime uptake of testing increased from 6% to 11% over a period of three years, but the authors note that uptake of testing in this population remained low, stating "although 88% of people said they wanted to know their HIV status at follow-up the majority had still not had a test, even when available, prompted, invited and—albeit at limited times— provided on site" (p. 858). One must question the logic of a strategy that both achieves low uptake and produces no net gain in terms of HIV infections averted. The authors warn that "increased sexual risk following receipt of a negative result may be a serious unintended consequence of VCT" (Sherr et al. 2007:851).

Another study in Zimbabwe, conducted in the capital of Harare, found that an intervention to increase testing rates also resulted in somewhat elevated HIV incidence compared to a control group (although the difference was not statistically significant). The authors concluded that these results supported a conclusion of "adverse behavioral consequences in some HIV-negative clients" (Corbett et al. 2007:483). The authors also noted that high-risk behavior after VCT was common and that behavior after VCT was not significantly different than that before VCT. In neighboring South Africa, AIDS expert Francois Venter noted the discouraging results from Zimbabwe and bluntly stated of South Africa:

> It's absolutely phenomenal how testing has been escalated over the last five years, but the argument that more testing will lead to more people on treatment earlier is not coming to fruition. . . . Donor projects want to know how many people tested and know their status. Who cares if they tested and know their status if they don't do anything with the information. (*PlusNews* 2009b)

What of high-risk groups? A study in Tanzania found that offering VCT as part of a prevention package to HIV-negative Tanzanian women who were at high risk of HIV infection (such as bar workers) did not reduce HIV incidence among these women. In fact, women who received VCT during the 30 months of the study had HIV incidence approximately *twice* that of women who refused VCT or were tested at the beginning of the study but did not seek additional tests (Watson-Jones et al. 2009). (The goal of this trial was to see if treating these high-risk women for herpes reduced HIV incidence; as will be discussed, it didn't.) In this trial, testing may have been sought by those felt themselves to be (and were) at particularly high risk of HIV acquisition, which would account for the fact that those who were tested had twice the HIV incidence of those who didn't.

Nonetheless, testing seems to have done very little to reduce risk among those who were tested. Counseling and testing may be most effective when a couple is tested together, and couples' counseling has been shown to increase condom usage among discordant couples (Allen et al. 1992). In one important study of discordant couples in Zambia, most condom usage was found to be imperfect (inconsistent), and the use of biological markers revealed that actual usage was often not as high as reported usage (Allen et al. 2003). Couples who were tested and found to be discordant increased their condom use over the course of a year to more than 80% of sexual contacts.[12] Yet most couples reported inconsistent condom usage, with less than 20% of couples reporting 100% condom use over the course of a year and having these reports corroborated by biological markers.[13] Condom use was associated with significantly reduced risk of pregnancy and HIV transmission.[14]

STI Treatment

Sexually transmitted infections (STIs), especially of the ulcerative variety, have long been recognized as cofactors and facilitators of HIV transmission; thus, it was believed for many years that treating the curable STIs ought to reduce HIV transmission. Green devoted much of his first book on African AIDS to finding ways to work with existing resources—notably indigenous healers—to find and treat cases of STIs (Green 1994).

Yet a number of randomized controlled trials that have been conducted to assess the affect of STI treatment (either syndromic treatment or mass treatment of a population) on HIV transmission have failed to find an effect. Randomized controlled trials (RCTs) are considered the gold standard of public health research: Like drug trials, they measure the effect of an intervention in an exposed (or intervention) group by comparing that group to an unexposed (or control) group. Although the first trial (reported in 1995) found a substantial reduction in HIV incidence in Mwanza, Tanzania, when STIs were treated syndromically, subsequent trials failed to find any impact of STI treatment on HIV incidence (Gray and Wawer 2008a).

Ronald Gray and Maria Wawer (2008a) recently raised the fact in the medical journal *The Lancet* that to date, seven out of eight RCTs had failed to find any effect of STI treatment on HIV incidence and questioned whether continuing to invest in STI treatment for HIV prevention was justified. When a number of other researchers protested in letters to *The Lancet*, Gray and Wawer insisted:

> In our Comment, we argued that it is "questionable" whether control of sexually transmitted infections (STIs) should be "promoted specifically for HIV prevention", and suggested that it is time to reassess policies on this matter. . . . If randomised trials are considered to be the gold standard of proof in medicine, we must, of necessity, openly debate the usefulness of current policies in the light of the negative trial findings. As indicated in our Comment, we strongly advocate STI control as an important public-health measure . . . [but] if such control cannot be adequately attained during a trial, it is likely to be even more difficult to achieve and sustain in a service programme. (2008b:1297–1298)

The evidence for the ineffectiveness of STI treatment to control HIV continues to amass. A recent trial testing an approach of "comprehensive" HIV prevention plus twice-daily herpes treatment (acyclovir) among young Tanzanian women at high risk of HIV infection failed to show any reduced risk over 30 months. This randomized controlled trial enrolled 821 women who were infected with herpes simplex virus (HSV) but not with HIV, and gave daily acyclovir (to suppress HSV) as well as comprehensive prevention services (free condoms, VCT, and treatment for other treatable STIs). Women receiving acyclovir did not avoid infection; they were infected with HIV at the same rate as women who received a placebo. This study also provided noteworthy data on alcohol use, with women who reported moderate alcohol consumption having twice the HIV infection rate of those without alcohol consumption, and women reporting 10 or more drinks per week reporting even higher HIV incidence (Watson-Jones et al. 2009).[15] Once again we note the need to address *behavior* (including alcohol use in the context of risky sexual behavior), and not rely on medical-technical solutions.

A similar randomized, placebo-controlled trial that attempted to use acyclovir to reduce HIV transmission among discordant couples also announced in early 2010 that the trial had failed. This massive trial followed 3,408 couples at 14 sites in Africa for two years. Twice-daily acyclovir reduced the viral load of HIV-infected individuals (all of whom were also coinfected with herpes) and genital ulcers, but did not reduce the transmission of HIV (Celum et al. 2010). Notably, 29% of the new infections (among the partners uninfected with HIV at the beginning of the study) appeared to be acquired *from outside the original discordant partnership.*

Effectiveness of Condoms in Generalized Epidemics

Condoms have been seen as *the* vital weapon against AIDS, even more so than access to HIV testing and STI treatment. AIDS programs and transnational agendas often seem myopic in their singular goal of increasing condom distribution and use, not just among vulnerable populations but among *all* populations. Of the seven behavioral indicators required by UNAIDS from the world's nations for annual reports on progress against AIDS, five indicators measure condom use. (The other two indicators measure sexual debut before age 15, and multiple partners in past year [UNGASS/UNAIDS 2010].) We wonder if this choice of indicators does not betray somewhat more passion (certainly not unique to UNAIDS) about increasing condom use, compared to changes in sexual behavior that we would argue are more fundamental and important for the majority of the populations at high risk of HIV infection. The UNAIDS executive director wrote in his 2010 letter to partners (while noting that the number of new infections has dropped 17% worldwide during the 2000s):

> Successful prevention means scaling up demand for and access to male and female condoms. One of the starting points for prevention has to be a concerted effort to increase condom use. . . . However, the supply of both male and female condoms is less than a quarter of the need. In sub-Saharan Africa, only four condoms were available each year for every adult male of reproductive age. We have not done enough in promoting this relatively inexpensive and highly effective tool for HIV prevention.[16]

We certainly agree that condoms are a vital prevention tool for certain most-at-risk populations (including those in generalized epidemics who practice risky sex), but we strongly disagree that AIDS prevention should have as its goal promoting condom use among everyone all the time. The assumption that no sexual relationship is safe and that every sexual encounter must be "protected" with a condom is, in our view, unrealistic, epidemiologically unsound, and deeply problematic. Such a norm certainly would not serve the needs of couples who were trying to conceive, and of course choosing to have children is a fundamental human right.[17] Given that few if any Western AIDS experts follow or want to follow a 100% condom policy in their personal lives, we should not be surprised that neither do most people around the world.

There are two questions to consider when it comes to condoms and HIV/AIDS. First, how effective are condoms in preventing the transmission of HIV at an individual level? Second, how successful have condoms been in curbing the spread of HIV within populations? There is considerable consensus that condoms have an estimated effectiveness of between 80% and 90% when used consistently and correctly—that is, they reduce HIV transmission by 80% to 90% compared to non-use.[18] Condoms can also reduce the risk of many other sexually transmitted infections, the presence of which can increase the transmission efficiency of HIV. These *in vivo* studies are usually done among discordant couples, when HIV status of both partners is known and condoms are supplied. In other words, these studies tend to be done under the ideal conditions for condom use.

The meaning of 80% to 90% effectiveness is often misinterpreted; it does *not* mean that condom use reduces risk of HIV infection to 10% to 20% per year (as it is often taken to mean). As discussed previously, many factors influence the risk of transmitting or becoming infected with HIV. A long-term discordant couple may have a risk of transmission of less than 10% per year, even without condom use, whereas sex with someone who is acutely infected may carry risk considerably greater than 10% per year, even if condoms are used. There is no single universally applicable figure for the risk carried in a single sexual act with an infected person, so decreasing that risk with condom use still results in a quite variable risk.

Although condoms can considerably lessen an individual's risk of infection with HIV and other STIs, promotion of condoms has not been shown to be an effective primary intervention strategy to lower infection rates at a population level in high-prevalence, generalized epidemics. John Richens and colleagues, in a 2000 article in *The Lancet*, stated that "it is hard to show that condom promotion has had any effect on the HIV epidemic" (p. 401). Researchers Norman Hearst and Sanny Chen, in a 2003 study commissioned by UNAIDS, stated (in the unpublished study report and in a 2004 published article), "No clear examples have emerged yet of a country that has turned back a generalized epidemic primarily by means of condom promotion" (Hearst and Chen 2004:41).

In 2008, a group of HIV prevention experts wrote in the journal *Science*, "condom use has not reached a sufficiently high level, even after many years of widespread and often aggressive promotion, to produce a measurable slowing of new infections in the generalized epidemics of Sub-Saharan Africa" (Potts et al. 2008:749).

Evidence for the effectiveness of condoms in reducing HIV rates at the population level comes from countries like Thailand and Cambodia, which have very different epidemic patterns than those found in Africa. In Thailand, which is considered the world's great condom success story, the HIV epidemic was largely fueled by contact with sex workers. During the early 1990s, the number of men reporting consistent condom use when visiting a sex worker increased from 36% to 71%. During this same time period, the number of men reporting premarital or extramarital sex was cut in half and the percentage visiting sex workers likewise declined by half (Phoolcharoen 1998). All of these trends, along with political support and increased STI control, likely contributed to Thailand's declining HIV incidence during the early 1990s. Data from antenatal clinics (ANCs) confirmed a decline in HIV prevalence from 2% in 1995 to 1.6% in 2001, following this decline in incidence (Phoolcharoen 1998). Condom use among non-sex workers remained relatively low. In Bangkok, where condom use among sex workers reached nearly 90% by 1996, only 18.9% of women in the general population reported condom use at last sex. Only 28.5% of Bangkok sex workers reported using condoms with non-paying sex partners, such as boyfriends (Family Health International 1996).

When HIV infections are concentrated among sex workers and their clients, condom promotion is an effective primary strategy, at least for these groups. This is *not* a population-wide strategy; it focuses on sex workers and their clients. However, the proportion of men in the population who regularly visit sex workers can be quite high in some countries (e.g., Thailand in 1990). In Africa, the vast majority of HIV infections occur outside high-risk groups, in the very groups in which condom usage remains stubbornly low. Even if sex workers, truck drivers, soldiers, and others at high risk consistently used condoms, generalized epidemics would continue because most infection occurs outside these defined high-risk groups. Few people are found to use condoms consistently outside of high-risk groups. Although those in the general population may use condoms for sex with a sex worker or "one-off" sex, such one-time sexual experiences are comparatively rare and do not add up to a substantial market for condoms. For example, only 1.6% of Ugandan men reported paying for sex during the last year, according to the last DHS (2006).

Many people in Africa seem to feel that condom use is advisable in short-term or casual relationships, but it is not common within marriage or other long-term relationships (de Walque 2009). There seems to be an inverse relationship between condom use and trust in a relationship, with condom use dropping off once a sexual partner becomes regular and trusted. Besides being felt to signal a lack of trust, condoms are felt to diminish the pleasure of sex or be unnecessary because there is no perceived risk within the relationship. A study in KwaZulu-Natal found that over 90% of respondents knew about condoms and where they could be obtained, but only 14% of men and 17% of women reported any condom use at all in marital and cohabiting partnerships (Maharaj and Cleland 2004). A study in Malawi found that only 2.3% of respondents had used a condom at last sex with a spouse, and qualitative interviews revealed that respondents felt condoms were an "intruder" into marriage (Chimbiri 2007).

Demand for condoms is simply low in Africa and, indeed, throughout the developing world. A Population Services International survey that analyzed data from six African countries concluded that the main reasons for not using condoms have to do with poor demand (Longfield et al. 2001). Condom social marketers who have worked in Africa (including Green) have faced this very real obstacle. After more than a quarter century of intense supply, marketing, and distribution of condoms, not to mention years of earlier condom promotion for family planning, it is amazing that much of the AIDS community continues to maintain that the problem is primarily lack of supply. One would think that Africans were begging for condoms and that the bottleneck was donor refusal to provide funds. There seems to be little acknowledgment of the reasons for the chronic *low demand* for condoms, especially in Africa.

Green remembers doing interviews at a clinic in the rural Qwa-Qwa area of South Africa. Short of furniture, the clinic had turned (full) crates of condoms into tables and chairs. The condoms were imported from Thailand and they were sized for Asians. Even if they had been stored properly (the clinic was very hot), these condoms were not usable because they were not the right size for Africans. The matron of the clinic commented that "someone" was sending too many crates of condoms, more than they could give away.

Condom quality is a serious concern in Africa. Condoms become less stable and more prone to break or burst when they are old (expired) or stored at high temperatures, both of which are common problems in Africa. A recent report noted problems with condom quality in a number of African countries (*PlusNews* 2009a). In Tanzania in 2002, the government stopped the UNFPA from importing 10 million condoms after laboratory tests found defects. In a much-publicized 2004 incident, Ugandans complained that a popular brand of government-subsidized condoms had signs of deterioration, and the condoms were subsequently withdrawn, leading to a purported condom shortage in the country. Mistrust of this brand has continued, and the Ugandan government reported in 2007 that 40 million of these condoms were likely to expire in medical stores because of low demand. In 2007, the South African government recalled 20 million government-distributed condoms amid allegations that a government official responsible for quality testing had been bribed. Both Zambia and Kenya had major condom brands fail safety tests in 2009. Keep in mind that all of these safety problems were discovered *before* distribution and that storage at high temperatures would only increase the likelihood of defects.

Consistent Versus Inconsistent Use

In Africa, condom usage rates at last intercourse with any type of partner remain relatively low, and consistent condom use is lower still. Although this issue has not been well studied, available data suggest that although *consistent* condom usage is protective against HIV and other STIs, *inconsistent* usage, which is the norm virtually everywhere, is not. A landmark study in Rakai, Uganda, which tracked new HIV infections and behaviors such as condom usage over a 10-year period, found that consistent condom use reduced risk of HIV infection by 63% (Ahmed et al. 2001). However, irregular (inconsistent) condom use did not reduce risk of HIV at all, even after adjusting for demographic and behavioral variables (such as the tendency among inconsistent condom users to have more partners and riskier sex). This is a very sobering finding, given the high rates of inconsistent use. In the Rakai study, 4.4% of the population reported consistent condom use in the last year and 16.5% reported inconsistent use (Ahmed et al. 2001).

An analysis of risk behaviors among South African youth stated that, "Inconsistent condom use is shown to be a *significant risk behavior for HIV infection*" (Katz and Low-Beer 2008:840; emphasis added). The authors note that in a national survey, only 19.7% of young men and 16.6% of young women reported consistent condom use (substantially fewer than reported condom use at last intercourse), and that inconsistent condom use among both genders was significantly associated with HIV infection.[19] Katz and Low-Beer further note the failure of inconsistent condom use to reduce infections of HIV and other STIs in Rakai, Uganda (Ahmed et al. 2001) and a study that showed inconsistent condom use to be associated with a higher rate of STIs among military conscripts in Thailand (Celentano et al. 1998). The authors conclude, "It is important to promote consistent condom use among South African youth, and stress inconsistent use as a risk behavior. *Standard indicators of condom use at last sex do not capture this key risk"* (Katz and Low-Beer 2008:840, emphasis added).

Unfortunately, the vast majority of data we have about condom use measure use during last sex *only* and tell us nothing about consistency of use. Available data suggest that a large percentage (probably the majority) of those reporting condom usage at last sex are inconsistent users, so we question whether increases in condom use indicate a reduction in risk, if that use is largely inconsistent. Yet there has been little if any movement within the international AIDS community to move to more reliable measures of condom usage, namely measures of consistent usage. In fact, much of the reporting done within AIDS programs does not even progress to monitoring usage but merely measures distribution. We can not assume that measuring the number of condoms distributed translates into prevention of HIV through correct and consistent condom use.

Even among known discordant couples, condom usage is not as consistent as we might expect. Two analyses by Allen and colleagues show high levels of condom use for discordant couples who had gone through couples counseling, although this usage was not necessarily consistent. In Rwanda, 9 of 53 couples reported using condoms every time (Allen et al. 1992). In Zambia, a similar study examined "compliance" (defined as no unprotected sex in 3-month period) and also used biological markers to confirm self-reports (Allen et al. 2003). Of couples who were "regular attenders" at follow-up meetings, 23% were perfect compliers (no unprotected sex) for all 12 months, another 26% reported unprotected sex in only one 3-month period, and another 24% reported unprotected sex in only two 3-month periods. However, there was sperm present in vaginal smears in 15% of "protected" intervals, confirming "substantial underreporting" of unprotected sex. Furthermore, consistent condom use was associated with only a 52% reduction in HIV transmission.

Although correct and consistent condom use may significantly reduce risk of HIV transmission, such usage does not seem to have reached high enough rates in any African country to impact HIV prevalence at a population level. In fact, we see an inverse relationship in Africa between condom usage and HIV prevalence; the countries with the highest prevalence also have the highest percentage of men who report condom use at last sex (Figure 6.1). The countries of southern Africa (such as Namibia, Swaziland, and Botswana) have the highest condom usage on the continent as well as the highest HIV prevalence. This is not to say that there is a causal relationship between condom use and HIV at a national level, but rather to note that even the countries with the highest condom usage do not seem to have reached high enough levels to have controlled their HIV epidemics. On the other hand, a number of countries seem to have

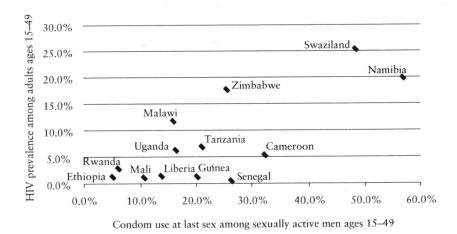

Figure 6.1 **National HIV prevalence by condom use at last sex among men.**
Sources: Demographic and Health Surveys, 2004–08.

successfully contained their HIV epidemics even without high levels of condom use.

There are several possible explanations for the observed relationship between condom use and more HIV infections. People who know they are HIV positive may be more likely to use condoms. People with riskier sexual behavior (such as having more partners) may be more likely to be HIV infected and to use condoms, whether they know they are HIV infected or not. Or people who use condoms may be more likely to take greater sexual risks out of a false sense of security (thus leading to higher HIV infection), another instance of risk compensation. There may also be other confounding factors, such as commercial sex, which is associated with higher condom usage but also higher HIV risk (Hulley et al. 2001).

We have recently undertaken a study to examine just these questions about the link between condom use and HIV infection, in collaboration with Norman Hearst and Esther Hudes of the University of California, San Francisco. Demographic and Health Surveys gather data on sexual behavior and recently have begun to test respondents for HIV infection, which allows us to link data on behavior with data on sero-status. These surveys also provide another valuable type of data, data on consistent condom usage. Consistent condom usage is the critical behavior, the "holy grail" of condom promotion, yet we have virtually no research about this type of usage in general populations. Although data on consistent condom usage have been collected by DHS for several years, to the best of our knowledge these data have not yet been analyzed and published. Therefore, we accessed the pertinent raw DHS data, which are in the public domain and available to researchers, and have begun to analyze them.[20] According to our preliminary results, consistent condom usage[21] is more often reported by men than women, suggesting that men may be overreporting, because if men are using condoms consistently with all partners, the reporting of consistent condom usage among their female partners should be similar. (It seems more likely that men would overreport condom usage than that women who were using condoms consistently would underreport this fact.) Consistent with previous research, consistent condom usage was far lower among married or cohabiting individuals than among never-married persons or those who were separated, widowed, or divorced (Table 6.1). However, in Swaziland, Tanzania, and Zambia, married persons were more likely to use condoms consistently if they had been tested and knew that they were HIV infected. This was generally not the case with unmarried men and women.[22] In fact, in Zambia and Swaziland married men who knew they were HIV positive reported consistent condom usage at nearly the same rate as unmarried men.

These data provide a powerful corrective to the common view that African men refuse to use condoms to protect their wives; in these data, it was *unmarried* men who did not increase their rates of condom usage when they knew themselves to be HIV positive. It should also be noted that in most cases having been tested and received a *negative* result did not result in higher condom use, compared to those who had never been tested, and in Swaziland unmarried women reported a significantly lower rate of consistent condom usage if they had been tested and found to be HIV negative.[23]

Our analysis of condom usage and its relationship to HIV infection has also yielded some surprising preliminary findings. We examined the HIV status of never, inconsistent, and consistent condom users who did *not* know their HIV status, to see if condom use resulted in lower HIV risk. (All analysis was among sexually active individuals.) As discussed, condom use might be higher among those who knew they were infected *because* they were already infected, whereas HIV prevalence among those who did not know their status would provide a better indicator of whether condom use actually reduced risk of infection. Among men and women in all countries, inconsistent condom users had an equal or higher HIV prevalence than never users, suggesting that inconsistent usage offers no protection (and consistent with previous research such as the Rakai study) (Ahmed et al. 2001).

Yet the more powerful finding, and one that to our knowledge has not yet emerged from other research, is that *there was no clear relationship between consistent condom use and HIV prevalence* (Table 6.2), except for Swazi men. We will again note that these data are for people who reported they had never had an HIV test and received the result,

Table 6.1 Consistent condom usage among those who did and did not know their HIV status.[a]

	Among those who did not know their HIV status, percent with consistent condom usage	Among those who knew status and were HIV+, percent with consistent condom usage	Among those who knew status and were HIV−, percent with consistent condom usage
Married men[b], Cote d'Ivoire	4.8% (78/1640)	0.0% (0/5)	2.5% (2/81)
Unmarried men[c], Cote d'Ivoire	35.5% (493/1390) ★	100.0% (6/6) ★	39.7% (31/78) ★
Married women, Cote d'Ivoire	1.1% (23/2187)	8.3% (1/12)	2.6% (4/153)
Unmarried women, Cote d'Ivoire	19.9% (227/1140) ★	53.8% (7/13) ★ ↑	34.2% (15/43) ★ ↑
Married men, Swaziland	14.7% (125/850)	40.8% (49/120) ↑	12.3% (24/195)
Unmarried men, Swaziland	46.8% (496/1060) ★	46.8% (29/62)	52.7% (68/129) ★
Married women, Swaziland	9.9% (111/1117)	25.1% (67/267) ↑	12.7% (65/510)
Unmarried women, Swaziland	36.0% (302/840) ★	40.2% (99/246) ★	28.6% (93/325) ★ ↓
Married men, Tanzania	3.0% (69/2268)	15.1% (8/53) ↑	5.5% (52/952) ↑
Unmarried men, Tanzania	36.0% (335/931) ★	25.0% (2/8)	51.0% (157/308) ★ ↑
Married women, Tanzania	2.1% (64/3088)	10.4% (11/106) ↑	2.9% (55/1906)
Unmarried women, Tanzania	30.1% (240/798)	34.1% (15/44)	34.0% (155/456)
Married men, Zambia	4.3% (103/2406)	16.7% (23/138) ↑	7.7% (35/455) ↑
Unmarried men, Zambia	30.0% (295/982)	18.5% (5/27)	32.7% (66/202)
Married women, Zambia	3.2% (82/2534)	14.7% (37/251) ↑	3.2% (36/1126) ↑
Unmarried women, Zambia	21.4% (128/598)	32.7% (32/98) ↑	24.6% (59/240) ↑

Sources: Cote d'Ivoire AIS 2005; Swaziland DHS 2006–07; Tanzania AIS 2007–08; Zambia DHS 2007.
[a] All data from Demographic and Health Surveys and AIDS Indicator Surveys, for adults ages 15–49. Note that as DHS and AIS are complex surveys, data are weighted. The data presented here therefore are not the actual numbers of respondents but are the weighted number of respondents, which were rounded to the nearest whole number for presentation.

[b] The DHS and AIS definition of married includes those who are "married or living together as if married" (i.e., cohabiting).

[c] Includes the never-married as well as those who are divorced, widowed, or separated.

★ = statistically significant difference (at $p < .05$) in consistent condom usage between married and unmarried.

↑ = higher consistent condom usage among those who knew HIV status compared to those who did not know HIV status, statistically significant at $p < .05$.

↓ = lower consistent condom usage among those who knew HIV status compared to those who did not know HIV status, statistically significant at $p < .05$.

Table 6.2 HIV prevalence among never, inconsistent, and consistent condom users who did not know their HIV status.[1]

	HIV prevalence among never condom users	HIV prevalence among inconsistent condom users	HIV prevalence among consistent condom users
Men, Cote d'Ivoire	2.4% (44/1819)	0.8% (2/256)	2.4% (10/413)
Women, Cote d'Ivoire	6.6% (171/2572)	7.1% (10/141)	3.2% (6/188)
Men, Swaziland	31.0% (244/788)	31.1% (103/331)	20.0% (103/514) ↓
Women, Swaziland	32.4% (381/1177)	41.4% (101/244)	37.5% (145/387)
Men, Tanzania	5.4% (123/2267)	7.0% (20/286)	4.68% (15/314)
Women, Tanzania	6.6% (216/3292)	9.0% (8/89)	12.3% (25/203) ↑
Men, Zambia	12.9% (250/1948)	15.3% (68/444)	10.7% (34/318)
Women, Zambia	14.3% (317/2215)	15.0% (15/100)	22.7% (41/181) ↑

Sources: Cote d'Ivoire AIS 2005; Swaziland DHS 2006–07; Tanzania AIS 2007–08; Zambia DHS 2007.

[1]All data from Demographic and Health Surveys and AIDS Indicator Surveys, for adults ages 15–49. Note that as DHS and AIS are complex surveys, data are weighted. The data presented here therefore are not the actual numbers of respondents but are the weighted number of respondents, which were rounded to the nearest whole number for presentation.

↓ = HIV prevalence lower than among never condom users, statistically significant at $p < .05$.

↑ = HIV prevalence higher than among never condom users, statistically significant at $p < .05$.

so condom usage cannot be an effect of knowing positive status and adopting condom use to avoid infecting others. We will also note that reported condom usage (consistent and inconsistent) decreases with age and HIV infection increases with age (up through the 30s or 40s), so that, all other things being equal, we would expect to see an inverse relationship between condom usage and HIV prevalence, whether or not condom usage reduced HIV infections, because of the confounding factor of age alone.

Among Swazi men (the only population for which consistent condom usage was significantly associated with lower HIV prevalence), there was a particularly strong inverse association between consistent condom usage and HIV prevalence among age cohorts.[24] Younger cohorts were much more likely to be consistent condom users and had lower HIV prevalence, compared to older cohorts. Further analysis will be required to assess whether the observed association between consistent condom use and lower HIV prevalence holds true when age and other factors such as sexual behavior are taken into account or is simply a result of decreasing condom use and rising HIV prevalence with age (see Table 6.2).

How are we to interpret the lack of association between consistent condom use and lower HIV prevalence? We know from a number of studies (mostly done among known discordant couples) that consistent condom use ought to reduce risk of HIV infection by approximately 85%, so, all other things being equal, consistent condom users should have significantly lower HIV risk compared to non-users. But several factors complicate this association. One is that these data are all cross-sectional, so they cannot be used to infer causality. In the words of AIDS expert David Stanton:

> The HIV testing technology used in these surveys is unable to establish time of infection. In other words, the result of the test reflects something that could have take place somewhere in an eight to ten year period. . . . I would be very cautious in drawing conclusions from the cross tabulation of HIV test result and survey responses. Even when the data are linked by respondent they are not linked in time let alone cause and effect.[25]

Another possible confounding factor is that condom users might differ significantly from non-users (e.g., they might have riskier sexual behaviors or other risk factors for HIV). Further analysis is needed to determine if there is a difference in HIV prevalence between consistent condom users and non-users, once other behaviors and risk factors were accounted for. If consistent condom users do engage in riskier behaviors than non-users (e.g., more sexual partners or commercial sex partners), we still need to determine what was the cause and what was the effect. If consistent condom users have greater numbers of partners, do they do so because using condoms makes them feel safer (risk compensation), do they use condoms consistently because they take more risks, or are the two behaviors unrelated?

Whether there is an association between condom use and riskier behavior or not, the lack of an association between consistent condom use and lower HIV prevalence is cause for thought about measuring success in HIV prevention by the number of people reporting condom use, even consistent condom use. An obvious but important point is that all of these data (as with all data on sexual behavior) are self-reported and may tell us more about who reports condom usage than about actual usage.

Those with riskier behavior may be more likely to report consistent condom usage, whether they actually practice it or not, because they know this is the right or expected response. Further, we would argue that the wording of the DHS question invites a "yes" response to the question of consistent condom usage. Rather than asking the question in the affirmative ("Was a male or a female condom used every time you had sexual intercourse with this person in the last 12 months?"), the question could be asked as, "Was there ever any time in the past 12 months when you did not use a condom with this person?"[26] The second wording might produce a far different response.

These findings are not dissimilar to a study conducted in Baltimore in the 1990s (Zenilman et al. 1995). This study was measuring STIs rather than HIV infection, and participants were divided into never, sometimes, and always users of condoms. There were no significant differences in STI infections among the three groups. These results became known as the Zenilman Anomaly and they generated a flurry of letters to the journal and considerable debate. Two years later, another article concluded that "fallibility in self-reports of condom use remains the primary suspect as the cause of these anomalous results" (Turner and Miller 1997). It is also possible that condoms were used consistently but often incorrectly, that there was product failure such as slippage or leakage, or that there was another mechanical problem such as condoms being the wrong size.

In sum, we have to be very careful about inferring causality, given that we are relying on self-reported data of unknown validity. The fact that those who report consistent condom usage do not have reduced HIV risk should make us very careful of how we interpret any data about condom usage, even consistent usage. We cannot assume that just because more of a population is reporting condom usage that HIV risk has been reduced. In fact, the opposite may be true. We simply do not know enough, and we need to continue to objectively evaluate the data about condom usage and HIV risk, to determine what effect condom usage has and how we should interpret increases in self-reported condom usage. Finally, the possibility that increased condom usage does not reduce risk warrants caution in how condoms are promoted. Reducing partners or mutual monogamy may in fact be an easier behavior change than consistent condom usage to adopt, and more effective.

Female Condoms

Female condoms present another challenge: Although there have been great efforts to introduce them in some parts of the world, they remain expensive, by many accounts rather awkward to use, and demand remains low. A recent news report about continuing low demand 15 years after female condoms were introduced profiled promotion efforts in various countries (*PlusNews* 2009b). Uganda is currently relaunching female condoms in the country, but the first launch failed not for lack of funding but for lack of uptake among women. In Namibia, women have reportedly been using the rubber rings of the condoms as bracelets, and the UNFPA country spokesperson commented that female condoms remain unpopular. Zimbabwe has the highest rate of female condom distribution per capita worldwide according to the UNFPA, with 5 million female condoms distributed in 2008. This translates into 1.6 female condoms per women per year (for a population of approximately 3 million adult women)—hardly a tremendous uptake.

Proponents of female condoms may point to studies that show favorable reactions to them among women, but Green's experience in 1998 suggests why this purported enthusiasm may not translate into significant uptake. A researcher at a major family planning organization hired several scores of women in Kenya to listen to a series of lectures about the benefits of the then newly available female condoms. At the end of this, but before they were paid for their time, the participants were asked to fill out a questionnaire. When they were asked questions such as, "Did you have a favorable impression of female condoms? Do you think you might use female condoms in the future? Would you recommend female condoms to their friends?" the great majority answered yes. Green had been hired to ensure the scientific credibility of the research, but when it became obvious that the process was anything but scientific, he resigned from the project.[27]

Microbicides, Vaccines, and Other Futures Therapies

We support the need for a female-controlled AIDS prevention technology, whether a barrier method, microbicide, or something else, although the search for an effective product has encountered many roadblocks.

Faced with the failure of standard prevention measures to control the AIDS pandemic, many in the AIDS prevention community have pinned their hopes on technological breakthroughs. Many believe that a vaccine is the only true solution, but so far trials have been disappointing, and it is estimated that we are at least 10 years from a viable vaccine. In late 2009, the first "successful" vaccine trial showed that two vaccines in combination can reduce risk of HIV infection by 30%. This is wonderful news, but such a vaccine is not yet ready to be distributed, may not be effective with the strains of HIV found in Africa, and, with a risk reduction effect of only 30%, is certainly no silver bullet.

Microbicides (gels that women could apply vaginally before sex without their partner's knowledge) have also received a major amount of research funding, attention, and excitement, as a woman-controlled method of HIV prevention. After a number of failed trials, it was announced in July 2010 that a microbicide had finally showed effectiveness in a clinical trial (CAPRISA 004), marking the first time that a biological intervention had ever shown efficacy in a large trial. In a very high-incidence population, women who used the microbicide (which required application before and after intercourse) had a 39% lower chance of becoming HIV infected than women who used a placebo. For women who used the microbicide more than 80% of the time, risk was reduced by 54% (Abdool Karim et al. 2010). In announcing the results of the trial, the researchers stressed that a microbicide gel was not yet ready for the market, that at least one more trial with a larger population was needed, and that they would continue to search for a more effective product. Microbicides may indeed one day give women an effective, available, and affordable tool, but it remains to be seen how this microbicide, or others that may be developed, will fare among women in other parts of Africa and the world.

Anti-retroviral drugs are also being explored as tools in prevention. Trials are currently underway to test pre-exposure prophylaxis, or PreP, low doses of ARVs that are taken as a prophylaxis. A trial known as Vaginal and Oral Interventions to Control the Epidemic (VOICE), begun in 2009, will enroll thousands of women across southern Africa to study two types of pre-exposure prophylaxis: daily vaginal application of a tenofovir gel and oral administration of an anti-HIV drug (Cohen 2010). Treating people infected with HIV as soon as they test positive, to lower their viral loads and make them less infectious to others, has also been proposed. Such strategies may work in theory, but we have serious doubts about their feasibility given the expense of ARVs and the reality that global resources for AIDS are already inadequate to provide treatment to all of the HIV-infected people who need it.

Risk Compensation

Condoms, or any prevention technology which promises to decrease the risk of risky sex, have the potential to create a false sense of security or make risky behaviors seem more attractive. We cannot discount the possibility that risk compensation or disinhibition may be causing condom users to take greater risks in their sexual behavior than they would in the absence of condoms.[28] The government of Uganda was aware of this possibility as early as 1988, when it advised, in what may be its earliest booklet on AIDS prevention, "Condoms give people a false idea they are totally safe from AIDS. The best way to avoid AIDS is to avoid causal sex and to stick to a faithful partner" (Government of Uganda 1988:33).

Any risk reduction measure has the potential to lead to risk compensation. Those who perform randomized controlled trials of male circumcision have been alert to the possibility of risk compensation and have monitored the sexual behavior of men after circumcision to see if riskier sexual behavior occurred post-circumcision.[29] Yet there seems to be reluctance to measure possible risk compensation or even discuss the matter in connection with condoms. In a 2003 presentation to USAID, Douglas Kirby prefaced his remarks on disinhibition by noting this seems to be a taboo word seldom spoken in public.

A recent prospective study of Ugandan men suggests that condom promotion might indeed encourage higher risk sex. A group of men in Kampala, Uganda, participated in a condom promotion program that taught condom technical use skills, encouraged condom use, and provided free condoms. Compared to a control group that received only a brief informational presentation about AIDS, the men in the intervention group did use more condoms. The men in the intervention group also increased their number of sexual partners by 31%, in comparison to those in the control group, who *decreased* their number of partners by 17%. The net result was an increase in sexual risk in the intervention group. The authors conclude:

> The increase in condom uptake that the intervention produced seems not to have been sufficient to counteract the increase in numbers of sex partners. Although this was not the result we intended or expected, it is consistent with the history of AIDS prevention efforts in Uganda. Uganda's success in AIDS control seems to have resulted from reductions in numbers of partners, with condoms playing a relatively minor role. (Kajubi et al. 2005:82)

Condoms can be promoted to anyone and everyone, but years of experience show that only those in high-risk groups are likely to use them consistently, especially in rural areas where a steady supply of condoms is problematic. As discussed above, *consistent* condom use in Africa is relatively rare and inconsistent use may actually be associated with higher HIV risk. Add to this a cross-sectional study of consistent condom use from four African countries showing no consistent evidence that even this type of reported condom use is associated with lower HIV infections and the outlook seems increasingly bleak for condoms living up to their promise of being the best weapon we have in the fight against AIDS, as is often said.

In their five-country study of "love, marriage, and HIV," anthropologist Jennifer Hirsch and colleagues voice concern that messages encouraging partner reduction may also lead to greater risk-taking. They state that in Nigeria and Uganda, "the barrage of communication campaigns associating the risk of HIV with illicit, immoral sex have made condoms something to be avoided, and thus 'safe sex' has come to mean sex that is presumptively and apparently monogamous rather than sex that is actually monogamous" (Hirsch et al. 2010:19). They additionally warn of "the iatrogenic consequences of HIV prevention programs . . . public health messages about monogamy interact with the rise of modern marital ideas to drive men's infidelity underground" (p. 21).

Certainly prevention programs must be sensitive to the way their messages are perceived. If a certain message about HIV risk strikes most people as talking about someone else and therefore makes them complacent about (or blind to) their own risk factors, it may do more harm than good. We should be concerned about any and all unintended consequences of HIV prevention programs, and more research is needed to make these links between how messages are intended and how they are understood. But in the absence of convincing data that messages stressing monogamy actually *are* leading to more male infidelity and less condom use, we question whether such great concern about possible unintended consequences is warranted. Furthermore, we should be concerned with the effect of these messages in total: Is it not possible that they will have a positive effect on many, even if they have a negative effect on a few? This reminds us of the specious argument that because not everyone might be able to abstain, abstinence should not be promoted to anyone (Tapiwanashe 2008).

Let us review the available evidence regarding risk compensation and HIV risk behaviors. We do have evidence linking inconsistent condom usage to greater risk taking and higher HIV prevalence and showing that even reported consistent condom usage is often not correlated with decreased HIV risk. On the other hand, reported abstinence and faithfulness are consistently associated with decreased HIV risk, as will be discussed in the next chapter.

Any self-reported data about sexual behavior (i.e., virtually *all* our data about sexual behavior) should be interpreted with caution, and self-reports should not necessarily be taken at face value. Positive trends in self-reported behavior may be more of a sign of changing social norms and what is considered acceptable and desirable behavior than of changed behaviors themselves. Increasing this "desirability bias" may be another unintended consequence of behavior change programs; behavior change programs may be teaching people the right answer to give to surveyors who come knocking on their doors, as well as (or instead of) influencing their behavior. Yet in our opinion these cautions do not mean that data on sexual behavior are useless. We should rather triangulate them with other sources of data, such as less subjective data on HIV infections. When we do so, the clear conclusion is that inconsistent condom usage may be associated with increased sexual risk taking and increased HIV risk, whereas abstinence and faithfulness are associated with less risk of HIV infection.

NOTES

1. For those who might remember estimated national prevalence being as high as 35% in some African countries, the explanation is not that HIV prevalence has substantially declined, but that estimates of prevalence have gotten better. In recent years UNAIDS has begun using population-based survey figures, resulting in substantially lower but far more accurate estimates of HIV prevalence.
2. See Shelton et al. (2006) for a discussion of incidence and prevalence trends in Africa.
3. Based on data from Rakai, Uganda, Hollingsworth et al. (2008) estimated that HIV-infected individuals were seven times as infectious during late-stage AIDS (10–19 months before death) as during the asymptomatic stage of infection, and that for the final 10 months before death the transmission rate was zero because the infected individual was too sick for regular sexual contact. Hollingsworth et al. estimated that late-stage infections were responsible for 20% of onward infections in a situation of serial monogamy.
4. Data from Rakai also show that HIV was transmitted during acute infection in 10 of 23 such couples in the observed cohort (Pinkerton 2007). Phylogenetic analysis of HIV-infected individuals in Quebec similarly found that acute infection accounted for half of all transmissions (Brenner et al. 2007).
5. See Boily et al. 2009. One evaluation of available evidence concluded that the risk in unprotected heterosexual sex between an infected and uninfected partner is one infection per 1,000–2,000 unprotected coital acts, although risk in male-to-male sex was considerably greater (see Royce et al. 1997).
6. Analysis of infections within discordant couples in Rakai, Uganda, found that subtype A viruses were associated with a significantly higher risk of transmission than subtype D viruses (see Kiwanuka et al. 2009).
7. Researchers recently discovered a genetic variation that may make Africans and those of African descent 40% more susceptible to infection while also delaying the onset of AIDS symptoms (see He et al. 2008).

8. MCP has been used to refer both to multiple and concurrent partnerships and to multiple concurrent partnerships, the latter being something of a redundant phrase as having concurrent sexual partners by definition involves having multiple sexual partners. At an April 2009 meeting, the UNAIDS Reference Group on Estimates, Models, and Projections recommended that MCP not be used, but rather the term "concurrent partnerships" or "concurrent sexual partnerships" (Consultation on Concurrent Sexual Partnerships: Recommendations from a Meeting of the UNAIDS Reference Group on Estimates, Modelling and Projections held in Nairobi, Kenya, April 20–21, 2009). However, programmatically the term MCP is still often used, as behavior change programs often target multiple and concurrent partnerships together.

9. See, for instance, Addressing Multiple and Concurrent Partnerships in Southern Africa: Developing Guidance for Bold Action (http://www.unaidsrstesa.org/files/u1/MCP_Meeting_Report_Gabarone_28-29_Jan_2009.pdf [accessed July 29, 2010]), a report of a January 2009 meeting convened by the Harvard AIDS Prevention Research Project, UNAIDS, and the World Bank in Gaborone, Botswana.

10. Generalized epidemics were called Type II or just African epidemics in the latter 1980s (see Green 1988).

11. Weinhardt and colleagues, in a 1999 meta-analysis of 27 studies from around the world, found that those who tested positive and sero-discordant couples increased their condom use, but that those who tested HIV negative did not change their behavior. A 2008 meta-analysis of seven developing-country studies concluded that VCT had no effect on number of sex partners. Four of the seven studies showed that VCT decreased unprotected sex, although this effect was mainly observed among HIV-positive respondents and sero-discordant couples and the overall rigor of these studies was low (Denison et al. 2008). See also Glick 2005 and Shelton 2008. However, a recent study in rural Zimbabwe did find that women who received VCT reduced their reported number of new partners more than those who did not test, with HIV-positive women reducing their number of partners even more than HIV-negative women. Both men and women who tested positive reported reduced levels of concurrent partnerships for 2–3 years following testing (Cremin et al. 2010).

12. In the beginning of the study, only 3% of couples had reported condom use (see Allen et al. 2003).

13. Twenty-three percent of discordant couples reported 100% condom use over the course of the year, but 17% of these had evidence of sperm when a vaginal swab was performed on the woman during a quarterly visit. This 17% may be an underestimate of the couples that had unprotected sex over the course of a year, as there were only four such visits to check for evidence of unprotected sex, and sperm can only be detected for a few days after unprotected intercourse.

14. Reported *consistent* condom use was associated with a 70% reduction in pregnancy and a 52% reduction in linked HIV transmission, but as the frequencies of these events were small, these results should be interpreted with caution (Allen et al. 2003).

15. In a multivariate model, HIV acquisition was independently associated with younger age, alcohol consumption at enrollment in the study, having paid sex in previous three months, and recent infections with gonorrhea, but was *not* associated with education and literacy. Women who reported no alcohol consumption had an HIV infection rate of 2.44 infections per 100 person-years, approximately

half the 4.53 infections per 100 person-years found among women who reported one to nine drinks a week. Women who had 10 or more drinks a week had even higher HIV incidence (8.34 infections per 100 person-years for women with 10–29 drinks a week, and 11.8 infections per 100 person-years for women with 30 or more drinks per week) (Watson-Jones 2009).

16. Sidibe, M. Letter to Partners, 2010. http://data.unaids.org/pub/BaseDocument/2010/20100216_exd_lettertopartners_en.pdf (accessed July 29, 2010).

17. We are indebted to Emily Chambers for this insight (personal communication).

18. Effectiveness, a measure of how well condoms work under normal conditions, is not the same thing as efficacy, which is the optimum success of condoms in an ideal or "best case" situation. Davis and Weller (1999) estimate based on a meta-analysis of multiple cohort studies that efficacy may be as high as 97%, but typical effectiveness was estimated to be 87%, or as low as 60% or high as 96%. See also Hearst and Chen 2004.

19. The survey was the 2003 loveLife survey, a nationally representative household survey of 11,904 youth ages 15–24 (Pettifor et al. 2004).

20. For this study, we used the four highest-prevalence African countries for which data were available: Cote d'Ivoire, Swaziland, Tanzania, and Zambia.

21. DHS surveys ask the following questions about up to three partners in the past year: If a condom was used at last sex and if a condom was used during every act of intercourse. If the respondent replies that he or she did not use a condom when last having sex with a partner, no other questions about condom use with that partner are asked. This then leads to the following definitions of condom use: "Never users" are defined as those who did not report using a condom at the last act of sex with any partner (up to last three partners in the past year) and thus have no evidence of condom use. It is possible that such respondents did use condoms with one or more partners at some point, but it is impossible to know because if a condom was not used at last sex, no other questions about condom use are asked. "Inconsistent users" are defined as respondents who replied that they did use a condom at last sex with at least one partner but did not use condoms consistently with all partners. This measure almost certainly underestimated inconsistent condom users, as any inconsistent condom user who did not happen to use a condom at last sex (and thus had no evidence of condom use within the DHS survey) was counted in this study as a never condom user. "Consistent users" were defined as respondents who reported using condoms consistently with all partners in the past year. In this study, over half of those who reported condom use reported consistent condom use, but it is likely that the number of inconsistent users was underestimated.

22. In Cote d'Ivoire, the numbers of men and women who knew their status were too small to determine whether knowing status was associated with higher or lower condom use, except for unmarried women, who were more likely to report consistent condom usage if they knew their status.

23. Because of the limitations of DHS data, knowing status was defined as having ever been tested and received the result, whereas HIV status itself was measured at the time of the survey. So, it is possible that a respondent had sero-converted after being tested and receiving the result and before being tested as part of the DHS survey. Such a respondent would be considered in our analysis as knowing his or her status and being *HIV positive*, while he or she believed, based on

the results of the last HIV test, that he or she was *HIV negative.* Those who knew their status and were HIV positive generally had higher rates of consistent condom usage than those who knew their status and were HIV negative. Had the first population not likely included a number of people who actually believed themselves to be HIV negative, the difference in consistent condom usage between those who were HIV positive and those who were HIV negative (and were counted as knowing their status) would have potentially been even greater.

24. When HIV prevalence and prevalence of consistent condom usage for 5-year-age cohorts were plotted, the best fit line had a slope of −1.03 (meaning that there was a nearly perfect inverse relationship between HIV prevalence and consistent condom usage, by age cohort), and R^2 equaled 0.75 (meaning that there was a high goodness of fit).

25. David Stanton, personal communication.

26. This was suggested to us by Daniel Halperin, personal communication.

27. Applied anthropologists often find themselves in dilemmas like this. On another occasion, Green was asked by an activist group in 1998 to "find the data that shows the increased HIV risks associated with female circumcision." Green replied that he would like nothing better than to end female circumcision, but he said he thought such data didn't exist, from what he had read. The group presumably went to another researcher willing to find data that would support a presupposition.

28. Risk compensation and disinhibition refer to the tendency for a perception of reduced risk to make risk-taking more attractive. People may take greater risks in response to the increased sense of personal safety that comes with protective behaviors such as wearing a seatbelt or using a condom.

29. The researchers in one trial discussed this issue explicitly, stating, "In the context of an RCT, circumcision does not appear to increase sexual risk or incident HIV" (Mattson et al. 2008).

Chapter 7

PRIMARY BEHAVIOR CHANGE AND HIV DECLINE

We have just shown that none of the standard technology-based prevention methods in global AIDS have thus far succeeded in changing the course of the world's worst epidemics. We believe that what is needed is not more of the same interventions, or more sophisticated evaluation systems, but rather a radically different approach. Effective HIV prevention requires primary behavior change, not just risk reduction measures to ameliorate the effects of risky sex and drug use. The risk behaviors themselves must be changed. At least, risk-avoidance behaviors that people are currently practicing should be encouraged and reinforced. But mention of fidelity or abstinence at global AIDS conferences is typically met with jeers and cat-calls.[1]

What is the evidence for this behavioral approach to AIDS? We cannot point to any randomized controlled trial (RCT) of abstinence and faithfulness interventions or any other clear study or piece of data that definitively proves that behavioral interventions are the key to HIV prevention. RCTs remain the gold standard of research, but as Nancy Padian and colleagues point out in a recent article reviewing 37 HIV RCTs for the prevention of sexual transmission of HIV, only five have decreased HIV transmission (Padian et al. 2010).[2] This includes all three male circumcision trials, which have been mentioned, as well as one STI trial and one vaccine trial. In other words, all the successful RCTs have been biomedical and none have been behavioral. Randomized controlled trials of primary behavior change interventions have not been carried out, nor has high-quality research using other research methods.

We agree with Judith Auerbach's recent assessment that the

> hegemony of RCTs is being challenged by social scientists who argue that experimental methods often are not appropriate for addressing social-level questions. They also note that declining HIV infection rates observed over the course of the pandemic in a number of diverse settings (e.g., San Francisco, Thailand, Uganda, and Senegal) resulted from community-driven behavioral and social change, not from experimental

interventions, and that such community-generated responses do offer observational evidence of effectiveness—even if it is not entirely clear to what specific actions the declining infection rates may be attributed. So, although RCTs remain valid and necessary for assessing the efficacy of some types of HIV prevention strategies, they will never produce the entirety of relevant evidence of what actually works in different modes, populations, and settings. Rather, the HIV prevention field must come to accept a range of "ways of knowing" in which evidence is derived from different methodologies appropriate to the question and level of analysis being addressed. (quoted in Mayer and Pizer 2008:xii)

The fact that a definitive RCT of behavioral interventions may never be feasible does not negate the need for high-quality research of behavioral prevention. It is possible that this research hasn't yet been carried out partly because behavioral research is tricky to carry out, but we and others would argue that it is more likely that the current dearth of evidence is because there has not been the will and financial resources to carry out the same kind of research about primary behavior change that has been invested in other methods of AIDS prevention.

So what do we know? We know that risky sexual behaviors, in particular greater numbers of sexual partners, are strongly and consistently related to HIV risk for both men and women. In other words, having fewer sexual partners is strongly protective at an individual level in a way that condom use or testing is not. (Infection with various STIs is also a strong risk factor for HIV infection, although as we have seen STI treatment has so far failed to reduce HIV risk in a number of experimental trials.) Li Chen and colleagues (2007), in a review of 68 studies of sexual behavior and HIV risk in Africa, concluded,

> [T]he key sexual risk factors for HIV infection in sub-Saharan African are a high number of lifetime sexual partners, engaging in paid sex, and having an STI- most notably HSV-2. We observed an approximately linear relationship between number of partners and HIV risk for both men and women that adjusted for potentially confounding variables. (p. s7)

Vinod Mishra and colleagues, in an analysis of Demographic and Health Survey data from four countries, also found a strong linear relationship between lifetime number of sexual partners and odds of being HIV-infected. This relationship persisted even when age, education, marital union, and a number of other demographic factors were accounted for, and was particularly strong for women (Mishra et al. 2009a). Men and women who reported two lifetime partners had double or more the risk of being HIV-infected compared to women who reported only one lifetime partner, and their odds of being HIV-infected continued to increase with each additional partner (Mishra et al. 2009a:12). But this clear connection between number of sexual partners and HIV risk is often all but ignored within the HIV prevention community.

There is also evidence to suggest that delay of sexual debut or abstinence (primary or secondary) can reduce HIV risk at an individual level. Delay of sexual debut delays the age at which a young person can become HIV infected, and a number of studies and meta-analyses have noted an association between later sexual debut, fewer lifetime partners, and less risky behavior once sex is initiated, and thus less HIV risk.[3] Even secondary abstinence (returning to abstinence after sexual initiation) has been associated with lower HIV risk, as in a 2005 national survey in South Africa that found an HIV prevalence of 3.8% among youth who reported never having had sex (primary abstinence), 11.3% among youth who were sexually experienced but had not had sex in the past year (secondary abstainers, who were over 20% of all youth), and 15.6% among youth who had been sexually active in the past year (Shisana et al. 2005).

At the population level, we have seen changes in risky behavior (primarily greater faithfulness and abstinence) associated with declines in HIV infections in a number of generalized epidemics. Perhaps these "natural experiments" do not tell us what brought about those changes in risky behavior or how to design programs that promote behavior change in the future. In one sense, they are the weakest type of evidence because it is impossible to prove causality and it is difficult to determine how to replicate their success. But in another sense, they are the best kind of evidence—not theoretical, abstract, or focused on what HIV prevention *could* achieve but actual evidence about actual successes. We believe that the epidemiological evidence strongly points to the fact that primary behavior change *must* occur for HIV to transmission to be stopped, so whatever programs and methods we use to get to these changes in behavior, the goal is clear.

The list of African success stories (i.e., countries that have shown prevalence decline and quite often measured behavior change) now includes Uganda (late 1980s), Kenya (late 1990s–early 2000s), Zimbabwe (late 1990s–early 2000s), Zambia (urban youth, 1990s), Ethiopia (Addis Ababa, late 1990s–early 2000s), Malawi (Lilongwe/central region, late 1990s–early 2000s), Rwanda (urban areas especially Kigali, late 1990s–early 2000s), Cote d'Ivoire (urban, late 1990s–early 2000s), urban Haiti (early 2000s), and possibly others. The common element in these HIV success stories has not been new or better technologies but simple changes in behavior. These successful responses to HIV have often arisen out of communities, been grounded in local cultures, and drawn on local knowledge rather than outside expertise. Furthermore, although extremely high rates of infection (upward of 20%) are seen in a handful of southern African countries, in most African countries HIV prevalence remains below 5% and in some it is as low as 1% or 2% (and even lower in North Africa). Even in the highest prevalence countries of southern Africa, the HIV epidemic appears to have stabilized. One analysis noted two associated trends: HIV prevalence among women attending ante-natal clinics had declined in Lesotho, Namibia, Swaziland, Botswana, Malawi, and Zimbabwe (achieving statistical significance at $p < 0.05$ in the last three), and young people in the region were reporting somewhat less risky behavior (Gouws et al. 2008).

The best available survey data indicates that sexual behavior on much of the continent is more conservative than outsiders typi-cally assume. Figures 7.1 and 7.2, which summarize data from the Demographic and Health Surveys, show that in any given year a majority of Africans practice abstinence or faithfulness. Therefore, behavior-based approaches to HIV prevention are not necessarily a matter of changing risky behavior (for many), but rather of reinforc-ing existing healthy and protective behaviors.

More than half of African youth ages 15–19 years report abstaining from premarital sex in the previous year, according to DHS data. For exam-ple, among unmarried youth 15–24, 77% of Zambian youth and 74% of Ugandan youth had no sex partner in the previous year, and in some coun-tries an even higher proportion reported abstinence. In only a handful of countries (all in west Africa) do more than half of unmarried adolescents report sex in the past year. In several countries, less than 10% of unmarried adolescent males or females report sex in the past year. Most sexually active adults, whether married or not, report having only one partner in the previ-ous year. In Uganda, this figure was 84%, whereas in Zambia it was 89% (see Uganda DHS 2006; Zambia DHS 2007). The number of Africans who practice abstinence or faithfulness in any given year is far greater than the number of Africans who practice consistent condom use.

These facts should make us question the validity of the assumption that consistent condom use is a realistic behavior, whereas abstinence and faithfulness are not. We are *not* saying that we should shift atten-tion and resources away from risk reduction programs for those who continue to practice high-risk behaviors. We are suggesting that donors and international health organizations reconsider which behaviors are realistic and which interventions are appropriate for most Africans, and apportion resources accordingly. In the few countries where abstinence and fidelity have been promoted at the national level and backed by resources, sexual behavior has changed and rates of HIV and other STIs have decreased. Let us now consider some country-level evidence.

Percent of unmarried youth ages 15–24 reporting premarital sex in past year

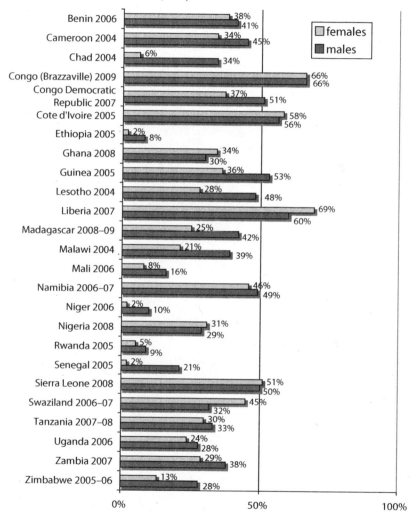

Figure 7.1 **Premarital sex among youth ages 15–24 in sub-Saharan Africa.**
Sources: Demographic and Health Surveys and AIDS Information Surveys.

Percent of adults ages 15–49 reporting multiple partners in past year, among those who had sexual intercourse in past 12 months

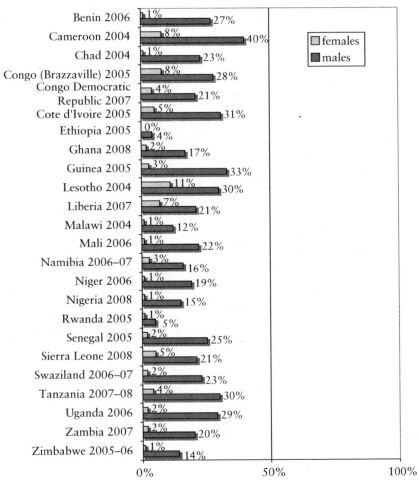

Figure 7.2 Multiple partnerships in sub-Saharan Africa.
Sources: Demographic and Health Surveys and AIDS Information Surveys.

UGANDA

Uganda's remarkable success in responding to AIDS has already been discussed, but here we will consider the epidemiological evidence in more depth. In Uganda, HIV prevalence declined from 18% to 6% between 1992 and 2002 (Wabwire-Mangen et al. 2009). No other country has ever seen such a dramatic decline. In the early 2000s, HIV prevalence stabilized between 6.1% and 6.5% (Wabwire-Mangen et al. 2009); as previously discussed, there is some reason to think that HIV may again be on the rise in Uganda.

The following behavioral changes occurred at the time of Uganda's decline in HIV prevalence (Figure 7.3). The proportion of young men age 15–24 reporting premarital sex decreased from 60% in 1989 to 23% in 1995. For women, the decline was from 53% to 16% (Global Program on AIDS, cited in Bessinger et al. 2003).[4] For all age groups, 41% of men reported higher-risk sex (sex with a non-marital or non-cohabiting partner) in 1989. This declined to 21% by 1995. For women, the decline was from 23% to 9% (Global Program on AIDS, cited in Bessinger et al. 2003). The proportion of men reporting multiple partners fell from 15% reporting three or more non-regular sex partners in the past year in 1989, to 3% reporting three or more non-regular sex partners in the past six months in 1995.[5] In the same period, the percentage of men who reported ever use of a condom increased from 15% to 30% for men and from 7% to 20% for women.[6] These data about condom usage do not tell us what percent of condom usage was consistent, so based on the

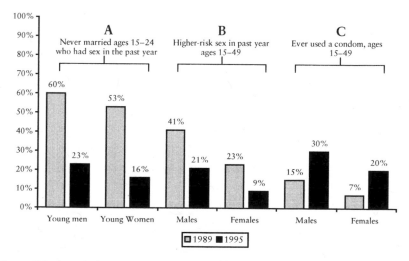

Figure 7.3 ABC behaviors in Uganda 1989 and 1995.
Sources: Global Programme on AIDS (GPA) Surveys, cited in Bessinger et al. 2003.

data we have reviewed about inconsistent condom usage, we believe it is not clear what impact these increases in condom usage had on new infections.

The primary factor that explains HIV incidence and prevalence decline in Uganda is reduction in the proportion of men and women who report more than one partner in the previous year. Green and colleagues argued this in a 2002 report for USAID (Green et al. 2002), and a 2004 peer-reviewed article by Stoneburner and Low-Beer drew the same conclusion. Although there has been considerable debate since then over the causes of Uganda's decline (or whether it happened at all), a consensus about the primary role of partner reduction has developed (Epstein 2007; Gray et al. 2006; Kirby 2008; Shelton et al. 2004).

Although AIDS prevention programs often focus on youth, evidence shows that it is reduction in the number of sexual partners among those who are sexually active—and not abstinence among youth—that is most critical to curbing an AIDS epidemic (Shelton et al. 2004). Most Ugandans ages 15–49 (the age group in which surveys typically measure both behavior and HIV status) were and are sexually active and faithful, not abstinent. Youth were given information on a range of AIDS prevention options, including condoms, with abstinence (often termed "delay of sexual debut") emphasized as the only 100% sure option. Adults were targeted with a "be faithful" message that included slogans such as "love faithfully" and "zero grazing."

When condom use and multiple partnerships in the mid- to late 1990s are compared across the region, it is in the latter that Uganda differs from neighboring countries (Stoneburner and Low-Beer 2004). As shown in Figure 7.4, condom use was not higher in Uganda than in other

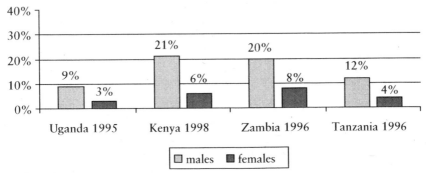

Figure 7.4 Condom use at last sex in four African countries.
Sources: Uganda DHS 1995; Kenya DHS 1998; Zambia DHS 1996; Tanzania DHS 1996.

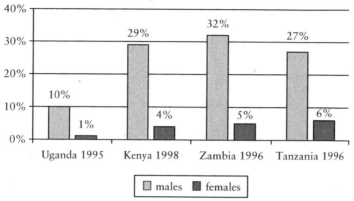

Sexually active men and women ages 15–49 who have had sexual intercourse with two or more partners in the last 12 months

Figure 7.5 Multiple sexual partnerships in four African countries.
Sources: Uganda DHS 1995; Kenya DHS 1998; Zambia DHS 1996; Tanzania DHS 1996.

countries. There was far less multi-partner sex reported in Uganda than in other countries, as illustrated in Figure 7.5.

KENYA

Kenya is a more recent example of a successful behavioral approach to HIV prevention. In Kenya, the major response to AIDS before 1999 was condom supply and promotion. There was little or no impact on the pandemic. Then the Kenyan government began to implement an approach more like that of Uganda. In addition, faith-based groups were mobilized. AIDS education was implemented in schools. Educators and officials emphasized the seriousness of the epidemic, and government officials were told that they must mention AIDS every time they had a public meeting (Green 2003). As illustrated in Figure 7.6, which compares Kenya DHS data from 1998 and 2003, there were declines in the proportion of youth reporting premarital sex in the past year and in the proportion of men and women reporting more than two partners in the past year. The proportion of men and women who reported using a condom at last higher risk sex (among those who reported having had higher risk sex in the past year) also increased. For men, the increase in condom use at last higher risk sex was from 44% to 47%, but the number of men having higher risk sex had shrunk enough between 1998 and 2003 that in 2003 there were actually *fewer* men reporting condom use at last sex, even as the percentage reporting condom use at last higher risk sex had increased.

What impact did this have? According to UNAIDS, Kenya's epidemic "peaked in the late 1990s with an overall prevalence of 10% in adults, and

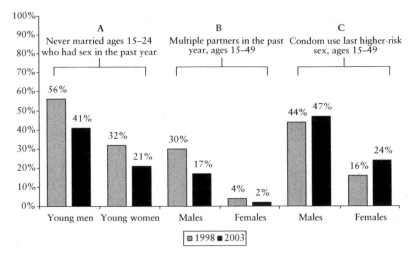

Figure 7.6 ABC behaviors in Kenya 1998 and 2003.
Sources: Kenya **DHS** 1998 and 2003.

declined to 7% by 2003" (UNAIDS 2005a). The "B" component again appears to be the crucial factor associated with national HIV prevalence decline, just as in Uganda. The 2003 Kenya DHS showed a national HIV prevalence of 6.7%, with the 2008–09 DHS showing a slight decline to 6.3%.

ZIMBABWE

Zimbabwe has also experienced changes in sexual behaviors, and, as in Uganda and Kenya, these changes seem to be the primary factors associated with a large decline in HIV prevalence. A 2010 review concluded that HIV prevalence fell in Zimbabwe from 29.3% in 1997 to 15.6% in 2007, a change accelerated by changes in sexual behavior (Gregson et al. 2010). ANC data showed a decline in HIV prevalence among pregnant women from 32.1% in 2000 to 23.9% in 2004 (Mahomva et al. 2006). DHS as well as other surveys have shown increases in faithfulness among men and women. For example, the 1999 and 2005 DHS showed a decline in the number of men and women reporting one or more non-regular (nonmarital, noncohabiting) sexual partners in the past year, from 57% to 47% for men and from 15.5% to 14% for women. Nationally there were no clear trends in abstinence among youth or condom use (Gregson et al. 2010); both age of sexual debut and condom use with non-regular partners were already quite high by the late 1990s.

A cohort study in Manicaland in rural eastern Zimbabwe also provides useful data on trends in HIV prevalence and behaviors. This study found that between 1998 and 2003 there was a decrease in overall adult HIV prevalence (from 23.0% to 20.5%), with steeper reductions of 23% and 49% in young men and women. During this same period, there were changes in reported sexual behavior. The proportion of sexually experienced men reporting a recent casual partner declined from 26% to 13%, and women reported a nonstatistically significant decline (from 7.5% to 5.9%). The proportion of 17–19-year-old men who reported having ever had sex decreased from 45% to 27%, and there was a similar decline from 21% to 9% for women (Gregson et al. 2006).

The data from Zimbabwe are strikingly similar to those of Kenya, shown above. In Zimbabwe, as in Kenya, there were increases in abstinence, faithfulness, and condom use behaviors between 1998 and 2003. As in Kenya, although the proportion of men and women reporting condom use at last high-risk sex went up slightly, the proportion of all men and women reporting condom use at last sex of any type declined somewhat, as the proportion of men and women engaging in high-risk sex shrunk. Mark Dybul, who was the U.S. Global AIDS coordinator at the time, observed about the evidence from Zimbabwe: "Perhaps one of the most interesting things is that the greatest behavior change was in abstinence and fidelity. The relative change in condom use was not as remarkable" (Check 2006). Gregson, the primary author of the study in Manicaland, remarked that "it is important to note that all three types of behavior change seem important in Zimbabwe. We need to be promoting all the different prevention possibilities" (Check 2006) (see Figure 7.7).

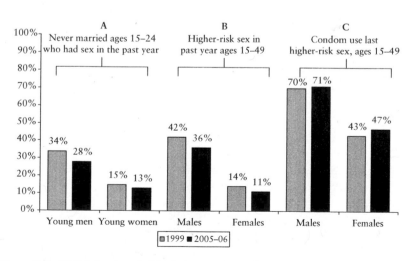

Figure 7.7 **ABC behaviors in Zimbabwe 1999 and 2005–06.**
Sources: Zimbabwe DHS 1999 and 2005–06.

Another remarkable part of the prevalence decline story in Zimbabwe is that it occurred during great economic decline, currency hyperinflation, increased employment and poverty, and political unrest. It is commonly believed that these factors drive or enhance HIV prevalence, yet some observers have even suggested that the economic decline may have helped to slow the rate of new infections as men could no longer afford to sustain extramarital affairs (Timberg 2007). A qualitative study involving dozens of interviews and focus group discussions also concluded that growing poverty had reduced casual and extramarital sex in Zimbabwe. This study found that the exposure to AIDS mortality (such as deaths of relatives and friends) led to increased perceived HIV risk and interpersonal communication about HIV/AIDS, and that this had a larger impact than AIDS prevention programs and services (Muchini et al. 2010).

Other Countries

Changes in sexual behaviors have also been associated with HIV decline in Zambia, Haiti, the central region of Malawi, urban Cote d'Ivoire, urban Rwanda, urban Ethiopia, and perhaps other countries or regions of countries.[7] In Zambia, there were significant declines in HIV among youth in the 1990s (Bessinger et al. 2003), but this was not sustained after about 1998. In Haiti, no stranger to poverty and social breakdown, prevalence in urban areas declined in the early 2000s from approximately 5.5% to 3% among women ages 15–44. This decline in HIV prevalence was preceded by a 20% decline in the reported number of sexual partners between 1994 and 2000. In addition, there was also a two- to three-fold increase in reported condom use between 2000–01 and 2003, although we do not know how much of this use was consistent (Hallett et al. 2006). Urban and semi-urban areas of Malawi's central region saw HIV prevalence decline from 1999 to 2003, although national prevalence remained stable, and in the capital city Lilongwe, HIV infections declined throughout the early 2000s (Bello et al. 2006).

In Cote d'Ivoire, the number of men and women reporting multiple partners in the past year declined between 1998 and 2005 (from 42.0% to 30.5% among males ages 15–49 and from 6% to 4.5% among females ages 15–49) (see Cote d'Ivoire DHS 1998, 2005), and between 2001 and 2005 HIV prevalence among antenatal clinic attendees also declined from 10% to 6.9%. Researchers of HIV/AIDS in Rwanda conclude that there may have been a decline in HIV prevalence in urban areas between 1998 and 2003, associated with low numbers of sexual partners and late sexual debut (Kayirangwa et al. 2006). Ethiopia experienced a decline in national HIV prevalence between 2001 and 2003 (from 14% to 12%), although one group of researchers argues these changes were not necessarily because of changes in sexual risk behavior (Hallett et al. 2006). Yet data from Addis Ababa showed a decline in HIV prevalence among women at ANC clinics, from 18.2% in 1997 to 11.8% in 2003. In addition, data from two VCT sites in Addis Ababa showed a decline in HIV prevalence from 29.1% in 2002 to 14.9% in 2004, for adults ages 15–44. There was an even greater decline for youth ages 15–24 attending the VCT sites, from 22.0% in 2002 to 9.0% in 2004. Along with declines in HIV prevalence, there was an associated decline in risky behaviors among VCT clients. The mean number of casual partners reported in the three months prior to testing declined among all clients between 2002 and 2004, from 1.0 to 0.6. Condom use did not increase, and, in fact, the proportion of clients ages 25–49 who reported never using a condom increased somewhat. More than 60% of clients reporting never using condoms consistently, and fewer than 35% of clients reporting having used condoms at their last sexual intercourse (Hladik et al. 2006).

NOTES

1. For example, according to one news report, during Bill Gates's opening remarks at the global AIDS conference in Toronto in 2006, "thousands of delegates violently booed one of the rare mentions of abstinence and sexual fidelity as possible solutions to AIDS, and enthusiastically cheered for latex, pharmaceuticals, and increasing acceptance of prostitution and hard drug use" (Jalsevac 2006).
2. This article was written before the results of the recent microbicide RCT, discussed in Chapter 6, were made available. We can now add that RCT to the list of successes (Abdool Karim et al. 2010).
3. The World Health Organization's Global Programme on AIDS (GPA), which conducted a number of surveys around the world in the late 1980s and early 1990s, found a "significant relationship between the level of pre-marital sex among youths and the level of 'casual sex'" for both men and women (see Caraël 1994a). Also using data from the GPA studies, White et al. (2000) found that for men, younger sexual debut, marriage to someone other than sexual debut partner, and higher number of sex partners before first marriage were associated with more extramarital partners in Cote d'Ivoire, Tanzania, and Lusaka. In an analysis of DHS and other population-based data from the late 1980s to the mid-1990s in six African countries, Bessinger et al. (2003) note that later sexual debut is associated with decreased number of lifetime sexual partners, and is predictive of "lower levels of future high-risk sexual behaviors and increased protective factors," including condom use. Most recently, a summary of DHS data from 19 countries concludes that earlier sexual debut (at an age less than 17 years) is generally associated with higher HIV prevalence, especially for women, and not surprisingly, HIV prevalence is consistently lowest among those who report never having had sex (Mishra et al. 2009b).
4. Data are from GPA surveys, as cited in Bessinger et al. 2003. The proportion reporting premarital sex in the 1989 GPA survey is among all respondents 15–24 years not *currently* married, whereas in the 1995 the denominator changed to

all *never* married respondents. Note also that the Uganda 1989 and 1995 GPA surveys were subnational and have a strong urban bias, and so provide somewhat different data than the DHS which were conducted in Uganda in the same years. Approximately 30% of the 1989 GPA survey sample was from Kampala (the capital and largest city in Uganda), compared to 6% of the sample in the 1989 DHS. Unfortunately, the 1989 DHS collected limited data on sexual behavior, particularly for men, and so when data for the critical period from 1989 to 1995 are not available from the DHS, we have used data from the GPA surveys. In the case of premarital sex, the 1989 and 1995 DHS surveys do provide data on premarital sex among women 15–24, which declined from 36% to 22% among never married women, a somewhat smaller decline than the 53% to 16% measured by the GPA surveys.

5. GPA surveys, as cited in Bessinger et al. 2003. These data are for adults ages 15–49.

6. GPA surveys, as cited in Bessinger et al. 2003. These data are for adults ages 15–49. In the 1989 GPA survey, respondents were asked if they had ever used a condom with their regular partner; the type of partner was not specified in the 1995 GPA survey.

7. See Green et al. (2009) and Shelton et al. (2006) for a discussion of incidence and prevalence trends in Africa.

Chapter 8

HIV PREVENTION AND STRUCTURAL FACTORS

Behavior-based HIV prevention approaches focus on what individuals can do to change (or maintain) behavior and thereby avoid or reduce risk of infection, while also recognizing that not all individuals have control over their sexual behavior. Many factors can limit or take away a person's ability to practice abstinence, faithfulness, or consistent condom use. These factors can include poverty, illiteracy, instability and displacement, and gender disparity. In countries such as Uganda where a behavioral approach has been successful, broader goals such as advancing women, increasing access to education, and decreasing poverty were also pursued. These broader social changes should be pursued in addition to—not instead of—an approach that addresses individual behavior. Policy-oriented HIV strategies may pursue social goals through political leaders, legislative bodies, and action at the level of civil society and communities. Yet most AIDS programs have a limited ability to bring about broad social changes, given their limited time-frames and the range of activities that can be funded under such programs. Further, although HIV prevention efforts may theoretically be strengthened by positive social changes, they are effective only when sexual behavior is changed.

In this discussion, it is useful to distinguish between direct and indirect factors that determine sexually transmitted HIV infection. The former (or proximate determinants) have to do with sexual intercourse itself. Indirect factors include things like increased access to VCT and treatment for HIV and other STIs, diminishing AIDS-related stigma, poverty alleviation, effective political leadership, open discussion about sexual behavior, and educating women and improving their status. These interventions should be promoted vigorously both because they are critical matters of justice and human rights and because they may create an environment that encourages positive changes in sexual behavior. But they themselves do not directly prevent the sexual transmission of HIV. For example, creating laws that protect women from sexual exploitation is critically important, but it is only when sexual behavior changes as a result that HIV transmission is directly impacted. It is widely assumed that these complementary measures have the *direct* impact desired, yet it is important to observe empirically which measures are effective (i.e., lead directly to measurable impact), through what mechanisms and to what extent.

Measures that empower women and alleviate poverty contribute to human health and dignity and may be protective on an individual level, but the evidence of an HIV prevention impact at a population level is somewhat more ambiguous. These realities should raise questions about the true relationship between many presumed HIV preventive measures and the transmission of HIV itself. The sexual transmission of HIV can be directly prevented in three basic ways: by avoiding the exposure to risk through sexual abstinence or mutual faithfulness with an uninfected partner; by reducing the risk of exposure through reducing number of sexual partners or avoiding risky partners (such as older men or sex workers); or by blocking the efficiency of transmission through condom usage, male circumcision, treatment of sexually transmitted infections, or use of microbicides.

Critics of HIV prevention approaches centered on changing sexual behavior often make statements such as: "The behavioral bias of the ABC approach is based on the assumption that all individuals have an innate and equal power to make perfectly correct decisions about every issue in their sexual and reproductive health lives" (Osborne 2003) or, "We all know that abstinence and couples being mutually faithful would be great if they were applicable to everybody's lives, but they're not" (Cohen 2005a:1002). Critics may argue that African culture is polygamous, that Africans have numerous partners, or that Africans start to engage in sex at an early age. According to this logic, A and B behaviors are not realistic and risk-reduction programs are justified by the alleged reality that Africans have many sexual partners and that women in particular can do nothing about their partners' infidelity. Many international health organizations have therefore put virtually all of their prevention resources for sexually transmitted HIV into risk-reduction measures, primarily condom promotion.

As to whether a behavioral approach is still an effective strategy in Africa, some of the strongest evidence for behavioral approaches comes from situations in which there were high levels of poverty, illiteracy, and instability. When Uganda began to respond to HIV/AIDS in the late 1980s and early 1990s, it was just emerging from two decades of war and extreme civil unrest. Far from being passive victims of forces beyond their control, Ugandans mounted an effective response to HIV/AIDS despite the difficult situations in which they were living. In Uganda and in other countries, HIV prevention has been successful even though broader societal goals such as gender equality, political stability, and poverty alleviation have not been fully met.

Rwanda provides another striking example. Many experts assume that strife, civil war, genocide, and breakdown of law and order—in short, social instability—would both limit AB behaviors and predict a high HIV sero-prevalence rate because of increased opportunities for casual and coerced sex. Nevertheless, a 2005 DHS found that Rwanda has a 3% national HIV prevalence, significantly lower than earlier estimates, which had been as high as 30% (Timberg 2006).

The data in Figures 7.1 and 7.2 show that Rwanda stands out in high level of protective A and B behaviors. In the 2005 DHS, only 9% of males and 4% of females ages 15–24 reported premarital sex in the past year. Likewise, only 4% of males and 1% of females of those sexually active, ages 15–49, reported multiple partners in the past year. Could other factors such as circumcision and condom use be responsible for low infection rates? In fact, male circumcision is not practiced widely in Rwanda and condom use is among the lowest in Africa. Among sexually active adults ages 15–49, 6% of males and 1% of females reported condom use at last intercourse with any type of partner. There seems to be no readily apparent explanation other than AB behaviors to explain why an impoverished east African population that has suffered great social instability should have an HIV prevalence rate of only 3%, less than half that of Uganda's rate at present.

POVERTY

It is increasingly recognized that there is an unexpected *inverse* relationship between poverty and HIV risk, at both national and individual levels. The countries in Africa with the most severe HIV pandemics (all in southern Africa) are also among the wealthiest countries on the continent. Even within countries, wealth is often associated with higher HIV prevalence, with wealthier persons being more likely to be HIV infected than poorer ones. As UNAIDS stated in its last report on the global epidemic (2008:89),

> In sub-Saharan Africa, for example, HIV prevalence is highest not in the poorest countries, but in two of the wealthiest—South Africa and Botswana—where prevalence is 18.8% and 24.1%, respectively [UNAIDS 2008b]. In this same region, a recent analysis of eight national surveys found greater HIV prevalence among adults with higher levels of wealth than among those with the lowest levels of wealth [UNAIDS 2008b]. This finding is tied to the fact that wealthier and better educated individuals tend to have greater sexual autonomy

and higher rates of partner change (due to their greater mobility) and greater likelihood of living in cities (where HIV prevalence is generally higher). (Gillespie et al. 2007)

Several analyses of poverty and HIV infection in Africa have found similar results. Mishra and colleagues (2007) analyzed DHS data from eight sub-Saharan African countries and found that in all eight countries, adults in the wealthiest quintiles had a higher prevalence of HIV than those in the poorer quintiles. This association was only partly explained by accounting for other factors such as place of residence, level of education, and behavioral factors. O'Farrell, who plotted HIV prevalence and per capita gross national product (GNP) in Africa and found a weak positive relationship, concluded:

> These results show that there is no correlation between a low GNP and a high HIV antenatal HIV prevalence. . . . Alleviation of poverty alone, however politically acceptable and justifiable, will divert attention away from biological risk factors such as male circumcision status and poor genital hygiene in core groups that may be the determining influences that drive high-prevalence HIV epidemics. (2001:627)

Poverty is believed by many to particularly affect women, stripping them of agency and forcing them into risky sexual behaviors out of economic need. The intersection of gender and HIV will be discussed more in Chapter 9. As this topic relates to poverty and wealth, we note that programs that aim to decrease women's risk through economic empowerment have so far failed to show any decrease in new infections among women. The most sophisticated randomized control trial to date to test structural interventions, the IMAGE (Intervention with Microfinance for AIDS and Gender Equity) trial in Limpopo, South Africa, used a microcredit scheme to increase earnings and empowerment among women and decrease gender-based violence and poverty. Women who participated in IMAGE reported a decrease in gender-based violence and an improvement in one out of five income generation indicators, but did not have fewer HIV infections compared to a control group (Pronyk et al. 2006). This was repeatedly overlooked at the 2008 International AIDS Conference, where IMAGE was hailed as a breakthrough in "structural interventions" for HIV reduction at no less than three separate sessions.

GENDER INEQUALITY

The argument is often made that women do not have the choice to abstain from sex or practice faithfulness. It is a tragic fact that some women who have practiced premarital abstinence and marital fidelity have become infected by unfaithful spouses or partners. Women may be victims of rape and sexual violence, including within marriage, and may be made vulnerable by poverty or other circumstances. Condoms are often proposed as the solution for these women, but condom use can be difficult if not impossible for a woman in a coercive situation to negotiate. And, as demonstrated by a number of studies and discussed in Chapter 6, condom usage rates are low among married couples and other regular partners (see also Agha et al. 2002).

The question of gender and HIV will be considered in considerable depth in Chapter 9, but for now we will note that African women exercise more freedom of individual choice than is often attributed to them. Last year, approximately two-thirds of unmarried girls and women in Africa (ages 15–24) practiced abstinence (see Figure 7.1). In all but a handful of countries in West Africa, a majority of men and women believe that a woman is justified in refusing sex if she believes her husband has other partners, or refusing sex or requesting that condoms be used if her husband has an STI (Mishra et al. 2009c). These beliefs are most widely held in East Africa. For example, over 80% of men and women in Ethiopia, Kenya, Tanzania, and Uganda and over 90% of men and women in Rwanda believed that a wife was justified in refusing sex if her husband has an STI, and over 70% of men and women (80% in Ethiopia and Rwanda) held this belief if a wife knew that her husband had sex with other women.

Yet even in countries in which a great majority of women report that a woman is justified in refusing sex with her husband, other data point to women's continued vulnerability. According to DHS data, a significant minority of women in Africa agree that a husband is justified in hitting or beating his wife for reasons such as burning the food, arguing with him, or refusing to have sex with him. In 2001 DHSs, over half of women in Zambia and Uganda believed that a husband was justified in hitting or beating his wife if she neglected the children.

STIGMA AND DISCRIMINATION

Even "stigma," one of the most frequently mentioned words in the global AIDS community, deserves a second look.[1] Is stigma in all forms always bad? In the world of AIDS we are conditioned to think so, and our condemnation of stigma is reflexive and immediate. Yet the wish to not be stigmatized or marginalized (two words that often go together in AIDS discourse) also serves to keep people from behaving in ways that invite censure from family and peers, or society as a whole. This could prevent some proportion of people from engaging in behaviors like seduction of young girls, or rape.

To use less extreme examples, fear of stigma can keep people from engaging in risky sexual behaviors, to their own benefit, if by that we mean decreased morbidity and mortality. This is so even if the "social price" for this is the continuing or even enhanced stigma and social marginalization of those who do engage in risky behaviors—assuming the social reference groups influencing behavior disapprove of the risky behaviors. It is another matter—and a great challenge for AIDS prevention—when such groups approve or even encourage certain behaviors, such as looking up to men who have made many sexual "conquests." The positive side of stigma is recognized by Reidpath and Chan as something that can serve a health promoting function, at the population level:

> When considered at a population level, stigma can be studied as an enduring social process, which inevitably produces negative outcomes for some individuals but might in some circumstances produce positive outcomes for a population. The orchestrated stigmatisation of smoking is a case in point. It appears to reduce the population burden of mortality and morbidity due to tobacco by encouraging some to quit (or never to smoke), although it leaves "recalcitrant" smokers more marginalised by their continued habit. (2006:1708)

Reidpath and Chan go on to mention the 2002 UNAIDS report that declared that the stigma associated with HIV was one of the "greatest barriers" to preventing new infections and alleviating the impact of the disease. Other publications soon began to pick up this assertion and repeat it as fact. Reidpath and Chan note, "For UNAIDS to make such a declaration, one would expect there to be a considerable body of evidence to back its position." Yet that it is one of those pieces of conventional wisdom for which the evidence is unclear or contradictory.

Many public health strategies promote healthy behaviors that not everyone in a population is capable of or willing to adopt. Although this may stigmatize and marginalize those who do not adopt those healthy behaviors, the benefit for those who do adopt them may outweigh the risks of stigmatizing some. Consider smoking. Even though the best public health campaigns about the dangers of smoking may not persuade all smokers to stop smoking and may, in fact, make some smokers feel stigmatized, antismoking campaigns have been effective. It is widely believed that the health, economic, and environmental benefits of decreased smoking justify some stigmatization of those who continue to smoke. In fact, antismoking campaigns in the United States have been largely successful, and rates of lung cancer have fallen. Similarly, to object to the promotion of abstinence and faithfulness because some will not or cannot abstain or be faithful denies information and support to the majority of the population that does practice AB behaviors.

Faith communities and their leaders have been accused of contributing to stigma toward PLHIVs, and some feel that it is inherently stigmatizing when faith leaders promote abstinence and faithfulness from a moral point of view. There have undoubtedly been times and situations in which faith communities and leaders have contributed to stigma toward PLHIV. Stigma is often a problem at all levels of society, and faith communities are not immune. But in many situations, faith communities have effectively addressed stigma, encouraged compassion, and effectively promoted A and B behaviors.

Uganda and Senegal stand out as African countries with relatively little AIDS-associated stigma. Both countries also promoted A and B behaviors and partnered with Christian and Muslim faith-based organizations (FBOs) in significant ways. Rather than being seen as part of the problem, faith communities were considered part of the solution, and their support was enlisted at a national level. In any case, FBOs run a great many health and educational services in Africa, thus it should not matter whether we (as Western outsiders) are religious or not; it makes practical sense to partner with powers that be and the resources that exist, including faith communities.

WAR AND CONFLICT

It has long been part of conventional AIDS wisdom that war and conflict fuel the spread of AIDS. This seems logical, as war often brings rape and sexual violence, displacement, dislocation of families, and other fragmentation of the usual social order. Rape is increasingly being used as a weapon of war, and soldiers and other rapists may be more likely to be HIV infected than members of the general population. In the aftermath of war and conflict there are often many accounts of women who were infected with HIV through rape, and these heart-wrenching stories make it seem obvious that times of strife and violence carry a high risk of HIV.

However, careful studies of the relationship between conflict and HIV challenge the notion that war and displacement lead to higher rates of HIV infection than times of peace. Paul Spiegel of the United Nations High Commissioner on Refugees (UNHCR) examined data from seven countries recently affected by some of the most brutal conflict in Africa (Democratic Republic of Congo, southern Sudan, Rwanda, Uganda, Sierra Leone, Somalia, and Burundi). He concluded that there was no increase in HIV prevalence during periods of conflict. Furthermore, most refugee camps studied had lower prevalence of HIV infection than their respective host communities (Spiegel et al. 2007). In a further analysis (Anema et al. 2008), Spiegel and colleagues modeled the affect on HIV incidence of a very extreme hypothetical situation in which 15% of the female population of a country was raped (not including intimate partner violence or partner rape), HIV prevalence among assailants was eight times the country population prevalence, and the HIV transmission rate was four times the average per sexual encounter. Even under such assumptions, HIV prevalence within a country would increase by only 0.023%—a minute amount. The study authors conclude (and we would agree) that:

> These projections support the finding that widespread rape in conflict-affected countries in SSA has not incurred a major direct population-level change in HIV prevalence. However, this must not be interpreted to say that widespread rape does not pose serious problems to women's acquisition of HIV on an individual basis or in specific settings. Furthermore, direct and indirect consequences of sexual violence, such as physical and psychosocial trauma, unwanted pregnancies, and stigma and discrimination cannot be understated. (Anema et al. 2008)

In a presentation at the 2008 International AIDS Conference, Spiegel discussed ways that assumptions can stand in the way of true evidence. At one time, it was thought that data about HIV prevalence among refugees should *not* be collected because it was assumed that prevalence among refugees would be higher and that this would lead to further stigma of refugees. When the UNHCR finally began collecting data on HIV infection among refugees, it was found that HIV prevalence was consistently *lower* than in surrounding populations. At the same time, reports of very high prevalence among refugees (often based on small samples or certain subpopulations, such as women treated for rape at a clinic) are often treated as being "typical" by journalists and others. For example, an organization serving women raped during Rwanda's 1994 genocide reported that 70–80% of their clients were HIV positive, and this was widely reported. But a 1997 nationwide sero-survey in Rwanda reported that 2.2% of the female population had been raped and that HIV prevalence in raped women was 15.2% versus 11% in non-raped women, which was not a statistically significant difference.[2]

At this session at the International AIDS Conference, Filippo Ciantia, a medical doctor with long experience working in conflict-torn northern Uganda, commented that accurately reporting HIV rates among refugees is very important for reducing stigma toward these groups. According to Ciantia, infection rates among internally displaced persons in northern Uganda (including escaped child soldiers) are often reported as being much higher than they actually are. This leads to stigma toward these groups and hinders their reintegration into their communities. Ciantia advocated for "a code of conduct from media and international organizations to be evidence-based in reporting, and not driven only by passion." Certainly we owe it to people affected by conflict—not to mention the rest of the world—to *accurately* report on conflict and HIV risk, no matter how high our passions over the tragedy of sexual violence during conflict.

Rachel Jewkes, a well-known expert on HIV and violence, comments that there are a number of reasons why HIV transmission may not be higher in conflict settings. Curfews or other restrictions on movement may reduce activities that can facilitate risky sex, such as drinking at bars. Refugee settings may have disproportionate numbers of women and girls, which might reduce sexual activity. She notes that postconflict settings might pose the highest risk, as "sexual activity is resumed in a context of economic recovery, infrastructure development, and renewed population mobility." She also notes that violence may have a long-term affect on children, such as causing them to engage in sexual violence and risk-taking years later. Of course, victims of rape and other forms of violence during times of conflict critically need appropriate care, whether that violence leads to increased HIV infection or not (Jewkes 2007:1241).

NOTES

1. "Stigma" means being devalued by individuals or communities on the basis of real or perceived health status. "Discrimination" refers to the legal, institutional, and procedural ways that people are denied access to their rights because of their real or perceived health status (see Gruskin and Ferguson 2009).
2. Ruark, personal notes, August 4, 2008.

Chapter 9

GENDER, MARRIAGE, AND HIV

Few topics stir up greater emotions and more impassioned debate within the AIDS world than that of gender and HIV. In the AIDS community, the word "gender" is usually employed to mean women; gender-specific causes of HIV vulnerability among men are much less often considered. WHO has a Department of Gender, Women, and Health; the UN has the United Nations Development Fund for Women (UNIFEM); and many other organizations particularly target women's health and HIV risk. Any health or AIDS conference will include an array of sessions dedicated to the particular health vulnerabilities of women.

The large numbers of women, particularly young women, infected with HIV/AIDS should be an urgent call to action for anyone committed to improving health worldwide. In most of the world, a preponderance of cases are among MSM and IDU and thus among men, but women account for 60% of HIV infections in Africa. In other words, there are three women infected for every two men, and a disproportionate number of these women are young women. Figure 9.1 shows HIV prevalence among young women in South Africa climbing steeply during the years of late adolescence and early adulthood, and this trend is typical for women across Africa. Young women in particular have much higher rates of infection than do young men, although HIV prevalence among men often surpasses that among women for adults in their 40s and 50s. But women do not report riskier behavior than men. So what accounts for women's great vulnerability?

Biological vulnerability, especially of young women, and age discrepancies between partners (with male partners tending to be older and more likely to be HIV infected) are certainly part of the puzzle of women's higher infection rates. Data on women's biological vulnerability are conflicting: Some data show that women sero-convert approximately twice as quickly as men;[1] other data show that women have a lower risk of infection within a discordant relationship than do uncircumcised men.[2]

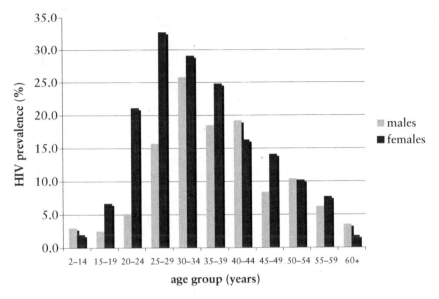

Figure 9.1 HIV prevalence by sex and age, South Africa, 2008.
Source: Shisana et al., 2005.

There is no straightforward answer to the question of whether men or women are more biologically susceptible to HIV infection, as a variety of factors can affect susceptibility in both men and women. The presence of STIs, particularly herpes simplex, increases risk, and pregnant women and uncircumcised men are also at greater risk. Evidence suggests that girls and young women, whose bodies have not fully matured, may be particularly vulnerable, although there is no real-world way to measure this conclusively. One cohort study in Uganda showed that among women with HIV-positive spouses, young women (under the age of 24) sero-converted at nearly twice the rate of older women (Carpenter et al. 1999), although more frequent sex among young women has also been suggested as a reason for higher rates of infection among young married women compared to older married women.

In recent years, scholarly articles, media reports, and major AIDS organizations have increasingly painted marriage as an institution that is highly risky to women in terms of HIV infection. Acclaimed *New York Times* columnist Nicholas Kristof wrote in a 2005 opinion piece that "what kills young women [in Africa] is often not promiscuity, but marriage. Indeed, just about the deadliest thing a woman in southern Africa can do is get married." In a 2006 *Newsweek* article, Melinda French Gates claimed, "Worldwide, 80 percent of women newly infected with HIV are practicing monogamy within a marriage or a long-term relationship. This shatters the myth that marriage is a natural refuge from AIDS."

More scholarly sources have been no less adamant about the risks posed by marriage. UNAIDS' 2004 annual report stated, "Marriage and other long-term, monogamous relationships do not protect women from HIV," and in 2005 the UN's special envoy for HIV/AIDS in Africa, Stephen Lewis, said in a speech at the Harvard School of Public Health that "one of the most dangerous environments for a woman in Africa is to be married." A 2004 joint UNAIDS/UNFPA/UNIFEM report claimed that: "In sub-Saharan Africa, 60 to 80 per cent of HIV-positive women report having had sexual relations only with their husbands" (without giving a source for the figure). The rationale given for women's risk in marriage, in this report and elsewhere, is that older and more sexually experienced partners put women at risk, that women are typically faithful but men are not, and that women have little power to negotiate condom use within marriage to protect themselves. Most recently, an article in *The Lancet* began with the bold statement: "Evidence suggests that a woman's greatest risk of contracting HIV lies within a marital relationship" (Dunkle et al. 2008:2183).

Are these claims justified? Virtually any discussion of HIV risk and marriage, in the popular media but also in the AIDS community, centers around the story of the innocent wife who was infected by a philandering husband and who had never engaged in any risky behavior herself. Actual data about risk in marriage are usually conspicuously absent, and the message seems to be that such innocent wives account for the vast majority of women infected with HIV in Africa and elsewhere. The question is not whether such tragic circumstances occur—they certainly do—but how *typical* such a scenario is among women who become infected with HIV. There are data about risk of HIV within marriage and they show that in some African countries, there are actually more men at risk of infection within marriage (from infected spouses) than women. There are rare stories in the news media about men who were infected by their wives, but the story about HIV risk in marriage has been told selectively and has focused on the infection of women by men.

We do not deny the tragic fact that many women are infected within marriage and that many had no other risk factor besides being married. But this scenario is not the whole story, particularly in the high-prevalence epidemics of Africa. If we are really serious about reducing women's HIV risk, we must admit the complexity of women's lives and HIV risk and the various ways that they become infected. Women are not always passive victims; they are also active agents in seeking sexual partnerships before and outside of marriage (for a variety of reasons), and in a significant minority of unions, it is the *woman* who brings infection into the partnership. By telling only one story about women's HIV risk, we have failed to learn very much about other situations in which women become infected (such as extramarital affairs), much less respond to these other situations with appropriate HIV prevention programs and messages.

Where have these assumptions about women, marriage, and HIV risk come from? Consider the following accounts, which are typical of the portrayal of African women in the media. In his 2005 column titled "When Marriage Kills," Kristof writes about a woman named Kero Sibanda, whom he met in a village in Zimbabwe. According to Kristof: "Mrs. Sibanda is an educated woman and lovely English-speaker who married a man who could find a job only in another city. She suspected that he had a girlfriend there, but he would return to the village every couple of months to visit her." Mrs. Sidanba tells Kristof, "I asked him to use a condom, but he refused. There was nothing I could do." Mrs. Sibanda's husband died of AIDS, and she fears that she and her 2-year-old daughter are also infected. Mr. Kristof also introduces the reader to a prostitute in Livingstone, Zambia, named Mavis Sitwala, "an orphan (probably because of AIDS) who is supporting her five siblings and one child." Ms. Sitwala tells Mr. Kristof that truck drivers pay $1 for sex with a condom or $4 for sex without. "At times, you need food or money to pay the rent," she says, "and so even if he won't use a condom, you agree."

The media is full of such stories of desperate women, infected by philandering husbands and forced into prostituting themselves (often without condoms) by dire economic need. But now let us consider Pretty (not her real name), who is a 17-year-old Grade 11 pupil at an elite private school in Durban, South Africa. She is, according to Saneka and colleagues (2007a), "bright, articulate and confident, [and] her knowledge of HIV/AIDS is considerable." She is also a "proud member" of the "High-Five club." According to Saneka and colleagues, "Entry is based on one simple requirement: You need to have five concurrent boyfriends." Pretty's boyfriends include a fellow high-school student as well as a married man and an engaged father of three. "When asked how she manages to combine school work with helping around the house, babysitting a young nephew, and cavorting with several boyfriends, Pretty describes a whirl-wind life of which only her friends, mostly fellow members of the High-Five club, are aware." Pretty confesses that not all of the boyfriends expect her to be faithful to them, although the younger ones apparently do. As she explains, "Boys my age are so insecure these days. That's why they expect you to love them" (Saneka et al. 2007a). Or consider Gladys from Zambia, who has her own reasons for having several concurrent boyfriends: "Having several partners is to me an advantage because when one disappoints you another comforts you. It reduces your stress. When I hear so-and-so is cheating I just don't worry myself as I'm doing the same. You can never trust men" (Saneka et al. 2007b).

Which of these four women is the real African woman? They all are, of course. A more difficult question is which woman's experience is more typical. There are some data (such as those from discordant couples; see below) that can shed light on "typical" HIV risk scenarios for women in Africa—or at least unsettle some of our common assumptions about what is typical. But there is no typical African woman any more than there is any typical woman from any other continent, country, or neighborhood. Why, then, is it only powerless and vulnerable women such as Kero Sibanda and Mavis Sitwala who are acknowledged in discussions about women and HIV? The discourse about why women in Africa are at risk and what can be done rarely if ever ventures into more controversial territory, such as discussions about women like Pretty and Gladys who *choose* risky sexual behaviors. The Western media and AIDS establishment has decided which stories will be told and which risk factors will be acknowledged. Women's vulnerability, lack of options, and infection through no fault of their own are acknowledged, whereas women's agency, control over their sexual lives, and sometimes risky and irrational choices are not.

A combination of quantitative and qualitative methods, including ethnographic methods, can help us understand common patterns in the lives of girls and women and ideally design HIV interventions that address their actual circumstances and account for the many scripts that describe their lives. But this goal is not helped by a simplistic, one-dimensional, and largely false view of women and what places them at risk of HIV infection. Until we are able to talk about women's lives and risk factors in more nuanced and realistic terms, we are doing little to help the great many women whose lives do not fit Western stereotypes, including women like Pretty and Gladys.

In a 2008 edited volume, a number of anthropologists describe the expected scenario of men infecting women within marriage or long-term unions, but not one of the writers considered that at times the tables can be turned. Teresa Swezey and Michele Teitelbaum, under a section titled "Marriage Does Not Mitigate Risk," tell us that in Africa "an estimated 60 to 80 percent of women infected with HIV . . . have had only one lifetime sexual partner" (2008:221). This is clearly *not* true, when in most countries (particularly the most AIDS-affected countries) there are not even this many women who have had only one lifetime sexual partner.[3] Furthermore, approximately one-third of the infections acquired by women in a union appear to come from an outside partner and *not* from the husband or primary partner. Oddly, Swezey and Teitelbaum cite data that actually show this (yet seem to fail to grasp the implications) when they note in the same paragraph that data from Masaka, Uganda, show that men bring HIV into marriage at twice the rate of women. In other words, for every two infections that men bring into marriage, women bring in one, or one-third of infections.

Swezey and Teitelbaum go on to claim that: "The idea that women who remain 'faithful' will be at less risk . . . is belied by gender power differentials within marital relations and other unions." But this is *exactly* what data show. Not only do data from across Africa show that women bring at least one-third of new infections into marriage (thus theoretically married women would reduce their HIV risk by one-third if they did not acquire infections outside marriage), but data consistently and powerfully show that women who report fewer sexual partners have less HIV risk, *regardless of their partner's behavior.* As discussed in Chapter 7, an analysis by Mishra and colleagues (2009b) found a strong linear relationship between African women's number of lifetime sexual partners and their odds of being HIV-infected, even when other factors including age, education, and marital status were accounted for.

Table 9.1 shows how HIV prevalence increases with number of lifetime partners, for four African countries for which we have DHS data. In Cote d'Ivoire and Swaziland, a majority of sexually active women report two or more lifetime partners. In Rwanda and Zimbabwe, a majority of sexually active women report only one lifetime partner, although the sample includes many young women who may presumably have other partners during their lifetimes. Another clear point to draw from these data is that HIV risk is still considerable for women who report only one lifetime partner, particularly (as we might expect) in the very high prevalence countries of Swaziland and Zimbabwe. But the risk of infection is considerably higher for those who report more partners.

As Figure 9.2 shows, there is also a clear correlation between behavior and HIV risk for women who report higher-risk sex in the last year (sex with a non-marital, non-cohabiting partner), compared to women who do not. Of course these data are cross-sectional and cannot establish causation; a woman's reported behavior in the past year may not be linked to her HIV-status. But they still provide persuasive evidence that *not* engaging in high-risk sex is protective for women.

Women's faithfulness cannot *eliminate* HIV risk if their partners are not also faithful. But it is false and dangerous to women to suggest that women are at no greater risk of HIV infection if they are not faithful. It is also dangerous for married African women to accept the myth that

Table 9.1   HIV prevalence by lifetime number of sexual partners, women.

Country and survey year	Number of lifetime partners	Percent of women 15–49 reporting this number of lifetime partners	HIV prevalence of these women
Cote d'Ivoire 2005			
HIV prevalence peaks	1	33.6%	**4.1%**
at 14.9%, among	2–3	43.1%	**5.6%**
30–34-year-old	4–5	16.0%	12.5%
women	6–10	6.0%	16.1%
	11 +	1.3%	18.3%
Rwanda 2005			
HIV prevalence peaks	1	69.6%	3.0%
at 6.9%, among	2	21.6%	8.1%
35–39-year-old	3–4	7.8%	12.1%
women	5–9	1.0%	9.1%
Swaziland 2006–07			
HIV prevalence peaks	1	35.4%	**22.9%**
at 49.2%, among	2	30.1%	**38.3%**
25–29-year-old women	3–4	26.6%	**46.9%**
	5–9	6.7%	**53.9%**
	10 +	1.2%	**57.9%**
Zimbabwe 2005–06			
HIV prevalence peaks	1	65.8%	**18.1%**
at 35.5%, among	2	21.9%	**37.1%**
30–34-year-old	3–4	10.3%	**42.2%**
women	5–9	1.9%	**43.9%**

Sources: Demographic and Health Surveys and AIDS Indicator Surveys: Cote d'Ivoire AIS 2005; Rwanda DHS 2005; Swaziland DHS 2006–07; Zimbabwe DHS 2005–06.

they are powerless victims. Of course we also fully support women doing everything they can to reduce risk *within* marriage, including using condoms or refusing sex if they suspect their partner of infidelity.

There has been little research on motivating factors for risky sex among women beyond the conventional explanations of economic need, powerlessness, and coercion. Anthropologist Suzanne Leclerc-Madlala has been bold in ascribing considerable agency to women in South Africa as well as well-defined reasons for engaging in risky sexual behaviors. She says about cross-generational ("sugar daddy") relationships: "Relationships

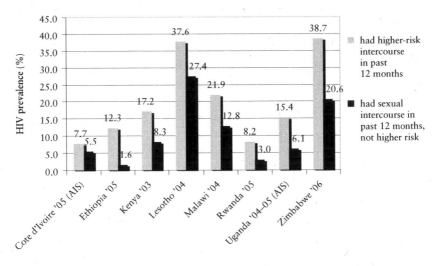

Figure 9.2 HIV prevalence by sexual behavior among women ages 15–49.
Sources: Demographic Health Surveys and AIDS Indicator Surveys.

with older men are a common and readily availably way through which young women gain materially, affirm self-worth, achieve social goals, increase longer-term life chances, or otherwise add value and enjoyment to life" (Leclerc-Madlala 2008:S17). Ethnographic research with Baganda women in Kampala, Uganda, revealed that although there were social norms against women having sex outside of marriage (norms that were considerably more relaxed for men), there were certain circumstances in which a woman might take other partners, including economic need, desire for greater sexual satisfaction, or revenge on a husband with other partners (McGrath et al. 1993).

Linda Tawfik and Susan Watkins present similar views in a fascinating article about women in southern Malawi entitled, "Sex in Geneva, Sex in Lilongwe, and Sex in Balaka" (2007). Tawfik and Watkins mince no words in stating that there are three interpretations of women and HIV risk in rural Balaka District:

> One is disseminated world-wide by institutions with a global reach such as the World Health Organization in Geneva and United States Agency for International Development (USAID); the second is provided by urban Malawians situated in the capital of Lilongwe, the seat of government and the site of the many international and national non-governmental agencies; the third is articulated by rural women and men in Balaka District, Malawi. . . . An implication of this study is that AIDS-prevention policies based on the view from Geneva and Lilongwe need

modification for Balaka, and by implication for rural Africa more generally. (2007:1090)

Although AIDS experts and program planners in Geneva and Lilongwe assumed that women engaged in extramarital sex out of dire economic need, women in Balaka talked about motivations such as lust, love, passion, and revenge. Dissatisfaction, sexual or otherwise, with a spouse was a prime reason for seeking an extramarital partner, and women also had affairs out of revenge when their husbands were unfaithful. The desire for money and gifts might play a role, but in most cases this desire to benefit materially through a sexual liaison was far from "survival sex." Overall, the women in Balaka saw themselves as "passionate and powerful." Tawfik and Watkins comment: "This perspective of women as poor, passionless and powerless is similar to that of academic feminists in the 1960s and 1970s; although now largely replaced in academia, it survives in Geneva and Lilongwe" (2007:1098).

While living in Swaziland in the early 1980s, Green noticed that the same Swazi women who were typically depicted as powerless, passive, and helpless pawns in a patriarchal society also showed considerable agency in forming *zenzele* (self-help) women's groups. These groups operated in rural areas and gave women the opportunity to sell handicrafts as a way of breaking the chain of peasant subsistence. A USAID project that supported these women found that after a few weeks of training in "leadership" and small business enterprise skills, some women's groups had gone on to build a roadside market or raise the down-payment for a gas station franchise (both projects requiring the equivalent of several thousand U.S. dollars) (Green 1992b).

Isn't it time we brought a fresh perspective to AIDS prevention, an acknowledgment that African women are as complicated in their needs, desires, and motivations as women anywhere? Not all African women are powerless; they are also active agents in their own lives. And like women anywhere who use tanning beds or smoke, eat too much dessert, or sleep with a man they don't know the first thing about (including HIV status), they do things that put their health at risk. African women, like *people* everywhere, can do irrational things that put their lives at risk, and one task of effective AIDS prevention must be to address that little-acknowledged reality.

WOMEN AND VIOLENCE

To quote WHO's Department of Gender, Women, and Health, "the HIV epidemic intersects in different ways with the epidemic of violence against women and girls" (2006:xi). This statement reflects a widespread consensus in the public health community. Violence is believed to fuel HIV infection through high-risk sexual encounters (including coerced sex and rape), and the threat of violence is felt to keep women from protecting themselves from HIV infection, for example, through condom usage and HIV testing. The same WHO report recommends that: "HIV counselors should engage in a discussion with women during the HIV testing and counseling process about fear of or experience with violence as a factor in their decision to disclose their HIV status to their partner."

The threat of violence for many HIV positive women is real, and the wife may be blamed for introducing HIV into the union, either when the husband is HIV negative or when he doesn't know his status or refuses to disclose it. Even when the woman does not face blame or violence, there is the potential for conflict and dissolution of the union. These factors should be considered when encouraging any woman (or man) to seek testing. On the other hand, there are millions of people across Africa who are at risk of infection from their spouses, and in a significant minority of these cases, it is the man and not the woman who is at risk (de Walque 2007).

Women globally, including in Africa, are experiencing a horrific epidemic of violence as well as a severe HIV pandemic. But what is the relationship between these two? As with other structural factors, it is much more complicated than we might assume. A 2005 WHO study of women's health and domestic (or intimate partner) violence that surveyed 24,000 women in 10 countries[4] found that between 15% and 71% of ever-partnered women reported they had experienced physical or sexual violence from an intimate partner (Garcia-Moreno et al. 2005). This study included data from four sites and three countries in Africa: Ethiopia (rural), Tanzania (urban and rural), and Namibia (urban). Ethiopia had the highest prevalence of sexual violence of any country in the study, with 58.6% of women reporting ever experiencing sexual violence. Yet Ethiopia is also notable for its low prevalence of HIV. Among rural women, HIV prevalence is only 0.6%.

We present the data from the three African countries (and four sites) included in this study in Figure 9.3. What emerges is an *inverse* correlation between violence and HIV prevalence. In Namibia, we see both high HIV prevalence (15.1% among urban women) and the lowest prevalence of violence for all three indicators. Even within Tanzania, for which we have data from urban and rural populations, this apparent inverse correlation holds true. Of course, *correlation* does not mean *causation*. We are not suggesting that HIV prevalence decreases when intimate partner violence increases. We submit, however, that these data suggest a far

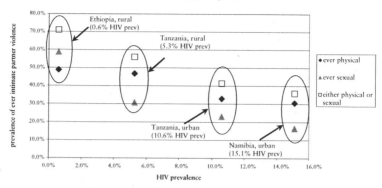

Figure 9.3 Intimate partner violence by HIV prevalence in three African countries.

Sources: Garcia-Moreno et al., 2005; HIV prevalence data from Ethiopia DHS 2005, Tanzania HIV/AIDS and Malaria Indicator Survey 2007–08, Republic of Namibia Ministry of Health and Social Services 2010.

Note: This figure was generated from the data in Garcia-Moreno et al. 2005. We included data from all African sites and countries included in the report. The goodness of fit lines are not shown in this figure, but R^2 values were very high, ranging between 0.87 and 0.97 (with 1.0 being a perfectly linear fit).

from clear relationship between gender-based violence and HIV infection in Africa. We also note the great diversity of prevalence of HIV and intimate partner violence, even in this small sampling of African countries. (Only three countries are shown because these were the only African countries and sites for which data were given in the WHO report.)

Any amount of *any* form of violence against women is unacceptable, whether HIV risk is increased as a result or not. Continuing HIV infections among women are equally unacceptable. Furthermore, it is indisputable that violence has increased risk of HIV infection for many individual women and probably for great numbers of women. This is no time to stop fighting gender-based violence or to stop educating women about gender-based violence and possible links to HIV.

However, the high prevalence of HIV infections in regions in which there are relatively low levels of gender-based violence suggests that there are more circumstances leading to HIV risk than just violence and the threat of violence. Conversely, the extremely high rates of violence in places such as Ethiopia that do not have high levels of HIV infections remind us that gender-based violence is a serious problem in its own right, not just because it can increase risk of HIV infection. Unfortunately, the disproportionate concentration of international health and development aid for the single disease of HIV/AIDS may mean that countries with serious gender inequalities and high rates of gender-based violence, but with low HIV prevalence, receive little attention from Western donors. Perhaps it is time to consider how failing to differentiate between the epidemics of HIV and gender-based violence (in funding priorities if nowhere else) may be causing us both to offer suboptimal HIV prevention and to fail to fight gender-based violence *for its own sake.*

It is experts within the AIDS world who are largely responsible for the oversimplification of the relationship between violence and HIV. Women with violent partners are assumed to be at greater risk of HIV infection primarily because they cannot insist on condom use. Perhaps we should be asking deeper questions about what kind of relationships put women at risk of both violence and HIV infection, what risk factors lead women into such relationships, and how we might help women to improve or leave such relationships or avoid them in the first place.

Might there not be an underlying constellation of risk factors, of which increased risk of violence and increased risk of HIV are but two? For example, we know that HIV risk increases with number of sexual partners and that the lowest HIV risk is within long-term, stable partnerships (particularly those in which both partners are uninfected and faithful to the relationship). If relationships characterized by violence also tend to be less stable and shorter in duration, not to mention that partners in such relationships may be less likely to know each other's status and less committed to sexual exclusivity, is it any wonder that HIV risk in such relationships is also higher? The bottom line is that the contributing factors may be much more complex than simply a lack of condom use.

Let us examine an important study that found a clear correlation between HIV infection and intimate partner violence (IPV), among women attending a prenatal clinic in Soweto, South Africa. Dunkle and colleagues (2004a) found that slightly over half (55%) of women reported a history of physical or sexual violence from a male partner, and physical violence (*although not sexual violence*) was associated with a higher likelihood of being HIV infected. This association between *physical* intimate partner violence and HIV remained even after controlling for demographic and behavioral variables, including women's risky sexual behavior. The researchers explain the relationship between physical violence and HIV by positing that "abusive men are more likely to have HIV and impose risky sexual practices on partners." Violent and controlling men are more likely to be HIV positive than other men, and in this study men who reported being perpetrators of partner violence were more likely to have concurrent sexual partnerships.[5]

But women with these multiple related risk factors seem to be at risk for more reasons than simply having an abusive and controlling partner. Being sexually assaulted as a child, having experienced forced first intercourse, and being sexually assaulted as an adult by a non-partner were correlated with increased sexual risk behavior. Sexual risk behaviors, including multiple partners and transactional sex, were associated with increased HIV risk. Transactional sex was more common among women who had a history of IPV, substance abuse, or living in substandard housing, and was less likely among women who were older when they first had sex and were more educated. In other words, having experienced sexual abuse (including childhood abuse) was associated with riskier sexual behaviors that were associated with increased HIV risk, and all of these things were associated with IPV. (And keep in mind that sexual violence did *not* seem to be independently associated with higher HIV risk; the correlation, much less causality, was not that simple.)

This same study also investigated transactional sex (sex in exchange for money or goods) among women in Soweto, finding that it was significantly associated with both HIV risk and having experienced violence (Dunkle et al. 2004b). Among women aged 16–44, 21.1% reported having ever had sex with a *non-primary* male partner in exchange for material goods or money. The researchers noted that gift-giving may be an "integral part of relationships, but may or may not be the principal motivating factor," and sought to distinguish this type of exchange from transactional sex. They hypothesized that non-primary relationships would have greater HIV risk as, by definition, they involved concurrent partnerships, and that those non-primary relationships that were transactional could be considered to be primarily motivated by material considerations. Transactional sex was associated with HIV infection even after controlling for other sexual behaviors, and also with IPV, substance abuse, and socioeconomic disadvantage.

None of these findings about the complicated linkages between abuse and vulnerability, risk behaviors, and HIV are surprising. Much previous research has explored the connection between childhood sexual abuse and transactional sex later in life, for instance, or between transactional sex and violence.[6] This latest study simply underscores these connections. The researchers also note broader implications to women's health, stating,

> It is useful to consider which women are most likely to engage in transactional sex. . . . Women with a history of violence may be more likely to subsequently engage in transactional sex, as has been demonstrated for a range of other risk behaviors [Maman et al. 2000], including having

multiple sex partners [Choi et al. 1998], having casual sex partners
[Kalichman et al. 1998], and trading sex for money or drugs [Beadnell et al.
2000; Gilbert et al. 2000; Kalichman et al. 1998]. . . . Abusive relationships can leave women impoverished [Lloyd and Taluc 1999] . . . abused
women are also more likely to suffer from depression, post-traumatic
stress disorder, and other psychiatric problems [Campbell 2002; Danielson
et al. 1998; Roberts et al. 1998], and may abuse alcohol or other sub-
stances [Kalichman et al. 1998], using transactional sex to sustain this
habit. Abused women in South Africa talk about the experience of abuse
changing the way they view relationships, reducing their ability to trust
men or expose themselves emotionally to men, and enhancing perceptions that a woman should get something tangible from relationships.
(Dunkle et al. 2004b:1589)

Dunkle and colleagues (2007) have also documented that it is not
only women who engage in transactional sex in South Africa, but also
men. A study of young men (aged 15–26) in rural Eastern Cape found
that 17.7% reported giving material resources or money to casual sex
partners, and 6.6% received resources from a casual partner. This study
was careful to distinguish between the giving of *gifts* within relationships and sexual partnerships that were based primarily on exchange of
goods or money. Young men were found to engage in both. In relationships with "main girlfriends," giving (14.9%) and receiving (14.3%)
were balanced. This study also revealed risk factors that were associated both with transactional sex and HIV risk, and, as with women,
these risk factors were interconnected in complex ways. Significantly, *all*
types of exchange were associated with more adverse childhood experiences, more lifetime sexual partners, and alcohol use. The researchers
further note:

> Men who were more resistant to peer pressure to have sex were less likely
> to report transactional sex with casual partners, and men who reported
> more equitable gender attitudes were less likely to report main partner-
> ships underpinned by exchange. The most consistent predictors of all
> types of transaction were perpetration of IPV and rape against women
> other than a main partner. . . . The strong association between perpetra-
> tion of GBV and both giving and getting material goods from female
> partners suggests that transactional sex in both main and casual relation-
> ships should be viewed within a broader continuum of men's exercises of
> gendered power and control. (Dunkle et al. 2007:1235)

Giving and receiving resources in exchange for sex was also associated
with higher socioeconomic status, leading the researchers to conclude:
"The association between perpetrating violence and getting money or

goods from sex partners suggests that simple financial empowerment of women may not decrease gender power dynamics or violence risk" (Dunkle et al. 2007:1246).

Our point is not that gender-based violence, particularly intimate partner violence, is not deplorable, or that there is not a nexus between violence and HIV infection, particularly (but not only) for women. But the roots of this connection may be quite complex, extending to adverse experiences in childhood, substance abuse, and patterns of risky sexual behavior such as earlier sexual debut, multiple partners, and transactional sex. The solution may be more complex, and more radical, than giving women greater economic resources or empowering them to negotiate condom use. These solutions may not go far enough, if women are already caught in patterns of risky behaviors, dysfunctional and dangerous relationships, and substance abuse. Girls and women who are engaging in substance abuse and transactional sex need help in breaking those patterns. And we need to do more, much more, to protect children (both boys and girls) from abuse, sexual and otherwise.

Maybe most importantly, women and men need to be empowered to form safe, stable, mutually respectful relationships with committed partners and to avoid partners who are unfaithful, violent, or otherwise abusive and untrustworthy. Some may argue that such a goal is unrealistic and that women do not have the choice or power to build such relationships. Yet many women across Africa have chosen their sexual partners and have stable and happy partnerships. Cultures everywhere are constantly changing, and in Africa they are certainly changing toward greater empowerment of women. Working to strengthen the social expectation that women should insist on respect, care, and faithfulness from their partners is not utopian and it is what we ourselves demand in our own relationships and societies.

To date two RCTs have endeavored to reduce gender-based violence and gender inequity, and test the impact of this on HIV incidence. The IMAGE trial, already described in Chapter 8, demonstrated decreases in gender-based violence although HIV incidence did not decline (Pronyk et al. 2006). A cluster randomized trial of the Stepping Stones HIV prevention program similarly found decreases in gender-based violence but no decrease in HIV incidence (Jewkes et al. 2008). Stepping Stones is a 50-hour participatory learning program which aims to build knowledge, risk awareness, communication skills, and to stimulate critical reflection, including about gender roles. Among participants in the Stepping Stones program, the incidence of herpes simplex (HSV-2) did decline by 33%, and men reported less intimate partner violence, less transactional sex, and less problem drinking. Women did not report the desired changes in casual sex, or problem drinking, or experience of intimate partner violence, and in fact reported increases in transactional sex. These trials have shown that promising models may exist for reducing gender-based violence, but we are still far from proving that such interventions can reduce risk of HIV infection.

MARRIAGE IS RISKY COMPARED TO WHAT?

The central question when examining HIV risk and marriage should be not whether HIV infections can happen within marriage (they certainly can), but whether marriage is *more* risky for women than other circumstances. Marriage is risky compared to *what*? Certainly marriage is risky compared to abstaining from sex, but the vast majority of adult men and women are sexually active. Secondary questions, also important, should be *who* is at risk in marriage (not always the woman), and what can be done about HIV risk within marriage, including known discordant couples.

The belief that marriage is *more* risky than not being married is largely based on the often-cited results from UNAIDS' landmark Multicentre study, which gathered data in the late 1990s in two low-prevalence African cities (Cotonou, Benin, and Yaoundé, Cameroon) and two high-prevalence African cities (Kisumu, Kenya, and Ndola, Zambia). This study found that married girls between the ages of 15 and 19 years and 20 and 24 years had higher HIV prevalence than their never-married *sexually active* counterparts. Never-married sexually active girls aged 15–19 in Kisumu were found to have an HIV prevalence of 22%, whereas married girls were found to have an HIV prevalence of 33%. In Ndola, prevalence was 17% and 27%, respectively (Glynn et al. 2001). Smaller differences in HIV prevalence were observed between married and unmarried young women aged 20–24 years.

These findings have been repeatedly cited as evidence that marriage is risky for young women. UNAIDS officials reacted to the study by stating that abstinence programs were an inadequate prevention approach for teenagers; that "the fact of being married carries significantly higher risk" for sexually active teenage girls; and that risk for young married women was due to age gaps between spouses and because "condom use in marriage has not been promoted" (Altman 2004). A 2004 UNAIDS/UNIFEM report commented that increased risk among married women was due to "older men's increased sexual experience and exposure to HIV, young wives' inability to make demands on older husbands, increased sexual relations and less use of means of protection." Shelley Clark identified similar risks in a 2004 article that examined the Multicentre data and argued that the protective effect of marriage (partner reduction) might be outweighed by these risks.

However, when the actual data are examined, some surprises emerge (Glynn et al. 2003). Sample sizes were quite small, so differences between married and unmarried girls were not statistically significant (at $p < .05$) in either city.[7] A more significant limitation was that both marriage *and* HIV prevalence rose sharply with age, and thus confounding between the two is likely, even within 5-year age cohorts. Clark (2004), using DHS data, identified other ways in which girls who married early differed from their sexually active but unmarried age mates. Married girls were under more pressure to get pregnant and thus had more regular sex, but were less likely to engage in risky transactional sex. Glynn and colleagues (2003) identified other possible confounders, such as the possibility that girls who get married younger engage in other risk behaviors such as younger sexual debut and more premarital partners. In fact, this was true in Ndola. In both Ndola and Kisumu, women who were virgins at the time of marriage had a significantly lower risk of HIV infection, leading Glynn and colleagues to conclude that "much of the HIV in women is acquired before marriage." The study found very similar rates of premarital sexual activity for young men and young women, and a higher number of lifetime partners among women was associated with higher HIV risk.

Perhaps the greatest surprise is that young married *men* in Ndola and Kisumu were also much more likely to be HIV infected than never-married, sexually active men of the same ages. The differences in HIV prevalence between married and sexually active never-married men were even *greater* than for women. For 20–24-year-old men in Kisumu and Ndola, the differences between married and never-married men *were* statistically significant (at $p < .05$). Never-married sexually active men aged 20–24 in Kisumu were found to have an HIV prevalence of 8%, whereas married men were found to have an HIV prevalence of 26%. In Ndola, prevalence was 10% and 29%, respectively (Glynn et al. 2001).

Glynn and colleagues pulled no punches in stating: "Many women enter marriage HIV-infected, suggesting that men may be predominantly infected by their wives." Almost twice as many women as men were estimated to be HIV infected at the time of their first marriage (Glynn et al. 2003). Furthermore, for both men and women, fewer than half of existing HIV infections were acquired from the spouse. Finally, there was a very high risk of HIV infection among the few women who never married, with 54% of women over 25 in Kisumu and 47% of women over 25 in Ndola who were never married being HIV infected.

What of other data that show higher risk among married girls and women? A study in Rakai, Uganda, also found higher HIV prevalence among women in a union, compared to never-married women, but these differences were also not statistically significant and are subject to the same confounding factors as the data from Kisumu and Ndola (Kelly et al. 2003). Another study, which used DHS data, reported that HIV prevalence was higher among married compared to nonmarried sexually active 15–19 year olds in only three of the 20 countries examined (Kenya, Tanzania, and Cameroon), and the difference was statistically significant only in Kenya (Clark et al. 2006).

However, another careful study of DHS data found that risk of HIV infection per year of exposure among sexually active women was higher *before* than *after* first marriage in Kenya as well as in Ghana (Bongaarts 2006). John Bongaarts surveyed DHS from a total of 33 African countries and concluded that marriage is protective for women. Furthermore, higher HIV prevalence among the 33 countries examined was associated with a longer interval between first sex and first marriage (in southern Africa this interval averaged 7.1 years), an interval in which a relatively high rate of partner change leads to higher risk of HIV acquisition. More infections do occur within marriage than without because over her lifetime, the average woman spends many more sexually active years within marriage than outside of marriage (Bongaarts 2006).

However, this report cautions that although marriage is protective *overall*, this does not negate the risk faced by young brides:

> The key issue is timing of first marriage in relation to timing of first sex. If a young girl marries before the age at which she would otherwise become sexually active (around 18 in much of sub-Saharan Africa), then she is exposed to an elevated risk of infection that would not occur in the absence of early marriage. (2006:10)

Clark and colleagues (2006) note that the youngest brides are more likely to be second or third wives and married to much older men. For virgin girls, marriage transitions them from virginity (no-risk) to frequent (probably unprotected) sex, and even for girls who are not virgins, marriage may mean more frequent unprotected sex. These early marriages are obviously of grave concern, and for more reasons than just HIV risk. Child marriage is a human rights violation, is considered as such by international bodies such as UNICEF, and most countries have laws against it.[8] These laws should be rigorously enforced and communities should be mobilized against the practice to reduce the number of girls who enter into high-risk early marriages. But saying early marriages are high risk is very different than saying that *all* marriages are high risk for women.

There are various definitions of marriage within Africa, ranging from traditional to legal to religious definitions, and surveys often count as "married" couples who are cohabiting.[9] However, data suggest that cohabitation is not as stable nor protective an arrangement as is marriage. The GPA studies conducted in Kampala and Lusaka in 1989/1990 found that individuals in "relatively informal" primary partnerships reported more non-regular sexual relationships than did married individuals (Caraël et al. 2001). A study of women in Nairobi slums found that cohabiting women were nearly *ten times* as likely to have multiple partners as married women, even after adjusting for education, ethnic group, religion, and age.[10]

Unmarried sexual partnerships, whether cohabiting or not, have now become the norm in certain countries of southern Africa. For example, the last national survey (2005) in Botswana showed that only 15% of people aged 10–64 were currently married (CSO, Botswana 2005). In the last DHS, the figure was 23% among Swazi men and 32% among Swazi women (CSO, Swaziland and Macro International 2008). It is striking that the two countries with the world's highest HIV prevalence have what may be the continent's lowest rates of marriage; where marriage is so rare, it can hardly be blamed for women's HIV risk. What is the implication for women, families, and cultures when AIDS experts consistently portray marriage as exceedingly risky for women? Could this not have an adverse affect, particularly in areas where the institution of marriage (and long-term, stable relationships generally) is increasingly fragile? It seems to us that the message that marriage is risky is not only false but irresponsible. The challenge, rather, is to make marriage as safe as possible, through programs such as the "zero grazing" campaigns in Uganda that encouraged fidelity of both partners.

The reasons for the decline of marriage in southern Africa are complex and have roots in labor migration (notably the cyclical migration of men from across southern Africa to South Africa's mines), oppressive political systems (such as South Africa's former apartheid regime), population shifts (including from rural to urban areas), and cultural changes including changes in gender roles as traditional cultures modernize and economies industrialize. In Chapter 2, we quoted a Zulu woman who lamented that "no one marries anymore," largely because people could not afford to. She also warned, "With so many people passing, we now worry that we will become [even] poorer . . . mak[ing] marriage even less likely." According to historian Benedict Carton, when asked whether she thought family life might disintegrate, she replied: "I don't know, truly" (Carton 2003:100). Hosegood and colleagues, in writing about modern KwaZulu-Natal, South Africa, note that marriage is in decline (while cohabitation increases somewhat), and they write, "For contemporary Zulu women '*doing without marriage*' is viewed by some commentators as a positive choice and indeed one of the survival strategies used by disadvantaged poorer women" (Hosegood et al. 2009:282). (They also note that other observers argue that marriage remains an ideal for most Zulu women, although one that is increasingly difficult to realize.) The reality is that many men and women in southern Africa never marry. The 2001 South African Census found that 27% of men and 18% of women in KwaZulu-Natal aged 50 and above had never married (Hosegoood et al. 2009).

Although the number of women who never marry is much smaller in other parts of Africa, data show that these women have very high rates of HIV infection. Once a woman is married, she is generally far safer staying married than leaving the marriage. (We are speaking of the average risks across populations of being married versus being unmarried and are not advocating that any woman should ever stay in a situation in which she is being abused or knows herself to be at risk of HIV infection.) Multiple studies have shown that married persons or others in long-term stable relationships have lower HIV prevalence than divorcees and widows of the same age (Caraël 1994b; Ntozi 1997; Spark-du Preez et al. 2004; Twa-Twa et al. 1997). Widowed, divorced, and separated women have by far the highest risk of multiple partnerships and HIV infection of any group of women (Hattori and Nii-Amoo Dodoo 2007).

Figure 9.4 shows HIV prevalence among never-married, married (or cohabiting), divorced or separated, and widowed women in Lesotho, Malawi, and Zimbabwe. As can be seen, divorced, separated, or

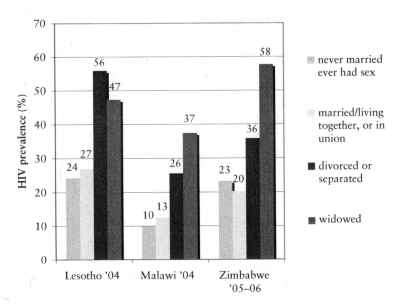

Figure 9.4 HIV prevalence by marital status among women ages 15–49 in three high-prevalence African countries.
Sources: Lesotho DHS 2004; Malawi DHS 2004; Zimbabwe DHS 2005–06.

widowed women have very high HIV prevalence. These data are also notable for the fact that sexually active never-married women have virtually the same HIV prevalence as married or cohabiting women. These data are not age adjusted, so we would expect never-married women, who as a group are much younger than married women, to have lower HIV infection rates, as HIV prevalence rises with age. Yet they do not, again suggesting that risk of HIV infection for married women is low, relative to being sexually active and unmarried.

The question is whether this increased HIV prevalence among widowed and divorced persons is primarily a result of infection before or after the dissolution of the marriage. A widow or widower who lost a spouse to HIV may have been infected by that spouse or, particularly for women, may become vulnerable due to divorce or widowhood and become infected with HIV as a result of risky behaviors after separation from or death of a spouse. A recent study of HIV infections in Rakai, Uganda, detected *recent* infections and established that widowed and divorced men and women had 2.5 and 1.5 times the risk of newly acquiring HIV infection, compared to married men and women.[11] (Never-married men and women had a significantly lower rate of new infections, but over half of them had never had sex.[12])

The same survey also provided data about married couples, which revealed some surprising facts. Of newly acquired infections, 38% occurred among men and women whose spouses had long-standing infections. In these discordant couples, one partner is clearly being placed at risk by the other's infection, and they need not only "be faithful" messages but also strategies such as testing and disclosure of status, anti-retroviral therapy to lower viral load and infectivity of the infected partner, and safer sex options such as condom use or nonpenetrative sex. (Such prevention strategies are often called "prevention for positives.")

However, even more incident infections among married people (49%) were among those whose spouses were *not* infected. These infections were obviously acquired not within marriage but outside of marriage, from an extramarital partner. An additional 14% of new infections among married people were among those whose partners were newly infected (obviously also through extramarital sex). Thus, nearly two-thirds of infections (63%) were attributable to sex outside of marriage, either directly or indirectly. Fewer than half of infections among married people were acquired from the spouse.[13] A study in Zambia among discordant couples found that 13% of new HIV infections among the uninfected partner were *not* acquired from the spouse (Allen et al. 2003). Similarly, a study of discordant couples that involved 14 sites in seven African countries found that 26% of new infections among the uninfected partner were acquired from outside the relationship—22% of new infections among women and 48% of new infections among men (Baeten et al. 2009).

Discordant couples are increasingly being seen as a key driver of the HIV epidemic in Africa, and testing plus condoms are usually proposed as the solution. But if a significant portion of new infections among discordant couples are actually acquired *outside* the relationship, this means "be faithful" messages are also extremely relevant for these couples, to prevent the uninfected partner from becoming infected outside the relationship as well as to prevent the infected partner from infecting others.

Encouraging condom use with outside partners is another potentially effective strategy. Data from Rakai, Uganda, showed that those who reported using a condom with at least one outside partner did not have a greater risk of HIV acquisition than those with no outside partners, although those with an outside partner who did *not* use condoms had a significantly higher risk of HIV infection.[14] The authors commented: "Many new HIV infections in Uganda could potentially be prevented if the risks associated with having multiple sexual partners, not using condoms with partners outside of marriage, and lack of circumcision were eliminated" (Mermin et al. 2008:544).

What of polygyny? Some research has found that polygyny leads not to greater risk to women within marriage but greater likelihood that women will seek and become infected by extramarital partners. Some researchers have found that men in polygynous unions are less likely to have extramarital sex (Caldwell and Caldwell 1993; Gregson et al. 1998). Other research has found that women in polygynous unions are more likely to seek partners outside marriage and bring HIV into marriage than women in monogamous unions (Nnko et al. 2004; Twa-Twa et al. 1997). DHS show that among infected couples, it is consistently more likely that the woman alone is infected in polygynous unions, compared to monogamous unions; in these cases, it is clearly the woman who introduced the infection.[15] In other words, being in a polygynous marriage seems to be a risk factor for women acquiring HIV outside the union.

This kind of complex, nuanced evidence about HIV risk within marriage is rarely discussed within the AIDS and anthropology communities, which continue to insist on the riskiness of marriage. For example, anthropologist Jennifer Hirsch and colleagues undertook a multiyear, National Institutes of Health–funded ethnographic study, "Love, Marriage, and HIV," in the countries of Papau New Guinea, Mexico, Vietnam, Nigeria, and Uganda. In their book about their findings, Hirsch and colleagues (2010) explain that this study had its genesis in the fact that "for most women in the world, their biggest risk of HIV infection comes from having sex with their husbands" (vii).[16]

Although their detailed research (involving 6 months of ethnography and many interviews and case studies in each of the sites) yields many fascinating insights about men's extramarital sexual behavior, the analysis is completely one sided. Nowhere in the book is women's extramarital sex discussed, and the fact that it exists is barely acknowledged. To the assertion that "men's behavior is a critical element of women's risk" (Hirsch et al. 2010:7), we would add the fact that women's behavior is also at times a critical element of men's risk; in heterosexual epidemics, there is no getting around the fact that the great majority of men are infected by women, and vice-versa.

Hirsch and colleagues argue that men and women collude to keep the "public secret" of men's infidelity: "[I]t seemed at times almost a secret that entire communities were trying to keep from themselves, insisting on the ideal of marital fidelity" (2010:3). Throughout the book, the authors insist that men's extramarital sexual activity is so common as to be normative. For example, they write, "[W]e gradually realized that in many settings, extramarital sex (particularly for men) is the socially determined 'default' option—the normal (though not perhaps the normative) behavior—and that the behavior that demanded explanation, in contrast, was marital fidelity" (2010:13).

A great many men (and women) around the world do have extramarital partners, but a great many also do *not* (or at least most of the time do not). Unfortunately, Hirsch and colleagues do not offer any data beyond the level of individual case studies to suggest how common and normative these extramarital relationships are. The authors are also very concerned with the gender inequalities and power differentials that are reproduced in extramarital sexual relationships. They write:

> [O]ur work explores whose interests are served and how inequality is reproduced through the keeping of these secrets . . . the collective consequence of these practices is to reproduce forms of social organization that provide men with greater access not just to the pleasures of extramarital sex but also to other valuable resources. (Hirsch et al. 2010:3)

An early outline of the study described it as a "comparative ethnographic study which explores the proposition that married women are placed uniquely at risk by the worldwide diffusion of an ideology of marriage as a relationship based on romantic love and companionship between equal partners" (Hirsch 2008). This seems to us to be a very biased proposition with which to begin a study, and we wonder what exactly the researchers are suggesting should *replace* these dangerous ideas of romantic love and companionship in marriage. Hirsch and colleagues seem to believe that their research upheld this proposition, but they give no indication of how many research subjects in their five research countries believed that the ideal of a marriage based on love and companionship was putting them at risk. In a summary report, the researchers recommend "defining married sex as risky sex," and discourage prevention approaches that promote monogamy among men and women (warning us that "extramarital sex needs to be addressed at the SOCIAL not the individual level") (Hirsch et al. 2005). In an article about marriage in Uganda, one of the coinvestigators warns that "being in a permanent relationship increases women's vulnerability for HIV infection" (Parikh 2007:1199). Is the author recommending that women pursue *impermanent* relationships, as if sex with multiple partners might be less risky? This article also takes aim at "be faithful" messages, warning that such messages, as well as "popular culture and religious discourses promoting monogamous marriages" (2007:1198) may increase the secrecy and denial around men's extramarital sex and contribute to "moral stigmatization" against people who are unfaithful. The author concludes: "[T]he current prevention message of 'be faithful' may be inadequate, unsustainable, and potentially counterproductive" (2007:1206).

More recently, an article by Dunkle and colleagues (2008) claimed that 92.7% of new heterosexually acquired HIV infections among adults in urban Rwanda (and 55.1% in urban Zambia) occurred *within* marital or cohabiting relationships, in spite of the fact that the number of infections acquired within marriage can never exceed the number of infections acquired from outside the union. Every infection passed on within marriage (or other long-term relationship) requires an incident infection acquired by one partner outside that relationship. Unless polygamy or other population dynamics cause, on average, more than one infection within marriage for every incident infection acquired outside of marriage, it is impossible that over time more than half of sexually transmitted infections could occur within marriage. In order for half of all infections to occur within marriage, the positive partner would always have to pass the infection on to the negative partner and the negative partner would never become independently infected—conditions that don't seem to occur in the real world.

Dunkle and colleagues (2008) admit in the article that by definition at least 50% of infections among married people (over time) must come from outside the union (for each infection transmitted within a union, an incident infection must first be acquired outside the union). Yet they still claim that, based on their model, over 90% of heterosexually transmitted infections in Rwanda occurred *within* marriage in a particular year. These data, which were based on modeling, have been widely misinterpreted to be actual findings. For example, Geeta Rao Gupta, president of the International Center for Research on Women, argued in a 2008 editorial in *The Washington Post* that marriage was not a "safe haven," and stated that 93% of new infections in Rwanda take place within marriage or cohabitation—missing the point that the researchers did not *find* this, but *modeled* it. She also claimed, erroneously, that in Uganda, "incidence rates are higher for married couples than sex workers." (A letter Ruark sent to the *Post* to correct these errors was not published.)

In the data analyzed by Dunkle and colleagues (2008), there were actually more female discordant than male discordant couples. In other words, in a majority of discordant couples it was the woman alone who was infected, and the man who was at risk of infection within marriage. However, the authors of this study seem determined to portray marriage as uniquely dangerous for women. In the article, they discuss the "cultural contexts" that "support men's extramarital sexual activities and prevent women from practicing HIV prevention within their relationships" (2008:2189). After a presentation of this research at the 2008 International AIDS Conference, Dunkle was heard to remark that marriage was "dangerous" and that "'Be faithful' is a horrible message to give to women."

WHO INFECTS WHOM IN MARRIAGE?

Data from across Africa show that a significant number of men are at risk of infection within marriage. An analysis of DHS data by Vinod Mishra found that in 4 of 11 African countries, a majority of discordant couples were female discordant, meaning that the woman was HIV infected (and had introduced the infection) and the man was uninfected and at risk. Mishra concluded: "[S]ubstantial proportions of female infections in discordant couples suggest infections within marriage from a non-spousal source" (2007b).

Damien de Walque of the World Bank also performed an analysis of DHS, this time from five African countries. This showed that among HIV-infected couples (including discordant couples and couples in which both were infected), the woman was infected in 30–40% of the couples and the man was not. There are two surprising things about these findings.

First, in over two-thirds of infected couples, one partner was still uninfected. This proportion ranged from 67% in Kenya to 85% in Burkina Faso. In all countries analyzed, *most* married or cohabiting women who were HIV infected had not been infected by their current partner (because their current partner was not infected), and, except for Kenya, *most* married or cohabiting HIV-infected men had not been infected by their current partner. In other words, most women (and men) were *not* being infected within marriage.

The second surprise is that in such a high percentage of cases, the woman had brought the infection into the relationship. The woman had introduced the infection in 30–40% of couples (varying by country) and likely also in some of the couples in which both were infected. De Walque (2007) notes that these high rates of female discordant couples are hard to reconcile with the fact that in these countries only 1–4% of women report extramarital sex in the past year. In an attempt to reconcile these realities, de Walque examined whether significant proportions of women might have been infected in a previous marriage or before marriage, but concludes that these two potential sources of infection are not driving factors for high rates of female discordancy.[17] De Walque concludes:

> In conclusion, the finding that a substantial proportion of HIV-infected couples in stable unions are discordant female appears robust to alternative explanations . . . it is extremely difficult to explain the sizable fraction (between 30 and 40 percent) of HIV-infected couples in which only the woman is HIV positive without female extramarital sex as a driving factor . . . it seems that self-reports of sexual behavior [among women] are not very reliable. (2007:519)

There is wide consensus that much of the data we have about sexual behavior is not very reliable. Sexual behavior data are nearly always self-reported, and men and women may have good reasons for not reporting accurately. In the case of a DHS-style survey, hundreds of questions are being asked by a complete stranger, and in any survey the respondent may feel that complete privacy is not assured. The problems with common survey methodologies are well understood, and other methodologies such as computer-assisted surveys or surveys that probe for information in more depth have been explored, although they have the obvious drawback of being more resource intensive.

Biological markers may also be used to confirm reports of sexual activity. For example, a prostate-specific antigen (PSA) test can confirm the presence of semen (and thus, recent unprotected sexual activity) in vaginal fluids. In a recent RCT that examined the effects of diaphragms plus lubricant gel in decreasing susceptibility among women in Zimbabwe, PSA test results were compared to women's self-reported sexual behavior. Nearly half (48%) of women who tested positive for recent semen exposure reported that they had not had sex in the previous 2 days (the window of sexual activity that would produce a positive PSA test). Of the 94 women whose self-reports did not match the objective measure of their recent sexual activity, 71 reported only having had condom-protected sex, and 23 reported not having had sex at all (Minnis et al. 2009).

Two examples demonstrate that different survey methods may yield remarkably different results. In Swaziland, a small 2006 survey found that 45% of men and 62% of women reported 2 or 3 partners in the past 3 months.[18] The 2006–07 Swaziland DHS, on the other hand, found that only 22.9% of men and 2.3% of women reported multiple partnerships in the past year. Although the first survey was not nationally representative and cannot be directly compared to the DHS findings, the difference between these survey findings is stark. We must ask whether, in a country with the world's highest HIV prevalence, the truth about men's and women's sexual behavior may not be closer to the first survey than to the DHS findings.

A 2007 study in Botswana used three different questions to ask about multiple sexual partnerships. When men and women were asked how many partners they had had sex with during the last 12, 6, and 1 months or how many different partners they had had by month for each of the last 6 months, approximately twice as many men as women reported concurrent relationships. However, when men and women were asked, "When did you first have sex with your last (up to) three sexual partners, and are you still having sex with that partner?" nearly identical numbers of men and women reported concurrency (more than one ongoing sexual partnership): 21% of men and 20% of women (Gourvenec et al. 2007). These findings also suggest that we should be cautious in how we interpret self-reported data, and mindful that different survey methodologies may yield widely different results.

Preventing HIV Infections within Discordant Couples

A recent series of national-level studies using a "modes of transmission" model developed by UNAIDS have described a very high proportion of infections occurring among monogamous couples or to people who are themselves monogamous (but who have a partner who has other partners). For example, 70% of new infections in Swaziland (Mngadi et al. 2009), 65% of new infections in Uganda (Wabwire-Mangen et al. 2009), and 58% of new infections in Zambia (Mulenga et al. 2009) were estimated to be among people who had only one sexual partner. These data are not empirical but are a result of a model, and the model uses self-reported sexual behavior data that are prone to all of the limitations described above. Most notably, the data used by the model probably greatly underestimate the prevalence of multiple partnerships, and the model does not account for the effect of concurrency (for which solid national-level data are generally not available).

214 • Chapter 9

Although these studies only claim to describe HIV infections occurring in the last year, *over time* no more than half of infections can occur within marriages. Many people in discordant relationships take a long time to become infected (as evidenced by the fact that there are so many discordant couples at any point in time), and some never do. In other words, it is probably an overestimate to say that even half of infections happen within marriage. Yet even if per-year risk of infection in marriage is low, the sheer number of married people means that infections within marriage are a significant proportion of all infections, even if not a majority.

Thus, halting the spread of HIV in the medium to long term requires increasing the length, stability, and mutual faithfulness of marriages or unions. At any given moment, there are quite literally millions of people who are at risk of infection from their spouse or partner. Stopping the spread of infection within these relationships is a unique challenge. Testing is often proposed as the solution, not just for those in committed relationships but for everyone who is sexually active. UNAIDS Director of Evidence, Monitoring, and Policy Paul De Lay said in 2008: "The importance of HIV testing in generalized epidemics cannot be discounted now that around half of all HIV infections occur between discordant couples." This statement reflects not only the priority of UNAIDS but of many AIDS organizations. A common assumption seems to be that marriages or long-term unions are fueling the spread of HIV (accounting for "around half" of new infections) and that the most effective weapon against these infections "within marriage" is increasing rates of couples' counseling and testing.

HIV testing for couples serves a number of important purposes, including giving couples the information needed to make decisions about their relationship, family, and HIV treatment, in case of infection. Being tested before entering a sexual relationship could minimize the number of couples who enter a relationship already discordant. But a new infection that is brought into the relationship has a high chance of being passed on during acute infection, before an HIV test could even detect the infection. How often must couples be tested to have some reasonable assurance that they are still uninfected, keeping in mind that no available test will reveal an infection in the critical first few weeks? Rather than advocating widespread testing as a means of reducing HIV infections in couples, a more realistic solution seems to be advocating faithfulness to that relationship to couples who are still uninfected, who make up the majority (in most countries, the vast majority) of couples in Africa.

By definition, all sexually transmitted HIV infections occur in a discordant couple—an HIV-positive man or woman infects an HIV-negative man or woman through sex. And, by definition, every infection passed on within a discordant relationship requires that one of those partners first become infected *outside* that couple. As discussed, the question is how risk varies by type of "couple"—whether long-term relationships (married or cohabiting couples, who may or may not be monogamous), one-off sexual encounters, or something in-between. Concurrent sexual partnerships, which may not seem particularly high risk as the total number of sexual partners may be low (for example, two or three over a period of years), are, in fact, extremely high risk, and discouraging these relationships must be a key prevention strategy in epidemics such as those in southern Africa.

We have noted that condom usage rates among married or regular partners are typically low. As already noted, couples' counseling has been shown to increase condom usage among discordant couples, but this usage is often inconsistent, and biological markers show that condom use is much more inconsistent than couples report. In Allen and colleagues' 2003 study of Zambian couples, discordant couples in which the woman was uninfected (and at risk of infection) reported significantly less frequent sex (both with and without condoms) than couples in which the man was uninfected (and at risk of infection). The researchers posit that this may reflect decreased libido in HIV-infected men, but also note that discordant couples in which the man was infected were more likely than couples in which the woman was infected to report 100% condom use. Contrary to common assumptions, these data do not support a view in which infected men insist on sex with uninfected wives, who are unable to refuse sex or sex without a condom. As Allen and colleagues state: "[M]any men who know they have HIV willingly use condoms to protect their uninfected spouses." (The data given in Table 6.1 about condom usage rates among married men who know they are HIV infected also support this statement.)

Sero-discordant couples also report abstinence from sex to avoid infection, and research has shown that many HIV-negative women would prefer abstinence had their partners not refused (Bunnell et al. 2005). A study of discordant couples in Kinshasa, Zaire in the late 1980s found that 25% of discordant couples in which the man was infected and 18.2% of couples in which the woman was infected reported sexual abstinence (Kamenga et al. 1991). However, a study in Zambia found that most discordant couples continued to have sex: 99% of couples reported sex at least once during the year, and 56% of couples did so in all four 3-month periods of the study (Allen et al. 2003).

Discordant couples clearly need the "be faithful" message. Even if every uninfected partner became infected, this would not perpetuate the epidemic unless infected people infected more than one partner. (For epidemics to be sustained, the "reproductive number"—the number

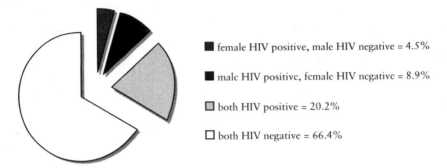

Figure 9.5 HIV infections among couples in Lesotho, 2004.
Sources: Lesotho DHS 2004.

of people infected by each infected person—must be greater than one.) Thus, the B message, if followed, has a strong protective effect at the broader population level. Even at the individual level, sex with multiple partners can lead to superinfection,[19] making AIDS worse and complicating the prospect of treatment for both individuals and populations. Therefore, even for serodiscordant couples, A and B messages can have great relevance.

Another crucial point is that even in the most severe HIV epidemics, a majority of couples are still uninfected. For example, even in Lesotho, which is one of the worst-hit countries in the world, two-thirds of couples are not HIV infected and will not become so as long as both partners (or all partners, in the case of a polygamous union) remain faithful to the relationship (Figure 9.5). A certain number of HIV infections among discordant couples may be inevitable, no matter how strenuously we promote "prevention for positives." But if there were not a continuous stream of new infections into unions, the hyper-epidemics of Africa would soon be ended.

CASE STUDY: TUKO CLUB

In July 2007, Ruark sat watching an elaborate wedding party taking pictures on the lush lawn of one of Kampala, Uganda's best hotels, and talking with the founder of an organization called the Tuko Club about modern marriage in Uganda. In a series of conversations with Ugandans that summer, Ruark had noticed a certain amount of concern over changing customs of marriage, particularly that the number of couples actually getting married was felt to be on the decline. Some Ugandans blamed the economy, explaining that many couples wanted to get married but did not have the financial means. This seemed to be exacerbated by the realities of modern urban life. For a man, mustering the money for a modern wedding and an urban abode seemed to be more of a challenge than the more traditional, rural process of acquiring a piece of land, building a house with locally found materials, and amassing enough cows to pay his bride's *lobola* (all things that might not take any money at all, given family support). One apparently deeply religious shopkeeper, after explaining that he had a partner of many years whom he had not yet married, burst out: "I pray to God for enough money to get married!"

Other Ugandans bemoaned the ever-increasing expectations of the wedding ceremony itself. As Uganda's economy stabilized and became more affluent during the 1990s, the explanation went, expectations changed, and have been increasing ever since. Television, glossy magazines, and other print media have made the lavish weddings of the well-off very visible. The urban and even rural poor have easy access to images of limousines, brides in Western-style white dresses, and bridesmaids in yards of satin. It seemed to be the new norm for wedding ceremonies to require years of saving and virtually bankrupt the families involved.

Many within public health and the AIDS community seem uncomfortable with the idea of AIDS prevention paying any attention to the institution of marriage. Marriage is, of course, a religious and cultural institution as well as being a context within which a sexual relationship is formed and HIV can be transmitted. Talking about marriage at all may seem to some to be veering dangerously close to promoting a religious or cultural agenda. Yet we argue that the practice and institution of marriage is exactly the type of cultural matter to which AIDS prevention should pay more attention. Whether people marry or not, when, and how has enormous implications for the spread of HIV.

From an epidemiological point of view, the spread of HIV in a population is driven by dynamics such as length and overlap of sexual partnerships, rate of partner turnover, frequency of sex, and frequency of condom use, and it matters not at all who has a marriage certificate and who doesn't. But all of the aspects of sexual relationships just mentioned have quite a lot to do with the cultural terms in which people define their relationships, including whether or not they are married. Thus, marriage matters.

So, how could marriage be supported from within an AIDS prevention paradigm? A Ugandan organization called the Tuko Club (standing for *Tukolere Wamu*, or "Let's work together" in the local Luganda language) is now in its third decade of promoting marriage and fighting AIDS, and provides an instructive example. The Tuko Club started in the late 1980s among a group of classmates who were leaving university and facing the demands of life. As this group of young men searched for jobs, raised money for their marriages, and paid medical bills, they bonded together into a club that was part social club, part self-help group, and part savings club. The club operated with a high level of commitment, trust, and mutual sharing of finances (e.g., members would pool their money to help one member with medical bills or other large expenses). The Tuko Club developed an executive board and a constitution, members were expected to pay dues, and new members were taken on very cautiously and only after a year-long trial period.

The group grew from the original four members and four girl-friends of members, and by 1998 there were twenty couples, most of them now married. In the words of Lawrence Sekimpi, one of the founders, "Our main focus was to marry legally so we could stay together [stay married]." They were keenly aware of the dangers of infidelity in a time of AIDS, and they also sought to find out what caused men to go outside their marriages so that they could avoid these pitfalls and AIDS. Before long, the women of the Tuko Club had formed their own weekly meeting, which focused on how they could strengthen their marriages, and they invited older women to come and talk with the group. (Among the Baganda, there is a tradition of paternal aunts, called *ssengas*, passing on advice about sex and marriage, so inviting older women to speak with the group was adapting this tradition.) In the same way, the men invited older men and church leaders to talk to them about marriage (adapting the somewhat less strong tradition of *kojjia*, or paternal uncles), although Mr. Sekimpi noted that the men were not always as open to this kind of discussion as were the women. The Tuko Club promoted communication, respect, and equal decision-making among couples as part of building strong marriages.

Around 2000, the Tuko Club began to spread their model of a social club that helped couples build strong finances, strong marriages, and avoid AIDS. In the words of Mr. Sekimpi, they saw that their fellow Ugandans, their "own brothers and sisters," were dying of AIDS. They began to visit churches and other meeting places to talk about the Tuko Club. In 2005, they received an HIV prevention grant that allowed them to travel throughout the country promoting faithfulness in marriage, using a "trainer of trainers" structure and relying on 375 model couples to spread the approach and form new Tuko clubs.

As of 2007, the Tuko Club could claim the following accomplishments. More than 6,000 people had received HIV testing as couples at the encouragement of the Tuko Club. Couples surveyed reported less fighting after involvement in a Tuko Club. And about two-thirds reported that they were faithful. (Interestingly, the Tuko Club found when it polled men and women about infidelity that as many women as men reported having had extramarital sex.) Although the Tuko Club defined marriage very broadly (including not only a ceremony in a church or mosque, but civil marriage or living together), Mr. Sekimpi emphasized that it was the Tuko Club's experience that having a formal or church wedding helped couples stay together, as it conferred public recognition and legal rights on them. The Tuko Club promoted the idea that couples did not need fancy or expensive weddings and even held a group wedding for eight couples who felt they couldn't afford individual ceremonies.

It is not the job of AIDS prevention to promote any particular agenda on marriage, other than the public health agenda of reducing new HIV infections as much as possible. If there are sound public health reasons for marriage—such as that the institution leads to longer, more stable, and more mutually faithful sexual relationships—then marriage can be considered a positive cultural practice and something that public health can support from within a culturally grounded and locally driven approach to AIDS. We should not minimize the power of such a long-standing and deeply held cultural practice as marriage to shape behavior and provide a culturally understood context for scientifically sound AIDS prevention.

NOTES

1. A cohort study in Masaka, Uganda, found that among those with HIV-positive spouses, age-adjusted HIV incidence in women was twice that of men (rate ratio (RR) = 2.2, 95% confidence interval (CI) 0.9–5.4) (see Carpenter et al. 1999). A cohort study in Mwanza, Tanzania, similarly found that the HIV incidence of women in discordant partnerships was twice that of men in discordant partnerships (RR = 2.0, 95% CI = 0.28–22.1) (see Gray et al. 2000).

2. A cohort study in Rakai, Uganda, found that HIV incidence among uncircumcised men in discordant relationships was 16.7 infections (95% CI = 12.0–21.4) per 100 person-years (compared to no infections among circumcised men), whereas HIV incidence among women in discordant relationships was 13.2 infections (95% CI = 9.6–16.8) per 100 person-years (see Hugonnet et al. 2002).

3. These data can be easily acquired from DHS, many of which report lifetime number of sexual partners for women. In the four countries for which data are given in Table 9.1, the percentage of sexually active women with exactly one lifetime partner ranges from 33.6% (Cote d'Ivoire) to 69.6% (Rwanda). These data capture a number of young women (the age range is to 15–49), so the proportion of women who have had two or more partners by later in their lives is likely much higher. Further, these data are self-reported and, as with all self-reported data about sexual behavior (particularly for women), may be underestimates.

4. The countries included were Bangladesh, Brazil, Ethiopia, Japan, Namibia, Peru, Samoa, Serbia and Montenegro, Thailand, and Tanzania.

5. HIV prevalence among women reporting no physical or sexual partner violence was 28.6%; for women reporting physical violence it was 37.9%; for women reporting sexual violence it was 26.7%; and for women reporting both physical and sexual violence it was 40.2%. In a multivariate model that accounted for demographic and behavioral variables, and for the frequency of IPV, experiencing "broad" IPV was significantly associated with HIV infection (OR = 1.48).

6. In their 2004 article in *Social Science and Medicine*, Dunkle and colleagues provide the following helpful references on transactional sex and violence: Beadnell et al. 2000; Cunningham et al. 1994; Gilbert et al. 2000; James and Meyerding 1977; Kalichman et al. 1998; Karim et al. 1995; Mullings et al. 2000; Nyanzi et al. 2001; Wojcicki and Malala 2001; Zierler et al. 1991.

7. See Ruark 2008. Statistical analysis performed using chi-squared statistics and Fisher's exact test.

8. There are many other reasons to discourage child marriage besides the risk of HIV. Too-early marriage denies girls other ordinary experiences of youth, such as schooling, good health, economic opportunities, and friendship with peers (see Mathur et al. 2003).

9. DHS ask respondents, "Are you married or living together as if married?" and DHS reports often group together everyone who answers this question affirmatively.

10. Widowed and divorced women were even more likely to report two or more partners in the past year, with the odds ratios as follows (all compared to women who were married and co-residing): not married and co-residing OR = 9.50; widowed OR = 15.56 (even accounting for the fact that 30% of widows abstained entirely in the previous year); divorced or separated OR = 31.33 (see Hattori and Nii-Amoo Dodoo 2007).

11. See Mermin et al. 2008. The weighted incidence (when adjusting for other confounding factors) was 2.0 infections per 100 person-years for married men and women, 4.8 infections per 100 person-years for widowed men and women, and 3.0 infections per 100 person-years for divorced men and women. These data were not separately reported for men and women, although women had a higher rate of new infections than men (2.1 infections per 100 person-years for women compared to 1.5 infections per 100 person-years for men).

12. See Mermin et al. 2008. The weighted incidence for never-married men and women was 0.7 infections per 100 person-years. In the sample, 2,610 men and women had never had sex, and, if they were all assumed to be never-married, they would comprise 53% of the 4,913 men and women who had never been married.

13. Although 51% of married people who were newly infected had an infected spouse, the data did not allow the researchers to establish whether these infections were actually acquired from the spouse. An uninfected man or woman with an infected spouse may have acquired his or her infection from an extramarital partner, and not from the spouse, meaning that even more than 49% of infections may have come from an extramarital source.

14. See Mermin et al. 2008. Incidence for those who did not have an outside partner was 2.4%; incidence for those with an outside partner who used a condom with at least one partner was 2.3%; and for those who had an outside partner and did not use a condom it was 7.8%.

15. Various DHS. The proportion of female discordant couples (in which the woman and not the man is infected) as a percentage of all infected couples for monogamous and polygynous unions, respectively, is as follows: Cote d'Ivoire (2005): 44%, 90%; Ethiopia (2005): 43%, 100%; Kenya (2003): 39%, 50%; Malawi (2004): 24%, 26%; Rwanda (2005): 19%, 43%; Uganda (2004–05): 18%, 26%; Zimbabwe (2006): 17%, 33%.

16. Other articles published by this team reinforce this view. Smith (2007) erroneously states that "data from around the world, including Nigeria, suggest that married women's greatest risk of contracting HIV is through sexual intercourse with their husbands" (p. 997). Smith also bemoans the fact that "both policymakers and ordinary citizens remain resistant to the idea that marriage must be understood as a risk factor for HIV infection" (p. 997).

17. See De Walque 2007. De Walque did this first by excluding from the analysis all couples in which the woman had been previously married; this caused the proportion of female discordant couples to decrease in Ghana (from 37.6% to 28.4%) and Tanzania (from 33.2% to 27%), but this proportion did not decrease significantly in Burkina Faso, Cameroon, or Kenya. Next, de Walque excluded from the analysis all couples who had been living together less than 10 years, under the assumption that in all couples who had been together more than 10 years HIV infection was not acquired prior to marriage, as the infected person would by then have passed away. This decreases the proportion of female discordant couples to 19.6% in Ghana and 22.0% in Tanzania, and to around 30% in the remaining three countries.

18. See James and Matikanya 2006. This survey involved 307 respondents and included a questionnaire, key informant interviews, and focus group discussions.

19. Superinfection occurs when a person becomes infected by two or more different strains of HIV.

Chapter 10

AN ENDOGENOUS RESPONSE TO AIDS

As Green wrote in 2004, we should not assume that all the solutions to the problems of the poor lie outside those communities and populations and can only be found in donor organizations. If the problem of global AIDS is seen primarily as an issue of transfer and adoption of technology, which is largely how the major players in global AIDS have treated the pandemic until very recently, then the need to understand sexual and related behaviors in a context of family, peer group, society, and culture is limited. However, if AIDS is seen primarily as a behavioral issue, then the need to understand behavior and culture becomes much more important.

A major mistake of standard, donor-driven AIDS prevention has been to ignore behavior and culture and to circumvent indigenous leaders, knowledge and beliefs, healers, institutions, and organizations rather than building on them. The mindset of Western development is against the indigenous approach; more accurately, working through this sector does not occur to those working in development and remains largely invisible to them. Thus, the multi-billion-dollar AIDS industry fails basic Anthropology 101, so to speak. Little has been learned from these mistakes. To quote Peter Piot (then executive director of UNAIDS) at the 2008 International AIDS Conference:

> Prevention needs to be innovative, using information communication technologies such as mobile phones and web based social networking applications—billboards will not appeal to the young people who need the information. . . . We need to use more *business-like methods* but ground these in community action and knowledge. (Piot 2008, emphasis added)

Piot continued, "[T]he epidemic is too serious to be left to cottage industry, improvisation and amateurism." This implicit disdain for indigenous knowledge and leadership has been typical of Western AIDS prevention organizations. The presumption is that Western experts know what is best for Africans and indigenous African leaders should be considered amateurs.

As William Easterly points out in *The White Man's Burden* (2006), this is paternalism at its most egregious. Easterly identifies two approaches to development. International development experts, whom he calls *planners*, follow a top-down approach based on "utopian social engineering." They see poverty as an engineering problem with technical solutions only they can concoct, and commodities as something only they can provide. In contrast, Easterly identifies as *searchers* those who go to Africa or elsewhere with humility, open minds, and an ability to learn and discern what works and what doesn't in different settings, before scaling up programs in a non-top-down approach.

As Green noted in his 2003 book *Rethinking AIDS Prevention*, populations in many parts of Africa and elsewhere have instinctively known how to respond to the threat of AIDS. They have responded by modifying risky sexual behaviors. Green writes,

> When people in majority populations of developing countries are asked about sexual behavior in surveys (such the DHS, and WHO/GPA or UN-AIDS surveys), they usually report that they have changed their behavior as a result of AIDS. When asked how their behavior has changed, the most common answers are as follows: fidelity to one's partner, reduction in the number of sexual partners, delay of sexual debut (among youth) and abstinence for a period. It is useful to refer to these actions as primary behavior change. Primary behavior change tends to be reported far more frequently than condom use, in fact between five and ten times more frequently in unprompted, open-ended questions. (2003b:9)

Yet, rather than building on these spontaneous, *effective* responses to AIDS, most donor-funded AIDS prevention programs have begun by trying to introduce a completely different set of behaviors, based in technology and products such as condoms and testing kits. Almost every country in Africa has a national strategic framework for HIV/AIDS, and they read largely alike. They emphasize professional and medical services, the integration of sexual and reproductive health and HIV services, and better access to services. These documents uniformly warn of consequences of *not* using clinical services. The current national strategic framework for HIV/AIDS for Uganda is titled *Achieving Universal Access to Services*. The national HIV policy of the first country that squarely addressed multiple and concurrent sexual partners (through "Stick to One Partner" and "Zero Grazing" messages) no longer contains visible objectives, goals, or program impact indicators related to what was the key intervention during Uganda's remarkable period of major behavioral change in the latter 1980s. Thus, Western professionalism has largely replaced an indigenous African model that worked far better than the global risk reduction model imposed by the West.

Public health is one of the few areas of broader development efforts that has achieved some genuine, sustained results. But we need only examine the Western response to AIDS, one of Africa's worst problems, to see replication of nearly every mistake made by planners in a variety of domains over the past half-century. To quote anthropologist Elizabeth Onjoro (2003):

> [P]revention strategies centered on providing large amounts of condoms have demonstrated very limited effectiveness in many African nations precisely because they do not take into account cultural factors. . . . It is no surprise that ABC has been at the center of effective HIV/AIDS prevention in Senegal and Uganda. The ABC strategy in each country is tailored to fit that country's cultural reality . . . effective HIV programs must integrate a cultural framework of health and healing, treatment and prevention messages. Prevention messages that are perceived as best and effective in the West may not necessarily be equally effective in the African context.

A growing number of African intellectuals, such as Ghanaian economist George Ayittey (2006a), present a very non-Western view of progress, arguing that the future of Africa lies in building on traditional political authorities and other indigenous institutions. They see that the economic and political failures of African governments have resulted from trying to plant European political models on African soil, to borrow a metaphor used by the Mozambican FRELIMO party when it reflected on its largely unsuccessful adoption of Marxism during the 1980s.

It is a matter of historical record that postindependence African governments, whether progressive, democratic, or Marxist-oriented, all tended to view indigenous leaders as holdovers from the past and obstacles to progress, economic development, and modernization. Most countries in southern Africa have policies regarding traditional leaders that might be characterized as "benign neglect." It has not been difficult for independence-era governments to justify policies of suppression or neglect as indigenous leaders are not democratically elected and are usually regarded by non-Africans as being authoritarian patriarchs lacking legitimacy. They are also sometimes regarded as guardians of dysfunctional cultural norms that serve to oppress women and exploit the poor.

Another perspective about indigenous leadership is that it provides a political alternative to the postindependence African governments that, at the centers of power, have often become as corrupt and despotic as the worst monarchs in Western history. The case can be made that these modern African politicians are far worse than traditional chiefs who operate within structures of regulation and cultural custom that serve to provide checks and balances (Ayittey 2006a, 2006b). Many postindependence governments have questionable legitimacy, having come to power through coups, violence, or burlesques of farcical democratic voting. It is currently estimated that $140 billion, or about 25% of Africa's total GDP, is lost annually to government corruption (Ribaudu 2009).

Maxwell Owusu, an anthropologist who participated in writing Ghana's constitution and in developing a decentralized district assembly model there, recently wrote that he sees potential in the "revival and proliferation of activist development-oriented civic organizations and mutual-aid societies based on village, town, ethnic, family membership, and similar affiliations" for creating a "grassroots participatory democracy" (1995, cited in Paley 2002:474). The system he describes "builds on indigenous political traditions of local self-government which assume the existence of consensual ethical and moral values shared within a community" (Paley 2002:474). These values are based on chieftaincy, which, "despite its inherent social inequality, embodies shared values and virtues of accountability, service, probity; the tradition of voluntarism and self-help; and a spirit that extols the committed and total involvement of all the members of a community in the formulation and implementation of policies for the community's welfare" (Paley 2002:474).

Viewed from the village level, civil servants assigned to rural areas and often not native to the area lack the respect, knowledge of local history and affairs, or even linguistic skills of the local traditional chief, even if they wield the official authority from the central government. *National* or modern leadership has been so disappointing (with a few exceptions, notably in Mandela's South Africa and in Botswana) as to make indigenous leaders look far better by comparison, at least to some. Ayittey (2006b) observes:

> The modern leadership in much of Africa is a despicable disgrace to black people. The exceptions have been trenchantly few. A leadership, characterized by arrant sloganeering, brutal repression and frenzied plunder, is a far cry from the type of leadership Africans have known under their chiefs and kings for centuries. Name one traditional African ruler who plundered the tribal treasury for deposit in Switzerland. The modern leaders have been a failure, not by Western or Eastern standards but by Africa's own indigenous standards.

Thus, there is at least a minority academic viewpoint that sees potential for a shift in the development paradigm, despite the problems inherent in collaborating with and perhaps thereby empowering indigenous leaders.

In economic, public health, and other development ventures, the approach of governments and foreign donors has tended to ignore the entire indigenous sector, from its knowledge and beliefs to its institutions, healers, and leaders (Reuee 2002). Western models and technology are typically implemented in vertical programs, conceived by Western technical experts in theoretical collaboration with their African, educated counterparts, and then implemented with little regard to local leadership, customs, knowledge, and structures. This model is justified based on the argument that indigenous systems of knowledge relating to sickness and healing have nothing in common with modern virus theories and that indigenous leaders are anti-democratic and male chauvinists.

In the area of AIDS, we advocate investigating new approaches to behavior change interventions through working with preexisting human resource and cultural assets such as traditional leaders. Green was involved in programs like this during the 1990s in South Africa, Swaziland, and Zambia, and in a contraceptive promotion program involving healers in Nigeria in the 1980s. The basic arguments for collaborating with traditional healers were that healers were ubiquitous while trained biomedical personnel were few, far between, and largely limited to cities. Furthermore, healers were eager to learn about Western medicine and to collaborate and cooperate with public health programs and could be trained quickly, easily, and cheaply (using peer education to achieve multiplier effect). Public health prevention programs working with healers could therefore potentially reach large numbers of people, some of whom might be effectively beyond the reach of the formal health care system.

Why collaborate with traditional healers in AIDS? Green's research and that of others found that traditional healers treat most of the cases of STIs in Africa. Indeed, they treat most cases of any disease or condition, but curiously, given the effectiveness of antibiotic therapy, STIs were widely believed to be an area of special competence among traditional healers (Green 1994, 1999a). Thus, there seemed to be potential for accessing large numbers of untreated or inadequately treated STI cases, if healers could be persuaded to refer their patients to biomedical health facilities.

Another reason to collaborate with healers in AIDS is that they could give advice to those infected with HIV about psychosocial problems; stigma and social marginalization; diet and exercise; how to avoid alcohol and tobacco, despair, and depression; how to maintain hope and spiritual faith; and how to avoid spreading the infection. Healers can, and often will, promote and distribute condoms or sell them in social marketing programs. But seeing them primarily as condom distributors is a minimalist approach, one that reflects Western donor priorities rather than cultural or epidemiological realties in Africa. It does not take advantage of great opportunities to do even more, to influence key behaviors such as avoiding multiple and concurrent partners and casual or commercial sex.

AIDS prevention programs could also collaborate with healers as partners in promoting male circumcision or reintroducing the practice in societies that do not (any longer) promote it. Early in the AIDS pandemic, some South African healers were actually promoting voluntary circumcision to adult males from ethnolinguistic groups that do not currently practice circumcision, such as the Zulu, Swazi, and Tswana. In the early 1990s, one South African healer organization, Traditional Doctors AIDS Project, wrote and distributed a pamphlet that advised: "To circumcise is the best remedy to reduce sexually transmitted diseases" (Koloko et al. 1993). It is fascinating that healers claim they were alerted to lack of male circumcision as a risk factor by their own "clinical" experience. They could not fail to notice that repeat male STI patients tended to be from noncircumcising groups, so on their own initiative they initiated a "campaign" (or an effort) to inform people, some 15 years before formal Western medicine began to gear up for such an intervention.

Once we can evaluate beliefs and practices on an objective scale according to what contributes to greater or lesser morbidity and mortality in a given health domain, we can encourage the useful, discourage the unhelpful or unhealthy, and leave the rest alone. Regarding training, information-sharing between public heath and traditional healers is best when it is not unidirectional, with the medical-scientific view promoted by "trainers," as if healers were blank slates, lacking their own ideas and practices. A typical rationale for this approach is that "we" (i.e., Western health professionals and donors) are right and "they" (i.e., healers) are wrong, and that there is no common ground between modern and indigenous theories of disease. But as discussed in Chapter 2, this is not true.

The model of collaboration with traditional healers that Green and his colleagues developed in several African countries was based on the public health arguments about the benefits of this collaboration, whether in HIV or STI prevention or some other area of health. This collaboration relied on the following principles: respect indigenous medicine, respect African cultures, discard preconceptions, and find and build on common ground. We know from experience that some compromise on both sides is possible and almost certainly necessary. We also recognize that the mobilization of African populations around behavior change and HIV prevention is only possible with the participation of traditional leaders.

Case Study: Mobilizing Chiefs for HIV Prevention[1]

In 2008, nearly 20 years after his work with traditional healers in southern Africa, Green embarked on a study of the role of traditional leaders in AIDS prevention in the same region. This research was undertaken with Cedza Dlamini of the Ubuntu Institute, a South Africa–based nonprofit organization investigating the role of culture, heritage, indigenous knowledge systems, and leadership in achieving the Millennium Development Goals in Africa.

The study was funded by the Ford and Kellogg Foundations and its purpose was to investigate the role that traditional leaders and African culture could play in reducing the spread of HIV and to explore the possibility that indigenous leaders and structures could become "levers for change" rather than obstacles to achieving "behavior change" objectives. The research also aimed to better understand cultural patterns related to sexual behavior, marriage, rites of passage, and other indigenous structures, and how HIV prevention could be built into existing cultural platforms such as rites of passage, customary law and traditional courts, cultural ceremonies, and festivals. The research focused particularly on rural populations for whom traditional structures and leadership remain important, who are often hardest to reach through mass media and other standard outreach campaigns, and who are still subject to traditional social controls.

Focus group discussions (FGDs) and in-depth interviews (IDIs) were carried out with chiefs and members of royal families in three provinces of South Africa (Eastern Cape, Mpulalanga, and KwaZulu-Natal), as well as in Swaziland, Botswana, and Lesotho. Most participants in the research were men, as the vast majority of indigenous leaders in the region are men, but female chiefs were included when they were available.

Chiefs fill a symbolic role, and many have real power within communities, but they also feel alienated from modern political parties and systems to varying degrees. They feel their power and authority have been diminished in recent generations and that they have been reduced to playing largely ceremonial roles by the government. Two of them said:

> The government uses us for ceremonial purposes but we have no nice houses, no salaries. We are exploited. Missionaries made us ashamed of our culture, made us "unlearn" our culture. (chief, KwaZulu-Natal, FGD)

> If you take a look before the new South Africa was formed, most nations were ruled by Kings. And there was a certain control of things and people—of how people should live their lives. I think what happened is that everything got disturbed after the existence of "politics," but traditional leadership is there to maintain that order. (chief, Mpumalanga, South Africa, FGD)

Green had an opportunity to discuss this matter with one of South Africa's newly recognized kings at a small dinner in September 2009.

(A few traditional kings are officially recognized by the South African government and they are provided protection and a few other perks.) This king, who must remain nameless, told Green that there is a movement afoot in Africa for traditional leaders to rise up and take a far more active role in national affairs. In early September, there was unrest in Uganda over just such a movement, when the Kabaka, or king of the Baganda (the largest of Uganda's many ethnolinguistic groups), clashed with the Ugandan government. The Baganda king told Uganda's *New Vision* newspaper: "We have realized that politics has greatly divided our country. We believe cultural leaders are the best people to spearhead the struggle for creating unity and oneness. Cultural leaders are our symbols of unity and heritage" (Mulondo 2009:1). Perhaps unfortunately for the credibility of any such movement, Muammar Gaddafi of Libya has been actively courting African kings with money and other support, after his attempt to rally the support of African presidents and prime ministers failed (Among 2009). His goal seems to be to establish himself as "King of Kings," and simultaneously minister of defense, for the entire continent.

Returning to the study, in all four countries, traditional leaders felt bypassed, marginalized, and circumvented by their respective governments in anti-AIDS efforts, and all seemed eager to become more involved. When the focus groups began, some traditional leaders wondered aloud why it had taken 25 years for those involved in AIDS prevention to systematically gather traditional leaders' opinions about the best ways to fight AIDS. In their view, foreign AIDS funds are channeled to NGOs that do not necessarily represent African values and priorities, bypassing traditional or genuine authorities. This fuels tensions that undermine effective and well-coordinated community-based responses to AIDS. Said one:

> They never came to talk to us about the National Strategic Plan at design phase. They always pretend to "consult with us" when in fact it's too late or they come and expect us to help at implementation level. Our participation needs to start at design level of the National Strategic Plan so that we can fully own it. (traditional leader, Mpumalanga, South Africa, FGD)

A number of traditional leaders were critical of the approach to HIV prevention they have witnessed in their home areas and suggested they could do a better job. Some remarked:

> There was a really big tent and they invited people like Mandoza [a popular singer] to entertain people after the speech about reducing HIV/AIDS and preventing it. After that meeting they gave people condoms and you

ask yourself: What are these condoms for? Then you see that they say [people] should continue having sex, while as their Chief, you say they should respect themselves and not practice sex before [a certain] age or before they get married. . . . If the government could give us [chiefs] power to do these things ourselves, we can do it. We will go back to the ways of our ancestors. (traditional leader, KwaZulu-Natal, South Africa, FGD)

We teach abstinence but outsiders promote condoms. A mixed message. Condoms actually encourage sex. Having one faithful partner is best. (traditional leader, KwaZulu-Natal, South Africa, FGD)

Preventing HIV/AIDS is all about discipline and nothing else. Discipline to either abstain, stick to one partner or consistent use of condoms. (traditional leader, Lesotho, FGD)

They also recognized many of the key risk factors for HIV in their communities, such as alcohol and labor migration:

Alcohol is a huge factor in disrupting culture and promoting HIV/AIDS and should be strictly controlled. Perhaps there should be only one central place in each village where it can be provided. (traditional leader, Botswana, FGD)

The textile industry in Lesotho is killing us! We have problems with urban/ rural migration fueling the spread of HIV/AIDS due to both men and women having multiple partners. (traditional leader, Lesotho, mixed gender FGD)

Traditional leaders often conceptualized the spread of AIDS in non-biomedical, sociocultural terms, explaining it within the paradigm of their own belief systems. At the core of this belief system is the idea that there is a clash between Euro American values, modernization, and African values, and that AIDS is spreading quickly *due to a breakdown in traditional family and social values* in African societies, leading to undesirable behavior. Current HIV prevention appeared to them to be strictly limited to the biomedical: condom promotion, voluntary counseling and testing, drugs, and other technological methods. Although these may be important, they felt, these interventions do not address the underlying sociocultural issues or factors motivating risk behaviors fueling the AIDS epidemic. In the words of two chiefs:

People today try to assume the norms and values of foreigners—they don't even know who they are any more. (chief, Botswana, FGD)

HIV/AIDS is a curse of God for losing our value and respect. It's a punishment from God! (chief, Lesotho, IDI)

The HIV prevention solutions offered by the leaders amounted to reviving and strengthening African values, traditional moral codes, and

232 ■ CHAPTER 10

social controls, such as those that encourage delay of sexual debut, discourage sex outside of marriage, and, in their view, protect women. Traditional leaders commented that most mass media campaigns do not reach the rural areas, and, if they do, they lack the cultural competence to educate African communities effectively about AIDS, at least in ways that translate into behavior change. The messages were viewed as being too medical and as not touching on the kind of solutions the traditional leaders propose.

Traditional leaders identified a number of traditional customs and practices that they said were "central to our traditional culture and way of life." One of the most important was traditional education about sexual matters and marriage. This often takes place (if still practiced) as part of initiation ceremonies. There was agreement among focus group participants that initiation schools and ceremonies prepare youth for adulthood, pass on traditional culture, instill proper values, and teach good behavior. They could also be an effective platform for AIDS education and for teaching boys respect for girls. Abandonment of initiation ceremonies was often blamed for crime, promiscuity, and in the words of one leader, "people perishing at present" from AIDS. In the view of one female chief:

> As a woman, *lebollo* [women's initiation rite] is an important stepping stone for me into womanhood. I learn about reproductive health issues, self-confidence, sexuality and cultural values. Cultural values directly have a link to my behavior and habits. (female chief, Lesotho, FGD)

During initiation ceremonies, information is provided to initiates that is deemed appropriate for their specific age and stage in life and is meant to prepare them for adulthood by furnishing them with the relevant information that they may require as they pass from childhood into the adult world. Both virginity testing and male circumcision were cited as important markers of a person's stage in life, clear indications of that person's readiness for marriage and reproduction as well as being a goal toward which young people strive. According to one chief:

> Once you have gone through the initiation ceremony, you are supposed to be a leader and lead by example. . . . You cannot even wear your old clothes any more after initiation. You need a new wardrobe, showing that you are a new man who is a responsible citizen. (chief, Lesotho, FGD)

Traditional leaders thought that traditions of education on sexual behavior have been undermined. Nowadays, young people are often discouraged from attending male and female initiation rites because they are seen by Westerners and modernists as backwards or infringing on individual human rights. This follows earlier disapproval of these rites by Christian missionaries in colonial times, and, more recently, by postcolonial Marxist governments, on the grounds that initiation rites perpetuated supernaturalism and "worship" of ancestral spirits (Green 1999a:108). Traditional leaders see the reestablishment of—or recommitment to—initiation rites as the first phase of redirecting society back to what they believe is a genuine, indigenous African way of living.

Traditional leaders discussed virginity testing with a considerable degree of fervor and conviction that this traditional practice is woefully misunderstood by outsiders, even educated Africans. Virginity testing worked this way: An elderly woman skilled in these matters would talk with a girl to find out if she was still a virgin, and there might be a digital examination to test the hymen. The practice was disappearing but has been revived in recent years among the Zulu and Swazi to protect girls from AIDS and other STIs by delaying sexual debut and encouraging "good behavior." The general viewpoint was that this traditional custom not only serves as a key tool of acculturation and socialization of young women but also has great potential to be used in HIV prevention. Said one female traditional leader:

> We love *Umcwasho*, the (Swazi) King's virginity promotion program. It preserves the pride of a girl. We want to revive that. But we see activists and NGOs attacking that. It is not right. (female traditional leader, Swaziland, IDI)

Respondents admitted that virginity testing can be associated with the public shame and dishonor of a girl who is found to have lost her virginity before marriage, but suggested that fear of shame and other negative sanctions might be a compelling factor to conform to tradition. Virginity testing also allows detection of rape, pedophilia, and other types of abuse and can lead to psychological and medical help for abused girls, and to the imposition of a fine on the rapist or seducer—or his family—under customary law. By South African law, virginity testing is not allowed for girls under the age of 16, which prompted one traditional leader to exclaim: "Where were Africans when this act [the Children's Act of 2005] was passed?" This points to the other side of stigma and individual rights, as discussed in Chapter 4. Regarding circumcision, traditional leaders from noncircumcising societies such as Tswana, Swazi, and Zulu for the most part knew that male circumcision was historically practiced in their societies. They also seemed quite well informed about the hygienic and HIV prevention benefits of male circumcision, as in the case of this chief:

> I heard a South African doctor say it's true that if a man is circumcised, it helps prevent AIDS. The initiation schools [used to] say, this is a

way to make you strong; it will help you avoid sexual diseases. (chief, Botswana, FGD)

One Tswana chief even seemed to have heard about the biological explanation of dendritic Langerhans cells on the foreskin providing a prime entry point for HIV. Traditional leaders in all countries seemed open to partnering with health officials in reviving—or initiating—programs of voluntary male circumcision. Some expressed concerns that male circumcision ceremonies could be unhygienic and unsafe if the same blade was used to circumcise more than one individual, facilitating the spread of HIV, although this has been a topic of AIDS education with African indigenous healers over the past 20 years (UNAIDS 2000). A traditional leader from Botswana gave the example of the recent institutionalization of male circumcision as a hospital procedure, as a way in which government and traditional leadership, or more specifically health interventions and customs, can cooperate in HIV prevention.

We [already] encourage it. Now because of HIV/AIDS transmission, you first have to go to the hospital for circumcision, then you go to the [initiation] school. In some villages the schools still exist. (chief, Botswana, IDI)

Traditional leaders also expressed their concerns about the changes they have witnessed in sexual cultures and sexual behavior. Some of these changes have been positive and necessary reactions to the risks posed by the epidemic, as noted by a traditional leader in KwaZulu-Natal.

Most people have changed because they know that they have to have one partner, not multiple partners and that when they have sex with their partner they have to use a condom. (traditional leader, KwaZulu-Natal, IDI)

In addition, traditional leaders commented that although they believe that people should behave according to traditional customs regarding sexual practice, some of these practices may not be realistic for young people today. They acknowledged that they would have to adapt their advice according to these changes in behavior and realize that in addition to promoting abstinence, they should also advocate the use of condoms if sex occurs.

Youths, you know, can go to initiation school and afterwards would want to go to a party. So I think with the youth, we just need to maybe throw them a batch [of condoms] and tell them about that and just hope that we tell them [soon enough] so that they at least "get it." (female traditional leader, Mpumalanga, South Africa, IDI)

Traditional leaders seemed well informed about the role of multiple sexual partners in driving the local HIV epidemic. However, the interviews and focus groups did not discover clear understanding of the special risk of *concurrent* partners, even though an anti-MCP campaign in Swaziland started in 2006 and one in Botswana (called "Break the Chain") was launched just months before our fieldwork there in February 2009. One Tswana chief commented that he regarded "small houses"—a euphemism for "kept women"—as part of the "evil" ways of modern society, which also included alcohol, premarital sex, rape, and a man having many sexual partners.

> It is all bad and we didn't do those things in the old days, when our initiation schools taught our African morals. The men cause the small houses, the divorce rate, and the main factor has been alcohol. Most are not married, their mobility is very high, so they can have the small houses. The unmarried also have HIV/AIDS. (chief, Botswana, IDI)

Traditional leaders were more likely to see risk in casual or occasional partners than in polygyny. Traditional leaders defended polygyny and regretted that it had been, in the words of one traditional leader, "declared something evil by Christian missionaries." He added: "But polygamy is an African custom, [found] all over." Whereas polygyny is culturally sanctioned, having casual and occasional partners is seen as a problem that has arisen from foreign influence. Most traditional leaders recognized that the practice of multiple and concurrent partnerships is a problem that will not be easily resolved. Two chiefs commented:

> 'It's difficult, because it [polygamy] is traditional. A person is just an animal; he's always thinking how can I satisfy myself? How can I get away with something that I want?' (chief, Swaziland, FGD).

> Nothing can be done. . . . If you have no self-discipline, you might get infected. But if you are self-disciplined, then (one is) not supposed to do it. It's only [by] preaching to people day and night. (chief, Swaziland, FGD)

Traditional leaders are not values neutral. They have strong opinions about what is right and wrong, African and foreign, proper and improper, and good and bad behavior. They expressed strong ideas and opinions about how to fight AIDS, primarily by reviving elements of culture such as moral codes, traditional values, and initiation rites, leading to changes in behavior. Because AIDS was often depicted as a part of a larger problem of a breakdown of family, traditional morals, values, and culture itself, it is not surprising that many discussants and respondents were strongly in favor of reviving traditional education through rites of passage or initiation "schools."

Initiation rites and rites of passage have historically been the most important platform for sexual education of young people. There is an opportunity to include innovative AIDS prevention education in these ritual occasions. In some areas, efforts have recently been made to revive them, for example, among the Swazi and Zulu. In other areas, they have been abandoned, for example among the Tswana, so there would have to be special efforts, possibly legislation, to reestablish them.

Traditional leaders may be important resources for spreading the message of the HIV risk posed by multiple and concurrent sexual partners. Beside awareness about the risks, another factor that might influence men's likelihood of having multiple sexual partners is the extent to which men are subject to traditional social control mechanisms that prohibit sex before marriage and extramarital sex, control mechanisms which come from being a member of a family, lineage, and ethnolinguistic group. In a study of men's multiple partnerships in 15 sub-Saharan African countries, Bingenheimer (2010) noted the existence of these controls and also that:

> [I]n many areas these traditional mechanisms of social control have been augmented in recent years by the growing popularity of Christian, especially Pentecostal and Charismatic, churches in Africa [Gifford 2004; Meyer 2004]. These churches have contributed to the spread in Africa of an ideology that equates personal respectability and success to behavioral adherence to a moral code that proscribes premarital sex, extramarital sex, and polygyny. (2010:3)

These social controls are also sustained by indigenous beliefs about appeasing the wishes of ancestral spirits and not offending them. Constraints on sexual behavior are implicit in indigenous theories of illness associated with sexual intercourse, such as the dangers of contamination or pollution through contact with death, funerals, or menstrual blood, or with wives who have been "protected" from extramarital sex through sorcery (*likhubalo*) (Green 1994; Murdock 1980).

There has not been much discussion of social controls in connection with sexual behavior in the AIDS literature because it is believed these have little influence today and possibly also because they are at odds with certain negative stereotypes that portray African men as operating without constraints in their pursuit of sex with multiple partners. Yet men who are more rural, less formally educated, more traditional in lifestyle, and more religious may be largely subject to the kind of social controls just mentioned. These men may also not be well reached by national mass media campaigns, so HIV prevention approaches that work through traditional leaders and local culture might have great potential.

We do not wish to idealize traditional leaders and their role in modern society, and traditional leaders themselves may idealize the past. Life was never as well ordered and regulated as often depicted by those who would like to return to a time when societies operated under time-honored familiar rules and when traditional leaders wielded more authority. Some South African anthropologists have depicted a mythical golden age in which members of the same moral or jural community behaved themselves under customary law and under the authority of the chief, and this was sometimes used to justify apartheid (Gordon 1989:46). Yet this ideal of traditional society may have the power to motivate indigenous leaders and others who still operate at least to some extent under traditional systems.

It is not clear how realistic it is to expect that traditional leaders could revive parts of the old social control system, or whether initiation rites could be reestablished in countries or societies where they are no longer practiced. Obstacles include modernization, Westernization, urbanization, party politics and democratic political systems, and the individual-centered approach to human rights and sexual freedom, which is predominant in HIV prevention. This approach can be contrasted to the set of values advocated by traditional leaders, which centers around responsibility to one's family and society. National governments are wary, at best, about ceding more power to indigenous authorities. Foreign donors and local AIDS activist groups would have to be convinced that such efforts might be worthwhile, and differences between values, approaches, and political agendas would have to be resolved. Certain pieces of national legislation, such as the Children's Act in South Africa, cited by several leaders as curtailing the rights of parents and traditional leaders (such as by outlawing virginity testing for girls under 16), would seem to present yet another obstacle.

We are not sure how to resolve this basic conflict between approaches, except to note that if we want to truly mobilize societies to fundamentally change behavior and prevent HIV, then we need to explore different types of interventions. In January 2009, the Harvard AIDS Prevention Research Project (with which we were both affiliated) sponsored a research meeting with UNAIDS and The World Bank that convened key experts in MCP-related prevention from the southern Africa region (UNAIDS 2009:13). Among the "bold actions" considered was an approach that appeals to clan and national pride (as well as personal gain) in attempting to change MCP behaviors. The regional experts present also considered the potentially constructive use of taking a values-based approach if it comes from credible local role models and leaders as well as the potentially creative use of fear-based messages in balance with messages that emphasized personal efficacy to change dangerous behaviors.

In sum, AIDS prevention in the future has much to overcome and improve on, and we see a crucial role for anthropologists to guide those who fund and direct interventions through the forest of culture, rather than around it. Recent research in southern Africa points to the need to target behaviors hitherto tiptoed around (such as multiple and concurrent partnerships) or simply ignored (such as male circumcision). Appropriate interventions in the hyper-epidemics of the region will require a certain kind of "social engineering" that addresses sensitive cultural and sexual matters. To be effective, this social engineering must be an "inside job," arising from key opinion and cultural leaders, such as traditional leaders, and then implemented with their active assistance.

We feel confident that the range and type of programs suggested by traditional leaders have potential to influence and change social norms and behaviors, in part because traditional leaders from four research countries diagnosed both problem areas and potential solutions in much the same way. Furthermore, interventions of the type recommended have scarcely ever been tried, and surely the sheer size and scope of the AIDS problem in southern Africa demands that we try every possible solution. The only wonder is—as traditional leaders themselves pointed out—that it has taken those on the donor or government side so long to try indigenous solutions that would have been available in the past, had they been sought.

As previously discussed, one reason that has been advanced to explain why HIV prevalence is so high in southern Africa is the relative late age of marriage and the high proportion of Africans who do not marry at all (Bongaarts 2007; Halperin and Epstein 2007). Evidence is clear that married women have lower HIV risk than women who are not in stable unions, as discussed in detail in Chapter 9. One idea that arose from this study is that traditional leaders could possibly lower bride-price (*lobola*) payments in their chieftaincies, thereby encouraging marriage at younger ages, which would also shorten the duration between sexual debut and first marriage. Research has shown that the longer this duration, the greater the number of sexual partners and the more likely HIV infection becomes (Bongaarts 2007). We are *not* speaking of child marriage, but rather encouraging marriage among young adults in a region where sexual debut occurs relatively late, but marriage occurs later still, if at all.

For example, Swazi men have a gap of 8.2 years between median age of first reported sex (19.5 years) and median age of first marriage (27.7 years) (Swaziland DHS 2006–07). South African women have a gap of 8.4 years between median age of first reported sex (18.6 years) and median age of first marriage (27.0 years) (South Africa DHS 2003). Among South Africans, 17.7% of women and 14.9% of men have never been married, in the oldest age cohort for which the South African 2003

DHS collected data (45–49 years for women and 55–59 years for men), and less than 30% of men and women were currently married.

Traditional leaders, like religious leaders, seem to be natural allies in potential efforts to encourage and strengthen marriage and discourage sexual behavior outside of marriage. Such an approach coincides with their values, and with their desire to see society return to where it was before the disruptions of modernity and the scourge of AIDS. Such an effort would animate and empower people who have largely remained on the sidelines, confused, unhappy, and perhaps feeling impotent, while death tolls rise and funerals accelerate in their home communities. It would direct them toward taking actions that have a chance of making a real difference.

NOTE

1. Some of the material in this section has been published in Green, Dlamini et al. 2009.

Conclusion

Where to from Here?

Building on What Has Worked

In this book, we have outlined what we believe to be an evidence-based anthropological approach to HIV prevention and have offered evidence that an AIDS prevention approach that focuses on fundamental changes in behavior can and has reduced HIV infections in real-world settings, especially in the African hyper-epidemics. We believe such a behavior-based approach also has much relevance to prevention in concentrated epidemics, as the same basic principles apply. We might summarize our proposed approach to HIV prevention by saying it is:

1. behavioral, rather than primarily technological or biomedical in nature;
2. evidence based and appropriate to the type of HIV epidemic (i.e., generalized or concentrated);
3. focused on avoiding risk, rather than solely reducing the risk of inherently risky behaviors;
4. innovative and oriented toward creative solutions that extend beyond the standard "main or common approaches" in prevention;
5. sensitive to the role of gender, including gender inequalities in sexual risk and behaviors, but does not succumb to various myths about HIV and gender;
6. cost effective and feasible; and
7. compatible with local cultures and built upon local and indigenous knowledge, structures, and leadership whenever possible, helping to ensure sustainability.

With regard to the last criterion, there are two basic approaches to development, an enterprise that includes public health and AIDS prevention. In one model, development is implemented through modern, formal structures, whether governmental or NGO. The second model

241

works through what might be called the indigenous sector. Such an approach builds on what already exists, namely indigenous knowledge, institutions, and leadership, including chiefs and traditional healers and spiritual and religious leaders. This second approach has been followed in a number of development success stories, notably in Uganda during its early, largely locally driven response to AIDS.

We recognize that there is some "Uganda fatigue" within the AIDS community, and many people are tired of hearing about Uganda's success (and various interpretations thereof). But we either learn from history or we repeat the same mistakes again and again. To summarize: Some of the distinguishing features of Uganda's prevention approach in the earlier years (1986–91) were bold leadership at the highest level and open discussion about AIDS and sexual behavior at the community level. President Museveni and others "sounded the alarm" and used fear arousal to engender perception of risk and behavioral change, particularly faithfulness and reductions in number of partners. PLHIV were involved, and AIDS-associated stigma was actively addressed. Religious leaders were brought fully on board in HIV prevention efforts. AIDS prevention focused on women and girls, and youth were especially targeted, with AIDS prevention education beginning at the primary school level. Women were empowered to be able to refuse unwanted sex and to not remain in marriages or relationships with men suspected of putting them at risk of HIV infection. During the 1990s, there was a tightening of laws concerning rape and seduction of minors (the latter known as "defilement laws"); with the result that many men started serving real prison time; and many women left marriages they thought to be dangerous, with many entering the labor market or cash economy (Carter 2003; Green 2003b; Murphy et al. 2006).

Some of these features are compatible with the prevailing Western prevention paradigm and its emphasis on human rights, such as advancing and protecting women, involving PLHIV, and fighting stigma. Other features are not compatible with Western priorities, such as use of fear appeals and involvement of faith communities. But, to reiterate, global AIDS prevention cannot continue to be driven only by those elements that we in the West approve of or favor, or by the *menus* of programs conceived and provided by the West. Regarding involving faith communities and traditional leaders in prevention, it only makes sense to work with the powers that be. This is especially true if what these leaders (religious and traditional) are "preaching" happens to be epidemiologically sound.

The Ugandan government recognized, for instance, that Catholics represented nearly 40% of the population and were major providers of treatment for PLHIV and of care and support for PLHIV, orphans, and vulnerable children. Catholics were also willing and able to effectively promote the abstain (A) and be faithful (B) components of HIV prevention, and the government realized that Catholics would be less likely to oppose condom promotion if they themselves were working collaboratively with major donors and NGOs in prevention. The Ugandan government, although not necessarily its foreign backers, also felt confident that promoting A and B behaviors was central to an effective AIDS prevention effort in Uganda.

Globally, effective HIV prevention will require this same kind of clarity about the need to fundamentally change the behaviors that spread HIV. In generalized epidemics (and we would suggest in MSM epidemics as well), this means discouraging the practice of having multiple and concurrent sexual partners, with condoms as a back-up strategy. Along with targeting adult behavior, we must discourage sexual initiation at an early age among youth and work to prevent and prosecute when necessary sexual violence such as rape, coercion, or seduction of minors.

We must put real resources into making treatment (detoxification) available to IDU as well as support programs (e.g. self-help groups) to help ex-addicts remain drug free. Such strategies should be pursued in addition to, not instead of, the distribution of needles and of substitute opioids for addicts who do not want to stop using drugs. Putting efforts into "reverse transition" from use of needles to inhalation methods for IDU and promoting serial monogamy among MSM and nonpenetrative alternatives to intercourse are other harm reduction measures that warrant attention and seem rarely to have been tried.

KEEPING AN EMPHASIS ON PREVENTION

As documented in this book, we have observed declines in HIV infections in a number of countries because of various combinations of epidemic dynamics, trends toward less risky behavior as a natural response to a deadly disease, and effective campaigns to discourage risky practices (most strikingly in Uganda). We have argued that whenever we have seen declines in HIV transmission, it has been because behaviors have fundamentally changed. In the case of Africa's heterosexually transmitted epidemics, declines in HIV have always been associated with a trend toward fewer sexual partners.

These successes notwithstanding, there is limited evidence about the effectiveness of behavior change *programs* or *interventions*. This is largely because the programs are quite new and little money has so far been spent to properly evaluate them. Yet this absence of evidence (which is not evidence of absence) has led much of the AIDS community to become profoundly discouraged about HIV prevention, especially behavioral approaches to prevention. Much of the prevention community has therefore turned its focus even more so to drug- and technology-based solutions.

In early 2010, the prevention strategy that is currently generating the greatest interest and traction is known as "test and treat," which proposes putting HIV-infected individuals on treatment as soon as they test positive. (This is opposed to the standard practice of not treating HIV-infected individuals with highly toxic and resistance-prone drugs until the onset of AIDS, which is typically 7–10 years after HIV infection.) Advocates of test and treat believe that the decreased viral loads among those who are infected but in treatment will prevent onward infections so effectively that the HIV epidemic could be ended within 5–10 years (*BBC News* 2010).

Although there is huge appeal to the idea of such a near end to AIDS (even if at great expense), the test and treat model has been controversial. It has never been tested in the real world, and some modelers have suggested that the increased viral resistance created by having people on treatment longer could lead to *increased* number of new infections (Wagner et al. 2010). We and many researchers are highly skeptical that a test and treat approach, which would require very high levels of testing and treatment adherence, would be able to overcome the huge barriers of cost, logistics, and acceptability. There are also serious concerns over the ethics of putting large numbers of people on a toxic treatment regimen that may have serious and negative health consequences for them personally—for a proposed yet uncertain population-wide prevention benefit.

Behavioral programs do not require large amounts of resources compared to interventions that rely on drugs or medical services, so we submit that the main challenge is not coming up with more money for prevention but rather orienting funds toward the *right* approaches. In 2005, while Green was a member of the Presidential Advisory Council on HIV/ AIDS (PACHA), the then CEO of Pfizer Pharmaceuticals Henry "Hank" McKinnel threw out a challenge to fellow members of PACHA. He said: "We all know we can never treat our way out of this epidemic, so let's put our heads together and figure out what we'd need to do to achieve zero percent new infections next year, *if politics and economics were not considerations.*" Green was amazed that the head of the world's largest drug company was asking the committee to think of non-drug solutions to prevention because drug solutions would not work. Green immediately seconded this suggestion and pointed out that instead of following the usual process of bringing in experts, there was already enough knowledge and experience to respond to this challenge among the membership of PACHA itself. PACHA's 36 members included scientists, physicians, gay men, HIV-positive men and women, black and Hispanic community leaders, and approximately equal numbers of men and women, progressives and conservatives, and scientists/physicians and lay persons.

The recommendations PACHA produced in response to McKinnel's challenge called for policy reforms, closer partnerships with recipient country leaders and health systems, working with and through major NGOs including FBOs, greater commitment to public health approaches, more evidence-based preventive education, increasing access to male circumcision in Africa, better data collection and reporting in order to replicate best practices, and basing prevention on proven success stories (PACHA 2005). (Uganda was the model for generalized epidemics and Thailand was the model for concentrated epidemics.) None of the recommendations was especially costly, even in an exercise where financial and political constraints could be ignored. Nor were the policy-related or political recommendations radical in any sense. The only drugs called for (in terms of HIV prevention) were for prevention of mother to child transmission, and the recommendations did not call for more approaches based on medical devices such as testing kits. There was an assumption that the United States would "maintain our commitment to those we helped place in care," but no special request for enrolling new patients in antiretroviral therapy (ART) programs. In short, all of the recommendations seemed highly achievable.

As we finish this book in early 2010, U.S. funds for global AIDS treatment programs are flatlining while the number of infected people needing ART increases. Globally, only about a third of those needing ART are receiving it (World Bank, UNAIDS 2009), and even if we suddenly acquired the means to stop new HIV infections entirely, there would still be millions of people newly in need of ART *every year* for several years to come; those needing treatment today are those who were infected 7–10 years ago. Furthermore, costs of treatment will increase as some of those currently on first-line treatment will inevitably have that treatment fail, and need more expensive second-line treatment.[1] Without curbing new infections, and in the absence of a truly massive increase in new funding for AIDS, the gap between those who need treatment and those who receive it will continue to grow rapidly and inexorably. In the words of Norman Hearst's March 2010 testimony before Congress, "We have labored to create the demand for antiretroviral treatment, and now we will inevitably find ourselves unable to satisfy that demand."[2] We must make prevention work.

A Move Toward More Evidence-Based Prevention in Africa's Hyper-Epidemics

There are encouraging signs of a movement toward more evidence-based AIDS prevention, at least in the hyper-epidemics of southern Africa. In recent years, the issue of multiple and concurrent partnerships has been an area of increasing focus in numerous meetings in the southern Africa region and in the AIDS strategies of many governments. There is a growing realization that changing patterns of multiple and concurrent sexual partnerships must be paramount and that condom promotion is not the most critical or effective intervention in these hyper-epidemics.

In January 2009, the Harvard AIDS Prevention Research Project sponsored a research meeting with UNAIDS and The World Bank that convened key experts in MCP-related prevention from the southern Africa region, including representatives from UNAIDS, World Bank, PSI, and several national HIV prevention initiatives (UNAIDS 2009). Participants reached a consensus that discouraging multiple and concurrent partnerships (MCP) must be the top prevention priority in the southern African region and that condom promotion must be secondary. As stated in a report on the meeting released by UNAIDS:

> First Priority [should be] a reduction in multiple and concurrent partnerships through social and behavioral change. . . . Second Priority [should be] a reduction in the transmission of HIV within multiple and concurrent partnerships as well as within known discordant relationships, including through consistent correct male or female condom use. (UNAIDS 2009)

The purpose of the meeting was not to debate these priorities, for which there was already consensus, but to develop action plans for immediate implementation and to review lessons learned to date from MCP programs already underway. Among the "bold actions" considered was an approach that appeals to clan and national pride (as well as personal gain) in attempting to change MCP behaviors. The regional experts present also considered the potentially creative use of fear-based messages in balance with messages that emphasized personal efficacy to change dangerous behaviors.[3] They also agreed that values-based prevention has a place in overall prevention, as long as the values are not imposed on Africans from the outside, as has too often been the case. By "values-based," we had in mind bringing chiefs and other indigenous leaders into AIDS prevention, knowing that they have their own ideas about right and wrong and about African and non-African values. The same is true for religious leaders, including not only Muslims and Christians but also leaders of indigenous religions (diviner-mediums) and African independent churches (syncretic sects blending Christian beliefs with elements of traditional religion and culture).

There is increasing acceptance by donors and NGOs of the need to work with indigenous and local leaders. Within a three-week period in early 2010, Green participated in four conferences in Swaziland and South Africa focused on MCP, male circumcision, and finding better ways to engage African culture and indigenous leaders. Three of these conferences were specifically for chiefs and "royals," traditional healers, and leaders of African independent churches, including the Zion Christian (*amazioni, mazioni*) and the Shembe churches, which allow divination and faith healing. Of all leaders that could be characterized as indigenous in southern Africa, the "Zionist" and related independent churches have probably been the most overlooked by AIDS program donors and implementers, even though they might be the numerically most powerful religious groups in the region.

One of these conferences[4] (The HIV/Culture Confluence: Changing the River's Flow), organized by the regional nonprofit organization SAFAIDS and funded by major AIDS donors (including DFID, SIDA, UNAIDS, USAID, and Oxfam), brought together NGOs and chiefs to discuss HIV, gender-based violence, and culture. There were a number of presentations showing ongoing, community-based programs that attempt to work in collaboration with local and traditional leaders to modify or change certain aspects of culture. There were fewer examples of identifying and reinforcing beliefs or practices that limit or reduce HIV transmission (namely changing risky sexual behaviors), but at least a start has been made in the right direction. PEPFAR and USAID are increasingly focusing on MCP and male circumcision in the southern African region. PSI is leading the way, at least in Botswana and Swaziland. In the former, there is a socially marketed condom with advice on the package itself to avoid MCP and to "Circumcise!" Green asked PSI/Botswana, which had played a very constructive role in the Harvard AIDS Prevention Research Project co-sponsored MCP conference in January 2009, whether both messages were also on the PSI condom promoted in Botswana. He was told, "We don't mix a condom message with our campaign to discourage MCP."[5]

Green recently met with USAID and PEPFAR officials in Swaziland and Botswana and found them very supportive of behavioral, evidence-based approaches. In some cases, they were young and relatively new in their jobs and did not seem to carry the baggage of having been personally embroiled in the bitter debates of the past over so-called abstinence-only versus condom-centered prevention approaches. Perhaps the most important explanation for what we regard as new thinking about prevention has been the failure of the Western technological and human rights approach to AIDS prevention to halt the spread of AIDS. It has been hard for even the most ardent supporters of this approach to contend that it has had an impact on HIV infection rates in southern Africa, where this last chapter is being written.

New Applications of Old Methods

The catastrophic hyper-epidemics of southern Africa are areas in which anthropologists and anthropological methods are urgently needed.

The oldest anthropological role, that of cultural expert (as discussed in Chapter 1), may, in fact, be the most important way in which anthropologists can contribute. Great strides have already been made in understanding the sexual behaviors that drive these epidemics, in particular patterns of concurrent sexual relationships. Anthropologists and others have written persuasively of the historical and cultural underpinnings of these relationships: the effect of long-term patterns of oscillatory labor migration; the economic inequality that has created desire for consumer goods that fuels many sexual relationships; cultural patterns of polygyny that have created contemporary expectations of multiple partners (among men) even when polygyny and the jural responsibilities and societal expectations that accompany it are no longer practiced; and a number of other factors that have created a unique culture of sexual relationships in southern Africa and a uniquely devastating AIDS epidemic.

We have made progress in understanding the behavioral patterns that must be addressed in the region, but we do not yet know what interventions will be effective in shifting these patterns and reducing the number of new HIV infections. We need to continue to learn about the "pressure points" that will change culturally imbedded and deeply complex behaviors such as concurrency, and how programs can leverage these pressure points. A number of governments in southern Africa have launched ambitious national-level initiatives to address MCP, including plans to evaluate those efforts. We commend these governments for their commitment to these national-level programs and hope that evaluation of these initiatives will show their effectiveness in changing behaviors and averting HIV infections.

Even more basic than learning from and evaluating the success of programs is continuing to evaluate and learn from the response of various cultures and societies to AIDS. How local communities respond to AIDS is at least as important as what programs are planned and funded by external donors. If donor interventions clash with local values, beliefs, and practices, they will have little impact. On the other hand, a very modest intervention could have major and sustained impact if communities respond as they did to Uganda's very modest (in terms of funding and technology) "zero grazing" campaign.

The irony of AIDS prevention in Africa (and probably elsewhere) is that so few AIDS programs have had an effect, whereas the successes we have seen have happened largely *without* the presence of an organized, donor-funded program. As we have seen, Uganda's pioneering approach to AIDS was centered in communities and neighbor-to-neighbor communication and did *not* come about because of any lavishly funded, high-tech effort from the AIDS industry. Kenya's success, approximately a decade after Uganda's, also seems to have been off the radar of what we can track and measure within the AIDS industry, and again we cannot take credit. Zimbabwe has been perhaps the biggest surprise of all; in a time in which the country was crumbling and Western-funded organizations were pulling out, behaviors changed and AIDS declined. Other AIDS prevention successes in Africa have been similarly mysterious; we have seen behaviors change and AIDS decline, but there is no program or initiative that can claim credit.

All of this points to the need for greater understanding and evaluation, not primarily of programs but of communities, cultures, and indigenous responses. If much of what constitutes an effective AIDS response is something beyond what we can control, a different, less choreographed approach to prevention is needed. Command prevention might work no better than "command economies." We need to look very carefully, humbly, and self-critically at how Africans and others react to interventions designed and implemented by outsiders—often, we must admit, without regard to the characteristics of that unique epidemic and culture. Unfortunately, there is little money available for monitoring those things that would be happening in communities and countries *anyway*, even without the investment of millions in AIDS money. AIDS programs are understandably motivated to demonstrate the efficacy of *their* activities, not that of community-based initiatives over which they have no control.

In our opinion, though, there is a critical need to better understand and monitor exactly those things that do not fall under the purview or radar of any particular program, but that may have more to do with the long-term trajectory of AIDS than all AIDS-industry programs put together. Such knowledge could help AIDS programs better understand the context of AIDS in a particular place and better address the behavioral and cultural factors that seem to have much more sway than externally funded programs, which are always going to be short-term and inherently have limited reach. Conversely, more study of these factors could help us know what "went right" in future AIDS successes (rather than trying to figure it out long after the fact, as in Uganda, Zimbabwe, or Kenya) and could help AIDS programs identify and support positive changes that were already happening in society.

As one example of a cultural factor that seems to be deeply enmeshed in the spread of AIDS but is rarely explored by AIDS programs, let us consider family structure. Anthropologists have much to offer in contributing to greater understanding of family structure, including changes over time and links to risky behavior and AIDS. Fragile family structure in southern Africa, particularly patterns of partner change among parents, and children growing up without one or both parents at home, has been implicated in the spread of AIDS. A 2009 report on AIDS in Swaziland produced by UNAIDS and the World Bank (NERCHA [Swaziland], UNAIDS, and World Bank) does not hesitate to identify the links between "fragile" families and behavioral norms that contribute to the epidemic. Absent and deceased parents and "fragile family structure because of migrant work patterns" are identified as factors influencing the AIDS epidemic (p. vii). The report continues:

> In Swaziland, little attention has been paid by researchers to the relationship between behavioural norms and the changing family structure and functions. . . . Studies on HIV and AIDS in Swaziland cite lack of behavioural change as the major barrier in combating the epidemic. The family remains an institution of prime importance in inculcating behavioural values, preparing the young for responsible adulthood, and giving a sense of belonging and identity to its members (p. 34). . . . However, traditional family values have been eroded by rapid urbanization and labour-related migration, leaving a void instead of an example for children to follow and learn conservative, traditional social norms for sexual behaviour. (NERCHA 2009:49)

The same report also identifies "adult choices in relationships" as creating changes in family structure, such as adults staying single longer, leading to "many single-headed households where the likelihood of concurrent multiple sexual partnerships is greater." Finally, the report calls for "reinforcing the family as a social institution" as an objective in Swaziland's response to AIDS. Although this call for a return to "family values" may strike American readers as an echo of our culture wars, this would be a false interpretation. The Swazi authors of this report, in putting forth one perspective on their country's HIV epidemic (the most severe in the world), offer explanations and solutions from within their own cultural context, a context in which changes in family structure are of great importance.

This discussion of family values and structure is similar to the perspective voiced by the indigenous leaders from southern Africa who were interviewed in the research discussed in Chapter 10. These indigenous leaders did not discuss what new technologies Americans or Europeans have come up with or how youth-friendly clinics have become. They *did* speak passionately about the erosion of traditional culture, of family structures, of respect for elders and for tradition, of men beating wives and alcohol abuse—all things they were ready to try to do something about in partnership with donor AIDS programs, if those programs were willing. The central question identified by these traditional leaders was how these problems within society and families could be fixed—for example, by confronting gender-based violence within their communities and strengthening marriages and family structure.

WHERE TO FROM HERE?

To date, far too much AIDS prevention has been based on myths, wishful thinking, and stereotypes derived from Western notions, values, attitudes, and the like and projected onto Africans and other non-Western populations. These mistaken ideas have taken on a life of their own supported by strongly held (and often unconscious and unexamined) ideologies, and as part of an entrenched paradigm that persists even in the face of ever-accumulating evidence to the contrary. With billions of dollars annually going to a single disease, perhaps it was inevitable that political agendas and ideologies would get in the way of science. The motives involved might be worthy, even noble, but if they constrain policies and programs that involve millions of human lives and billions of dollars, they must be reexamined and held up to the standard of what actually works to prevent HIV infections. There is no logical, scientific, or moral/ethical justification for overlooking risk elimination approaches based on the ideas that because not everyone can change certain behaviors, no one should be expected to change any behaviors, and that everyone has a right to engage in whatever behaviors he or she wishes, no matter how risky.

We are not arguing for a morals police, but simply for the development and implementation of interventions that inform people very clearly the true risks involved in certain behaviors, along with guidance on how to avoid potentially fatal risks. Surely it is a violation of human rights to withhold life-saving information about how to prevent a disease that is incurable and still usually fatal in the medium term for most people in the developing world.

In our view, the problem is not so much that behavioral prevention has been tried and found lacking but that it has not been seriously tried on a large scale, with resources for adequate implementation and evaluation, and with time to learn from mistakes and improve approaches. At a time when the world's massive spending for AIDS has essentially flatlined, it is more essential than ever that we reorient our efforts toward prevention and that prevention be in line with existing evidence. With investment in the careful evaluation of behavioral programs, we can develop a solid evidence base for knowing which programs and interventions work and which do not.

It is tempting to think that we are doing all we can to prevent AIDS when we improve health systems, create demand for HIV technologies and services and make them widely available and youth- and women-friendly, stock clinics with drugs and devices, and demand universal access to all that AIDS prevention dollars can buy. Such a medical services oriented approach certainly has a role in HIV prevention, but it also omits the behavioral and cultural forces that shape the epidemic.

This medical-technological approach does not require us to really understand the behaviors and norms we are trying to influence, in the ways anthropologists usually try to gain a comprehensive understanding of person, society, and culture. We should develop our thinking beyond bringing people to a clinic and providing services. How much better to facilitate risk avoidance and health promotive behavior, so that these norms take root in local communities and organizations and become locally "owned". It should be remembered that in much of rural Africa, local communities lack any sort of health facility and many people still operate within a paradigm of indigenous health knowledge and beliefs. Yet global AIDS prevention continues to be focused on the "bricks and mortar" (building facilities and providing drugs and services), rather than on issues of culture, behavior, or community.

Future historians will look back on the first quarter century of AIDS prevention and marvel how so little attention should have been given to primary prevention, to developing risk elimination strategies that address the underlying behavior itself rather than only reduce the risk. The techno-fixes that involve export of commodities from donors to recipients, from north to south, have not been effective in generalized epidemics. In these hyper-epidemics, which still account for two-thirds of all HIV infections, we must address sexual behavior head-on. In IDU and concentrated epidemics, we must similarly move beyond risk reduction *only* approaches to offer people a real choice and real support if they want to quit high-risk activities such as sex work and drug use. It is time we begin admitting what has not worked, recognize what has, and allow for a major realignment of prevention priorities (and dollars) toward behavioral solutions.

NOTES

1. A recent study from South Africa showed that second-line ART was 2.4 times as expensive as first-line treatment. Perhaps even more sobering, of the respondents in this study, only 58% remained in care and responding after 1 year; 15% were in care but not responding (to second-line ART); and 26% were no longer in care (see Long et al. 2010).

2. Hearst also warns of the ethical dilemmas that will be introduced if treatment cannot meet demand, stating:

   Remember that many PEPFAR priority countries have tremendous disparities between rich and poor, between men and women, between the capital city and rural areas. Many have poorly functioning governments and serious problems with corruption. We will need mechanisms to ensure that treatment funded by PEPFAR goes equitably to those who need it most. This will prove a tremendous challenge in countries where nothing else is distributed equitably. (Hearst 2010)

3. Self-efficacy is defined as knowing what to do to avoid unwanted or feared consequences (see Green and Witte 2006; Witte and Allen 2000).
4. The conference involved the 10 countries of southern Africa plus Senegal, and was held in Johannesburg, South Africa, April 12–13, 2010.
5. Toby Kasper, personal communicaction.

References

Abdool Karim, Q. A., S. S. Abdool Karim, J. A. Frohlich, et al. 2010. Effectiveness and safety of tenofovir gel, an antiretroviral microbicide, for the prevention of HIV infection in women. *Science*. doi:10.1126/science.1193748.

Agha, S., T. Kusanthan, K. Longfield, et al. 2002. Reasons for non-use of condoms in eight countries in sub-Saharan Africa. Washington, DC: Population Services International. http://www.aidsmark.org/resources/pdfs/sub-saharanafrica.pdf (accessed August 3, 2010).

Ahmed, S., T. Lutalo, M. Wawer, et al. 2001. HIV incidence and sexually transmitted disease prevalence associated with condom use: A population study in Rakai, Uganda. *AIDS* 15:2171–79.

AIDS and Anthropology Research Group (AARG). 2003. AIDS Prevention and Paradigms: An Electronic Discussion. http://groups.creighton.edu/aarg/prevention.html (accessed August 6, 2010).

Allen, A. 2002. Sex change; Uganda v. condoms. *The New Republic* May 27:14–15.

Allen, S., J. Meinzen-Derr, M. Kautzman, et al. 2003. Sexual behavior of HIV discordant couples after HIV counseling and testing. *AIDS* 17:733–40.

Allen, S., J. Tice, P. Van de Perre, et al. 1992. Effect of serotesting with counselling on condom use and seroconversion among HIV discordante couples in Africa. *British Medical Journal* 304:1605–9.

Allen, T. and S. Heald. 2004. HIV/AIDS policy in Africa: What has worked in Uganda and what has failed in Botswana. *Journal of International Development* 16:1141–54.

Altman, L. 2004. HIV risk greater for young African brides. *New York Times*, February 29. http://www.nytimes.com/2004/02/29/world/hiv-risk-greater-for-young-african-brides.html (accessed August 2, 2010).

Among, B. 2009. How Museveni fell out with Colonel Gadaffi. *Sunday Vision* (Kampala, Uganda), September 29, p. 1.

Amory, D. n.d. Society of Lesbian and Gay Anthropologists: A brief history. http://www.uvm.edu/~dlrh/solga/history.html (accessed March 12, 2010).

Anema, A., M. R. Joffres, E. Mills, and P. B. Spiegel. 2008. Widespread rape does not directly appear to increase the overall HIV prevalence in conflict-affected countries: So now what? *Emerging Themes in Epidemiology* 5. doi:10.1186/1742-7622-5-11.

Ankrah, E. M. 1992. AIDS in Uganda: Initial social work responses. *Journal of Social Development in Africa* 7:53–61.

Arroyo, M. A., W. B. Sateren, D. Serwadda, et al. 2006. Higher HIV-1 incidence and genetic complexity along main roads in Rakai District, Uganda. *Journal of Acquired Immune Deficiency Syndromes* 43:440–45.

Auvert, B. 2002. UNAIDS multi-site study analysis. In *The "ABC" of HIV Prevention: Report of a USAID Technical Meeting on Behavior Change Approaches to Primary Prevention of HIV/AIDS*, p. 3. Washington, DC: USAID.

Auvert, B., A. Buvé, E. Lagarde, et al. 2001. Male circumcision and HIV infection in four cities in sub-Saharan Africa. *AIDS* 15:S31–S40.

Auvert, B. and B. Ferry. 2002. Modeling the spread of HIV infection in four cities of sub-Saharan Africa. In *"ABC" Experts Technical Meeting*. Washington, DC: International Conference of AIDS.

Auvert, B., D. Taljaard, E. Lagarde, et al. 2005. Randomized, controlled intervention trial of male circumcision for reduction of HIV infection risk: The ANRS 1265 trial. *PLoS Medicine* 2:298.

Ayittey, G. 2006a. A broken and dysfunctional continent. Washington, DC: The Free Africa Foundation. http://www.freeafrica.org/president.htm (accessed August 3, 2010).

Ayittey, G. 2006b. *Indigenous African Institutions*. Ardsley, NY: Transnational Publishers.

Baer, H. A. 1997. The misconstruction of critical medical anthropology: A response to a cultural constructivist critique. *Social Science & Medicine* 44:1568.

Baer, H. A., M. Singer, and I. Susser. 2003. *Medical Anthropology and the World System*. Westport, CT: Praeger.

Baeten, J., D. Donnell, M. Inambao, et al. 2009. Male circumcision and male-to-female HIV-1 transmission risk: A multinational prospective study. Program and abstracts of the 5th International AIDS Society Conference on HIV Pathogenesis, Treatment and Prevention, July 19–22. Abstract LBPEC06. Cape Town, South Africa.

Bailey, R. C., S. Moses, C. B. Parker, et al. 2007. Male circumcision for HIV prevention in young men in Kisumu, Kenya: A randomised controlled trial. *The Lancet* 369:643–56.

Bailey, R. C., F. A. Plummer, and S. Moses. 2001. Male circumcision and HIV prevention: Current knowledge and future research directions. *The Lancet Infectious Diseases* 1:223–31.

Ball, J. C. and C. D. Chambers. 1970. *The Epidemiology of Opiate Addiction in the United States*. Springfield, IL: Charles C. Thomas.

Bancroft, J. 2004. Alfred C. Kinsey and the politics of sex research. *Annual Review of Sex Research* 15:1–39.

Bannerman, R. H., J. Burton, and C. Wen-Chieh. 1983. *Traditional Medicine and Health Care Coverage*. Geneva: WHO.

Baryarama, F., R. Bunnell, W. McFarland, et al. 2007. Estimating HIV incidence in voluntary counseling and testing clients in Uganda (1992–2003). *Journal of Acquired Immune Deficiency Syndromes* 44:99–105.

BBC News. 2010. Anti-retrovirals could halt AIDS spread in five years. February 21. http://news.bbc.co.uk/2/hi/8526690.stm (accessed July 31, 2010).

Beadnell, B., S. A. Baker, D. M. Morrison, and K. Knox. 2000. HIV/STD risk factors for women with violent male partners. *Sex Roles* 42:661–89.

Bello, G. A., J. Chipeta, and J. Aberle-Grasse. 2006. Assessment of trends in biological and behavioural surveillance data: Is there any evidence of declining HIV prevalence or incidence in Malawi? *Sexually Transmitted Infections* 82(Suppl_I):i9–i13. doi: 10.1136/sti.2005.0.

Bessinger, R., P. Akwara, and D. Halperin. 2003. *Sexual behavior, HIV and fertility trends: A comparative analysis of six countries; Phase I of the ABC Study.*

Measure Evaluation, USAID. http://www.cpc.unc.edu/measure/publications/pdf/sr-03-21b.pdf (accessed July 30, 2010).

Bingenheimer, J. B. 2010. Men's multiple sexual partnerships in 15 sub-Saharan African countries: Socio-demographic patterns and implications. *Studies in Family Planning* 41:1–17.

Boily, M-C., R. F. Baggaley, L. Wang, et al. 2009. Heterosexual, risk of HIV-1 infection per sexual act: Systematic review and meta-analysis of observational studies. *The Lancet Infectious Diseases* 9:118–29.

Bolin, A. and P. Whelehan. 2004. *Perspectives on Human Sexuality*. Boston: McGraw-Hill.

Bolton, R. 1992. AIDS and promiscuity: Muddles in the models of IV prevention. *Medical Anthropology* 14:168.

Bond, G. and J. Vincent. 1997. AIDS in Uganda: The first decade. In *AIDS in Africa and the Caribbean*, G. Bond, J. Kreniske, I. Susser, and J. Vincent, eds., pp. 85–97. Boulder, CO: Westview.

Bongaarts, J. 2006. Late marriage and the HIV epidemic in sub-Saharan Africa. *Policy Research Division Working Paper* No. 216. New York: Population Council. http://www.popcouncil.org/pdfs/wp/216.pdf (accessed July 26, 2010).

Bongaarts, J. 2007. Late marriage and the HIV epidemic in sub-Saharan Africa. *Population Studies* 61:73–83.

Bongaarts, J., P. Reining, P. Way, et al. 1989. The relationship between male circumcision and HIV infection in African populations. *AIDS* 3:373–77.

Boster, F. J. and Mongeau, P. 1984. Fear-arousing persuasive messages. In *Communication Yearbook* 8, R. N. Bostrom, and B. H. Westley, eds., pp. 330–75. Newbury Park, CA: Sage.

Brenner, B. G., M. Roger, J. P. Routy, et al. 2007. High rates of forward transmission events after acute/early HIV-1 infection. *Journal of Infectious Diseases* 195:951–59.

Brown, K., R. Burdon, K. Casey, et al. 2007. *Treatment and Care for HIV Positive Injecting Drug Users: Drug Use and HIV in Asia Participant Guide*. Jakarta: The Association of Southeast Asian Nations and Family Health International.

Bruneau, J., F. Lamothe, E. Franco, et al. 1997. High rates of HIV infection among injection drug users participating in needle exchange programs in Montreal: Results of a cohort study. *American Journal of Epidemiology* 146:994–1002.

Buchbinder, S. P., J. M. Douglas, Jr., D. J. McKirnan et al. 1996. Feasibility of human immunodeficiency virus vaccine trials in homosexual men in the United States: Risk behavior, seroincidence, and willingness to participate. *Journal of Infectious Diseases* 174:954–61.

Buckingham, R. and E. Meister. 2003. Condom utilization among female sex workers in Thailand: Assessing the value of the health belief model. *Californian Journal of Health Promotion* 4:18–23.

Bunnell, R. E. and P. Cherutich. 2008. Universal HIV testing and counselling in Africa. *The Lancet* 371:2149–50.

Bunnell, R. E., J. Nassozi, E. Marum, et al. 2005. Living with discordance: Knowledge, challenges, and prevention strategies of HIV-discordant couples in Uganda. *AIDS Care* 17:999–1012.

Busulwa, W. R. 1995. Abstinence for AIDS control: A study of adolescents in Jinja District. Dissertation submitted as partial fulfillment for the award of the degree of Master of Medicine (community practice), of Makerere University, Kampala, Uganda.

Buve, A., M. Caraël, R. Hayes, et al. 2001. Multicentre study on factors determining differences in rate of spread of HIV in sub-Saharan Africa: Methods and prevalence of HIV infection. *AIDS* Suppl_15:S5–S14.

Cáceres, C., K. Konda, M. Pecheny, et al. 2006. Estimating the number of men who have sex with men in low and middle income countries. *Sexually Transmitted Infections* 82:Siii3–Siii9.

Cahn, P. 2008. Opening session. Paper read at the 17th International AIDS Conference at Mexico City, Mexico City, August 3.

Caldwell, J. and P. Caldwell. 1993. The nature and limits of the sub-Saharan African AIDS epidemic: Evidence from geographic and other patterns. *Population and Development Review* 19:817–48.

Caldwell, J., P. Caldwell, and P. Quiggin. 1989. The social context of AIDS in sub-Saharan Africa. *Population and Development Review* 15:185–234.

Campbell, J. C. 2002. Health consequences of intimate partner violence. *The Lancet* 359:1331–36.

Caraël, M. 1994a. Pre-marital sexual behaviour in the developing world: Results of 17 AIDS-related surveys. International Conference on AIDS, August 7–12.

Caraël, M. 1994b. The impact of marriage change on the risks of exposure to sexually transmitted diseases in Africa. In *Nuptiality in Sub-Saharan Africa: Contemporary Anthropological and Demographic Perspectives*, C. Bledsoe and G Pison, eds., pp. 255–73. Oxford: Clarendon Press.

Caraël, M. 2006. Twenty years of intervention and controversy. In *The HIV/ AIDS Epidemic in Sub-Saharan Africa in a Historical Perspective*, P. Denis and C. Becker, eds., pp. 30–39. Online edition. Réseau sénégalais "Droit, éthique, santé"/Senegalese Network "Law, Ethics, Health," October.

Caraël, M., M. Ali, and J. Cleland. 2001. Nuptiality and risk behaviour in Lusaka and Kampala. *African Journal of Reproductive Health* 5:83–89.

Caraël, M. and K. Holmes. 2001. Dynamics of HIV epidemics in sub-Saharan Africa: Introduction. *AIDS* Suppl_4:S1–S4.

Carpenter, L. M., A. Kamali, A. Ruberantwari, et al. 1999. Rates of HIV-1 transmission within marriage in rural Uganda in relation to the HIV sero-status of the partners. *AIDS* 13:1083–89.

Carter, R. W. 2003. Uganda leads by example on AIDS. *Washington Times*, August 28, p. A13.

Carton, B. 2003. The forgotten compass of death: Apocalypse then and now in the social history of South Africa. *Journal of Social History* 37:199–218.

Carton, B. 2006. Historicizing the unspeakable: Legacies of bad death and dangerous sexuality in South Africa. In *Historical Perspectives on HIV/AIDS: Lessons from South Africa and Senegal: The HIV/AIDS Epidemic in Sub-Saharan Africa in a Historical Perspective*, P. Denis and C. Becker, eds., pp. 97–112. Online edition. Réseau sénégalais "Droit, éthique, santé"/Senegalese Network "Law, Ethics, Health," October.

Celentano, D. D., K. E. Nelson, C. M. Lyles, et al. 1998. Decreasing incidence of HIV and sexually transmitted diseases in young Thai men: Evidence for success of the HIV/AIDS control and prevention program. *AIDS* 12:F29–F36.

Celum, C., A. Wald, J. R. Lingappa, et al. for the Partners in Prevention HSV/ HIV Transmission Study Team. 2010. Acyclovir and transmission of HIV-1 for persons infected with HIV-1 and HSV-2. *New England Journal of Medicine.* doi: 10.1056/NEJMoa0904849.

Centers for Disease Control (CDC). 2008. Trends in HIV/AIDS diagnoses among men who have sex with men—33 States, 2001–2006. *Morbidity and Mortality Weekly Report* 57(25):681–86.

Centers for Disease Control (CDC). 2009. *Sexually Transmitted Disease Surveillance, 2008.* Atlanta, GA: U.S. Department of Health and Human Services. November.

Central Statistical Office (CSO) [Botswana]. 2005. *The Botswana AIDS Impact Survey II, 2004.* Gaborone: Central Statistical Office.

Central Statistical Office (CSO) [Swaziland], and Macro International Inc. 2008. *Swaziland Demographic and Health Survey 2006–07.* Mbabane, Swaziland: Central Statistical Office and Macro International Inc.

Central Statistical Office (CSO), Ministry of Health (MoH), Tropical Diseases Research Centre (TDRC), University of Zambia, and Macro International Inc. 2009. *Zambia Demographic and Health Survey 2007.* Calverton, Maryland, USA: CSO and Macro International Inc.

Chamberlain, E. 2009. Harm reduction and pleasure maximisation—are they the same thing? International HIV/AIDS Alliance. http://www.ahrn.net/index.php?option=content&task=view&id=2824 (accessed July 30, 2010).

Chambers, D. L. 1994. Gay men, AIDS, and the code of the condom. *Harvard Civil Rights—Civil Liberties Law Review* 29:353–85.

Check, E. 2006. HIV infection in Zimbabwe falls at last. *BioEd Online,* February 2. http://www.bioedonline.org/ncws/news.cfm?art=2318 (accessed March 2, 2006).

Chen, L., P. Jha, B. Stirling, et al. 2007. Sexual risk factors for HIV infection in early and advanced HIV epidemics in sub-Saharan Africa: Systematic overview of 68 epidemiological studies. *PLoS ONE* 2:e1001. doi:10.1371/journal.pone.0001001.

Chimbiri, A. M. 2007. The condom is an 'intruder' in marriage: Evidence from rural Malawi. *Social Science & Medicine* 64:1102–15.

Chin, J. 2007. *The AIDS Pandemic: The Collision of Epidemiology with Political Correctness.* Oxford: Radcliffe Publishing.

Choi, K.-H., D. Binson, M. Adelson, and J. A. Catania. 1998. Sexual harassment, sexual coercion, and HIV risk among US adults 18–49 years. *AIDS and Behavior* 2:33–40.

Clark, S. 2004. Early marriage and HIV risks in sub-Saharan Africa. *Studies in Family Planning* 35:149–60.

Clark, S., J. Bruce, and A. Dude. 2006. Protecting young women from HIV/AIDS: The case against child and adolescent marriage. *International Family Planning Perspectives* 32:79–88.

Coghlan, A. 2009. First HIV vaccine trial success confirmed. *New Scientist,* October 20. http://www.newscientist.com/article/dn18011-first-hiv-vaccine-trial-success-confirmed.html (accessed July 22, 2010).

Cohen, J. 2005a. Prevention cocktails: Combining tools to stop HIV's spread. *Science* 309:1002–5.

Cohen, J. 2005b. The less they know, the better: Abstinence-only HIV/AIDS programs in Uganda. Human Rights Watch. http://www.hrw.org/reports/2005/uganda0305/ (accessed July 30, 2010).

Cohen, J. 2010. At last, vaginal gel scores victory against HIV. *Science* 329:374–75. doi:10.1126/science.329.5990.374.

Cohen, J., R. Schleifer, and T. Tate. 2005. AIDS in Uganda: The human-rights dimension. *The Lancet* 365:2075–76.

Committee on the Prevention of HIV Infection among Injecting Drug Users in High-risk Countries. 2006. *Preventing HIV Infection among Injecting Drug Users in High Risk Countries: An Assessment of the Evidence.* Washington, DC: Institute of Medicine.

Conant, F. P. 1988. Evaluating social science relating to AIDS in Africa. In *AIDS in Africa: The Social and Policy Impact*, N. Miller and R. Rockwell, eds., pp. 197–209. New York: Mellen Press and the National Council for International Health.

Corbett, L. E., B. Makamure, Y. B. Cheung, et al. 2007. HIV incidence during a cluster-randomized trial of two strategies providing voluntary counselling and testing at the workplace, Zimbabwe. *AIDS* 21:483–89.

Creese, A., K. Floyd, A. Alban, et al. 2002. Cost-effectiveness of HIV/AIDS interventions in Africa: A systematic review of the evidence. *The Lancet* 359:1635–42.

Cremin, I., C. Nyamukapa, L. Sherr, et al. 2010. Patterns of self-reported behavior change associated with receiving voluntary counselling and testing in a longitudinal study from Manicaland, Zimbabwe. *AIDS and Behavior* 14:708–15.

Cunningham, R. M., A. R. Stiffman, P. Dore, and F. Earls. 1994. The association of physical and sexual abuse with HIV risk behaviors in adolescence and young adulthood: Implications for public health. *Child Abuse and Neglect* 18:233–45.

Dalrymple, T. 2000. All sex, all the time. *City Journal*, Summer 2000. http://www.city-journal.org/html/10_3_urbanities-all_sex.html (accessed March 17, 2010).

Danielson, K., T. E. Moffitt, A. Caspi, and P. A. Silva. 1998. Comorbidity between abuse of an adult and DSM-III-R mental disorders: Evidence from an epidemiological study. *American Journal of Psychiatry* 155:131–33.

Davis, D. L. and R. G. Whitten. 1987. The cross-cultural study of human sexuality. *Annual Review of Anthropology* 16:69.

Davis, K. R., and S. C. Weller. 1999. The effectiveness of condoms in reducing heterosexual transmission of HIV. *Family Planning Perspectives* 31(6):272–79.

De Bruyn, M., H. Jackson, M. Wijermars, et al. 1995. *Facing the Challenges of HIV, AIDS, STDs: A Gender-Based Response.* Amsterdam: Royal Tropical Institute Southern Africa AIDS Information Dissemination Service World Health Organization, Global Programme on AIDS.

Delamater, J. D. and J. Shibley Hyde. 1998. Essentialism vs. social constructionism in the study of human sexuality. *The Journal of Sex Research* 35:10–18.

DeLay, P. 2008. Tailoring AIDS prevention (letter). *Science* 321:1631.

Denis, P. 2006. Towards a social history of HIV/AIDS in sub-Saharan Africa. In *The HIV/AIDS Epidemic in Sub-Saharan Africa in a Historical Perspective*, P. Denis and C. Becker eds., pp. 13–26. Online edition. Réseau sénégalais "Droit, éthique, santé"/Senegalese Network "Law, Ethics, Health," October.

Denison, J. A., K. R. O'Reilly, G. P. Schmid, et al. 2008. HIV counseling and testing, and behavioral risk reduction in developing countries: A meta-analysis, 1990–2005. *AIDS and Behavior* 12:363–73.

de Walque, D. 2007. Sero-discordant couples in five African countries: Implications for prevention strategies. *Population & Development Review* 33:501–23.

de Walque, D. and R. Kline. 2009. *Comparing Condom Use with Different Types of Partners: Evidence from National HIV Surveys in Africa (Policy Research Working Paper 5130).* Washington, DC: The World Bank.

Des Jarlais, D., C. Casriel, S. R. Friedman, et al. 1992. AIDS and the transition to illicit drug injection—results of a randomized trial prevention program. *British Journal of Addiction* 87:493–98.

Douglas, M. 1992 [1966]. *Purity and Danger: An Analysis of Concepts of Pollution and Taboo.* London: Routledge and Kegan Paul.

Dover, K. J. 1978. *Greek Homosexuality.* Cambridge: Harvard University Press.

Drain, P. K., D. T. Halperin, J. P. Hughes, et al. 2006. Male circumcision, religion, and infectious diseases: An ecological analysis of 118 developing countries. *BMC Infectious Diseases* 6:172. doi:10.1186/1471-2334-6-172.

Duh, S. V. 1991. *Blacks and AIDS: Causes and Origins.* London: Sage.

Dunkle, K. L., R. K. Jewkes, H. C. Brown, et al. 2004a. Gender-based violence, relationship power, and risk of HIV infection in women attending antenatal clinics in South Africa. *The Lancet* 363:1415–21.

Dunkle, K. L., R. K. Jewkes, H. C. Brown, et al. 2004b. Transactional sex among women in Soweto, South Africa: Prevalence, risk factors, and association with HIV infection. *Social Science & Medicine* 59:1581–92.

Dunkle, K. L., R. Jewkes, M. Nduna, et al. 2007. Transactional sex with casual and main partners among young South African men in the rural Eastern Cape: Prevalence, predictors, and associations with gender-based violence. *Social Science & Medicine* 65:1235–48.

Dunkle, K. L., R. Stephenson, E. Karita, et al. 2008. New heterosexually transmitted HIV infections in married or cohabiting couples in urban Zambia and Rwanda: An analysis of survey and clinical data. *The Lancet* 371:2183–91.

Easterly, W. 2006. *The White Man's Burden: Why the West's Efforts to Aid the Rest Have Done So Much Ill and So Little Good.* New York: Penguin Press.

Echenberg, M. 2006. Historical perspectives on HIV/AIDS: Lessons from South Africa and Senegal. In *The HIV/AIDS Epidemic in Sub-Saharan Africa in a Historical Perspective*, P. Denis and C. Becker, eds., pp. 89–96. Published Online at Academia-Bruylant (Louvain-la-Neuve) and Karthala (Paris).

Elovich, R. 1998. Four percent and counting. *The Body: The Complete HIV/AIDS Resource*, Feburary. http://www.thebody.com/content/whatis/art31016.html (accessed July 27, 2010).

Elovich, R. and E. Drucker. 2008. On drug treatment and social control: Russian narcology's great leap backwards. *Harm Reduction Journal* 5:23. doi:10.1186/1477-7517-5-23. http://www.harmreductionjournal.com/content/5/1/23 (accessed July 27, 2010).

Emrick, C. D., J. S. Toniga, and H. Montgomery. 1993. Alcoholics Anonymous: What is currently known? In *Research on Alcoholics Anonymous: Opportunities and alternatives*, B. S. McCrady and W. R. Miller, eds., pp. 41–76. New Brunswick, NJ: Rutgers University Press.

Epstein, H. 2007. *The Invisible Cure: Africa, the West and the Fight against AIDS.* New York: Farrar Straus & Giroux/Macmillan.

Family Health International. 1996. *AIDS Control and Prevention Project: Final Report for the AIDSCAP Program in Thailand November 1991 to September 1996.* http://www.fhi.org/en/HIVAIDS/pub/Archive/aidscapreports/finalreportAIDSCAPthailand/index.htm (accessed January 3, 2010).

Farley, M. 2004. Bad for the body, bad for the heart: Prostitution harms women even if legalized or decriminalized. *Violence against Women* 10:1087–125.

Farley, M. 2006. Prostitution, trafficking, and cultural amnesia: What we must not know in order to keep the business of sexual exploitation running smoothly. *Yale Journal of Law and Feminism* 18:109–44.

Farley, M. and S. Seo. 2006. Prostitution and trafficking in Asia. *Harvard Asia Pacific Review* 8:9–12.

Farmer, P. 1996. On suffering and structural violence: A view from below. *Daedalus* 125.

Farmer, P. 2003. AIDS: A biosocial problem with social solutions. *Anthropology News.* http://www.stwr.org/health-education-shelter/dialogue-on-aids-prevention.html (accessed March 1, 2010).

Fauci, A. 2009. A policy cocktail for fighting HIV. *Washington Post*, April 16. http://www.washingtonpost.com/wp-dyn/content/article/2009/04/15/AR2009041503040.html (accessed August 6, 2010).

Feldman, D. 2004. Creating a viable AIDS program for Africa: Condoms, condoms, and more condoms. Paper presented at the 2004 Society for Applied Anthropology meeting, Dallas, Texas, March 31–April 4, 2004. http://www.sfaa.net/sfaa2004/SfAA2004Program.pdf http://groups.creighton.edu/aarg/ewsletter/aarg_vol_16_no_2.pdf (accessed January 17, 2010).

Foulkes, J. R. 1992. Traditional health workers [letter]. *Tropical Doctor* 22:121–22.

Freeman, D. 1986. *Margaret Mead and Samoa: The Making and Unmaking of an Anthropological Myth.* Cambridge, MA: Harvard University Press.

Freeman, M. and M. Motsei. 1990. Is there a role for traditional healers in health care in South Africa? The Center for the Study of Health Policy, Department of Community Health, University of the Witwatersrand, Paper No. 20, Johannesburg.

Fumento, M. 1990. *The Myth of Heterosexual AIDS.* New York: Basic Books.

Garcia-Moreno, C., H. Jansen, M. Ellsberg, et al. 2005. WHO Multi-country study on women's health and domestic violence against women: Initial results on prevalence, health outcomes, and women's responses. Geneva: World Health Organization.

Gates, M. F. 2006. What women really need. *Newsweek*, May 15. http://www.newsweek.com/id/47744 (accessed July 28, 2010).

Gausset, Q. 2001. AIDS and cultural practices in Africa: The case of the Tonga (Zambia). *Social Science & Medicine* 52:509–18.

Gelfand, M., S. Mavi, R. B. Drummond, and B. Ndemera. 1985. *The Traditional Medical Practitioner in Zimbabwe.* Harare: Mambo Press.

General Assembly. 2001. *Declaration of Commitment on HIV/AIDS.* Special Session 26, S-26/2. Agenda item 8, points 11, 13, 14, 16.

Genuis, S. J. and S. K. Genuis. 2005. HIV/AIDS prevention in Uganda: Why has it worked? *Postgraduate Medical Journal* 81:615–17.

George, E. R. 2007. Virgin territory: Virginity testing as HIV/AIDS prevention: Human rights universalism and cultural relativism revisited. Social Science Research Network Working Paper, 2007. http://ssrn.com/abstract=995851 (accessed September 30, 2009).

Giddens, A. and M. Duneier. 2000. *Introduction to Sociology.* 3rd ed. New York: W. W. Norton.

Gifford, P. 2004. Persistence and change in contemporary African religion. *Social Compass* 51:169–76.

Gilbert, L., N. El-Bassel, R. F. Schilling, et al. 2000. Partner violence and sexual HIV risk behaviors among women in methadone treatment. *AIDS and Behavior* 4:261–69.

Gillespie, S., S. Kadiyala, and R. Greener. 2007. Is poverty or wealth driving HIV transmission? *AIDS* 21(Suppl_7):S5–S16.

Glick, P. 2005. *Scaling up HIV voluntary counseling and testing in Africa: What can evaluation studies tell us about potential prevention impacts?* Strategies and Analysis for Growth and Access (SAGA) Working Paper. Ithaca, NY: Cornell University.

Global HIV Prevention Working Group. 2008a. *Behavior Change and HIV Prevention: (Re)Considerations for the 21ˢᵗ Century*. Global HIV Prevention, August. http://www.globalhivprevention.org/pdfs/PWG_Executive%20Summary_FINAL.pdf (accessed July 30, 2010).

Global HIV Prevention Working Group. 2008b. *Bringing HIV Prevention to Scale: An Urgent Global Priority—Press Release*. Global HIV Prevention, August 5. http://www.globalhivprevention.org/pdfs/PWG_Executive%20Summary_FINAL.pdf (accessed July 30, 2010).

Gluckman, M. 1956. *Custom and Conflict in Africa*. New York: Barnes and Noble.

Glynn, J. R., M. Caraël, B. Auvert, et al. 2001. Why do young women have a much higher prevalence of HIV than young men? A study in Kisumu, Kenya and Ndola, Zambia. *AIDS* 15(Suppl_4):S51–S60.

Glynn, J. R., M. Caraël, A. Buvé, et al. 2003. HIV risk in relation to marriage in areas with high prevalence of HIV infection. *Journal of Acquired Immune Deficiency Syndromes* 33:526–35.

Good, C. M. 1987. *Ethnomedical Systems in Africa: Patterns of Traditional Medicine in Rural and Urban Kenya*. New York: Guilford Press.

Gordon, R. 1989. The Ehie Man's burden: Ersatz customary law and internal pacification in South Africa. *Journal of Historical Sociology* 2:13.

Gorna, R. 1996. *Vamps, Virgins and Victims: How Can Women Fight AIDS?* London: Cassell.

Gourvenec, D., N. Taruberekera, O. Mochaka, and T. Kasper. 2007. *Multiple Concurrent Partnerships among Men and Women Aged 15–34 in Botswana: Baseline Study*. Population Services International (PSI) Botswana: PSI.

Gouws, E., K. A. Stanecki, R. Lyerla, and P. D. Ghys. 2008. The epidemiology of HIV infection among young people aged 15–24 years in southern Africa. *AIDS* 22(Suppl_4):S5–S16.

Government of Uganda, National Resistance Movement Secretariat. 1988. *Control of AIDS: Action for Survival*. Kampala, Uganda, p. 33.

Gowan, A. and P. Reining. 1988. Resource guide to non-governmental organizations concerned with AIDS in Africa based in North America. In *AIDS in Africa: The Social and Policy Impact*, N. Miller and R. Rockwell, eds., pp. 311–26. New York: Mellen Press.

Gray, G. and T. Page. 2009. International Network of People Who Use Drugs (INPUD). *An Overview of Advocacy Activities*. http://www.worldaidscampaign.org/en/content/download/87626/865174/file/INPUDAdvocacyReportPrintingFinal.pdf (accessed August 6, 2010).

Gray, R., G. Kigozi, D. Serwadda, et al. 2007. Male circumcision for HIV prevention in men in Rakai, Uganda: A randomized trial. *The Lancet* 369:657–66.

Gray, R., N. Kiwanuka, T. C. Quinn, et al. 2000. Male circumcision and HIV acquisition and transmission: Cohort studies in Rakai, Uganda. *AIDS* 14: 2371–78.

Gray, R. H., D. Serwadda, G. Kigozi, et al. 2006. Uganda's HIV prevention success: The role of sexual behavior change and the national response. *AIDS and Behavior* 10:347–50.

Gray, R. and M. Wawer. 2008a. Reassessing the hypothesis on STI control for HIV prevention. *The Lancet* 371:2064–65.

Gray, R. and M. Wawer. 2008b. Control of sexually transmitted infections for HIV prevention—Authors' reply. *The Lancet* 372:1297–98.

Greeley, E. 1988. The role of non-governmental organizations in AIDS prevention: Parallels to African family planning activity. In *AIDS in Africa: The Social and Policy Impact*, N. Miller and R. Rockwell, eds., 175–96. New York: Mellen Press and the National Council for International Health.

Green, E. C. 1986. Themes in the practice of development anthropology. In *Practicing Development Anthropology*, E. C. Green, ed., pp. 1–9. Boulder, CO: Westview.

Green, E. C. 1988. AIDS in Africa: An agenda for behavioral scientists. In *AIDS in Africa: The Social and Policy Impact*, N. Miller and R. Rockwell (eds.), pp. 175–96. New York: Mellen Press and the National Council for International Health.

Green, E. C., T. Tomas and A. Jurg. 1991. A Program in Public Health and Traditional Health Manpower in Mozambique. Mozambique Ministry of Health and the European Community. Maputo, March 30. (English and Portuguese versions available). Summary at http://www.hst.org.za/update/37/policy2.htm (accessed March 10, 2010).

Green, E. C. 1992a. The anthropology of sexually transmitted diseases in Liberia. *Social Science & Medicine* 35:1459.

Green, E. C. 1992b. Women's groups and income generation in Swaziland. *Practicing Anthropology* 14:19–23.

Green, E. C., ed. 1993. The involvement of African traditional healers in the prevention of AIDS and STDs. In *Anthropology in Public Health: Bridging Differences in Culture and Society*, R. A. Hahn, ed., pp. 63–83. New York: Oxford University Press.

Green, E. C. 1994. *AIDS and STDs in Africa: Bridging the Gap between Traditional Healing and Modern Medicine*. Boulder, CO: Westview.

Green, E. C. 1998. Report on the situation of AIDS and the role of IEC in Uganda. Entebbe, Uganda: Ministry of Health; Reston, VA: Social Impact.

Green, E. C. 1999a. *Indigenous Theories of Contagious Disease*. Lanham, MD: AltaMira.

Green, E. C. 1999b. The involvement of African traditional healers in the prevention of AIDS and STDs. In *Anthropology in Public Health: Bridging Differences in Culture and Society*, R. A. Hahn, ed., pp. 63–83. New York: Oxford University Press.

Green, E. C. 2000. African men, circumcision, HIV/AIDS and anthropology. Paper presented at the American Anthropological Association Annual Meeting, November 18. http://www.stwr.org/africa/african-men-circumcision-hiv/aids-and-anthropology.html (accessed July 31, 2010).

Green, E. C. 2003a. Faith-based organizations: Contributions to HIV prevention. Washington, DC: USAID/Washington and The Synergy Project, TvT Associates, Washington, DC. http://www.usaid.gov/our_work/global_health/aids/TechAreas/community/fbo.pdf (accessed July 30, 2010).

Green, E. C. 2003b. *Rethinking AIDS Prevention*. Westport, CT: Praeger.

Green, E. C. 2004a. Indigenous or Western responses to African AIDS? In *Indigenous Knowledge: Local Pathways to Global Development*, R. Woytek, P. Shroff-Mehta, and P. C. Mohan, eds., p. 18. Washington, DC: World Bank, Africa Region Knowledge and Learning Center.

Green, E. C. 2004b. Youth, empowerment and support: The YES! Project, Final evaluation. Washington, DC: Africare and the Bill and Melinda Gates Foundation. http://www.usaid.gov/our_work/global_health/aids/TechAreas/community/fbo.pdf (accessed July 26, 2010).

Green, E. C. 2009. Risk elimination and harm reduction in AIDS prevention. *Russian Journal of AIDS, Cancer and Public Health* 13:33–56.

Green, E. C. n.d. Field notes from Senegal and The Gambia, January 2007. Unpublished.

Green, E. C., C. Dlamini, Z. Duby, et al. 2009. Mobilizing indigenous resources for anthropologically designed behaviour change interventions. *African Journal of AIDS Research* 8:389–400.

Green, E. C., D. T. Halperin, V. Nantulya, et al. 2006. What happened to reduce HIV prevalence in Uganda? *AIDS and Behavior* 10:347–50.

Green, E. C., P. Kajubi, S. Kamya, et al. 2010. Current perceptions of HIV prevalence and multiple partner sex in Uganda. Paper presented at the 18th International AIDS Conference, Vienna, July 18–23.

Green, E. C., T. L. Mah, A. Ruark, and N. A. Hearst. 2009. A framework of sexual partnerships: Risks and implications for HIV prevention in Africa. *Studies in Family Planning* 40:63–70.

Green, E. C., V. Nantulya, R. Stoneburner, and J. Stover. 2002. *What Happened in Uganda? Declining HIV Prevalence, Behavior Change, and the National Response.* Washington, DC: USAID. http://www.usaid.gov/our_work/global_health/aids/Countries/africa/ uganda_report.pdf (accessed April 8, 2006).

Green, E. C. and A. H. Ruark. 2008. AIDS and the churches: Getting the story right. *First Things* 18:22–26.

Green, E. C. and K. Witte. 2006. Fear arousal, sexual behavior change and AIDS prevention. *Journal of Health Communication* 11:245–59.

Green, E. C., B. Zokwe, and J. D. Dupree. 1993. Indigenous African healers promote male circumcision for prevention of STDs. *Tropical Doctor* October:182–83.

Green, E. C., B. Zokwe, and J. D. Dupree. 1995. The experience of an AIDS prevention program focused on South African traditional healers. *Social Science & Medicine* 40:503–15.

Gregson, S., R. Anderson, T. Zhuwau, and K. Chandiwana. 1998. Is there evidence for behaviour change in response to AIDS in rural Zimbabwe? *Social Science & Medicine* 46:321–30.

Gregson, S., G. P. Garnett, C. A. Nyamukapa, et al. 2006. HIV decline associated with behavior change in eastern Zimbabwe. *Science* 311:664–66.

Gregson, S., E. Gonese, T. B. Hallett, et al. 2010. HIV decline in Zimbabwe due to reductions in risky sex? Evidence from a comprehensive epidemiological review. *International Journal of Epidemiology* 2010:1–13. doi:10.1093/ije/dyq055.

Grund, J. P. 1993. *Drug Use as a Social Ritual.* Rotterdam, the Netherlands: IVO. http://www.drugtext.org/library/books/grund/chasdra4.htm (accessed July 27, 2010).

Gruskin, S. and N. Daniels. 2008. Justice and human rights: Priority setting and fair deliberative process. *American Journal of Public Health* 98:1573–77.

Gruskin, S. and L. Ferguson. 2009. Using indicators to determine the contribution of human rights to public health efforts. *Bulletin of the World Health Organization* 87:714–19. doi:10.2471/BLT.08.058321.

Gruskin, S., E. J. Mills, and D. Tarantola. 2007. History, principles, and practice of health and human rights. *The Lancet* 370:449–55.

Gruskin, S. and D. Tarantola. 2008. Universal access to HIV prevention, treatment and care: Assessing the inclusion of human rights in international and national strategic plans. *AIDS* 22:S123–S132.

Gupta, G. R. 2008. Facing facts on HIV in Africa. *Washington Post*, July 5. http://www. washingtonpost.com/wp-dyn/content/article/2008/07/04/AR2008070402127. html (accessed August 6, 2010).

Hallett, T. B., J. Aberle-Grasse, G. Bello, et al. 2006. Declines in HIV prevalence can be associated with changing sexual behavior in Uganda, urban Kenya, Zimbabwe, and urban Haiti. *Sexually Transmitted Infections* 82(Suppl_1):i1–i8.

Halperin, D. T. 1999. Heterosexual anal intercourse: Prevalence, cultural factors, and HIV infection and other health risks, part I. *AIDS Patient Care* 13:717–30.

Halperin, D. T. 2008. Putting a plague in perspective. *New York Times*, January 1. http://www.nytimes.com/2008/01/01/opinion/01halperin.html (accessed August 6, 2010).

Halperin, D. T. and A. Allen. 2000. Is poverty the root cause of African AIDS? *AIDS Analysis Africa* 11:1, 15.

Halperin, D. T. and R. C. Bailey. 1999. Male circumcision and HIV infection: 10 years and counting. *The Lancet* 35:1813–15.

Halperin, D. T. and H. Epstein. 2004. Concurrent sexual partnerships help to explain Africa's high HIV prevalence: Implications for prevention. *The Lancet* 364:4–6.

Halperin, D. T. and H. Epstein. 2007. Why is HIV prevalence so severe in southern Africa? The role of multiple concurrent partnerships and lack of male circumcision. *Southern African Journal of HIV Medicine* 26: 19–25.

Halperin, D. T., K. Fritz, W. McFarland, G. Woelk. 2005. Acceptability of adult male circumcision for sexually transmitted disease and HIV prevention in Zimbabwe. *Sexually Transmitted Diseases* 32(4):238–39.

Halperin, D. T., M. J. Steiner, M. M. Cassell, et al. 2004. The time has come for common ground on preventing sexual transmission of HIV. *The Lancet* 364:1913–15.

Harm Reduction Coalition. n.d. Mission & History of Harm Reduction Coalition. http://www.harmreduction.org/section.php?id=63 (accessed April 24, 2010).

Hattori, M. K. and F. Nii-Amoo Dodoo. 2007. Cohabitation, marriage, and "sexual monogamy" in Nairobi's slums. *Social Science & Medicine* 6:1067–78.

Hayes, R. and H. Weiss. 2006. Enhanced: Understanding HIV epidemic trends in Africa. *Science* 311:620–21.

He, W., S. Neil, H. Kulkarni, et al. 2008. Duffy antigen receptor for chemokines mediates trans-infection of HIV-1 from red blood cells to target cells and affects HIV-AIDS susceptibility. *Cell Host & Microbe* 4:52–62.

Hearst, N. 2010. Testimony to House Foreign Affairs Committee, Subcommittee on Africa and Global Health. Washington, DC, March 11.

Hearst, N. and S. Chen. 2004. Condom promotion for AIDS prevention in the developing world: Is it working? *Studies in Family Planning* 35:39–47.

Herdt, G. 1999. Clinical ethnography and sexual culture. *Annual Review of Sex Research* 10:100–19.

Hirsch, J. S. 2008. Love, marriage and HIV: A multisite study of gender and HIV risk. http://www.mailman.hs.columbia.edu/sms/chsg/lmhiv/html (accessed February 22, 2008).

Hirsch, J. S., S. Parikh, H. Phinney, et al. 2005. Love, marriage and HIV: Summary and recommendations. Presentation at Natcher Center, National Institutes of

Health, December 1. http://www.cumc.columbia.edu/dept/sph/sms/cgsh/presentation/Love,%20Marriage%20and%20HIV%20-%20Summary.pdf (accessed October 9, 2009).

Hirsch, J. S., H. Wardlow, D. J. Smith, et al. 2010. *The Secret: Love, Marriage, and HIV.* Nashville, TN: Vanderbilt University Press.

HIV & AIDS and STI Strategic Plan for South Africa 2007–2011. 2007. South African National AIDS Council.

Hladik, W., I. Shabbir, A. Jelaludin, et al. 2006. HIV/AIDS in Ethiopia: Where is the epidemic heading? *Sexually Transmitted Infections* 82(Suppl_1): i32–i35.

Hollingsworth, T. D., R. M. Anderson, and C. Fraser. 2008. HIV-1 transmission, by stage of infection. *Journal of Infectious Diseases* 198:687–93.

Hong Kong Community Planning Process on HIV/AIDS MSM Working Group. 2002. *Draft Situation Analysis, Part 1: Review of Research and Prevention Programs.* http://ihome.cuhk.edu.hk/~b102103/cpp/doc/repmsm.pdf (accessed October 9, 2009).

Hosegood, V., N. McGrath, and T. Moultrie. 2009. Dispensing with marriage: Marital and partnership trends in rural KwaZulu-Natal, South Africa 2000–2006. *Demographic Research* 20:279–312.

Hospers, H. and C. Blom. 1998. HIV prevention activities for gay men in the Netherlands 1983–93. In *The Dutch Response to HIV Pragmaticism and Consensus*, T. Sandfort, ed., pp. 40–60. New York: Routledge.

Hugonnet, S., F. Mosha, J. Todd, et al. 2002. Incidence of HIV infection in stable sexual partnerships: A retrospective cohort study of 1802 couples in Mwanza Region, Tanzania. *Journal of Acquired Immune Deficiency Syndromes* 30:73–80.

Hulley, S. B., S. R. Cummings, W. S. Browner, et al. 2001. *Designing Clinical Research: An Epidemiologic Approach.* 2nd ed. Philadelphia: Lippincott, Williams & Wilkins.

Hunter, M. 2002. The materiality of everyday sex: Thinking beyond "prostitution." *African Studies* 61:105.

Hunter, S. 2004. *Black Death: AIDS in Africa.* New York: Palgrave Macmillan.

Hunter, S. 2006. *AIDS in America.* New York: Palgrave MacMillan.

Imperato, P. J. and D. A. Traoré. 1979. Traditional beliefs about smallpox and its treatment in the Republic of Mali. In *African Therapeutic Systems*, D. M. Warren, Z. Ademuwagun, J. Ayoade, and I. Harrison, eds., pp. 15–18. Los Angeles: Crossroads Press for the African Studies Association.

Ingstad, B. 1990. The cultural construction of AIDS and its consequences for prevention in Botswana. *Medical Anthropology Quarterly* 4:28–40.

Institute of Medicine. 2006. *Preventing HIV Infection among Injecting Drug Users in High Risk Countries: An Assessment of the Evidence Committee on the Prevention of HIV Infection among Injecting Drug Users in High-Risk Countries.* Washington, DC: Institute of Medicine.

Institute of Medicine. 2007. *PEPFAR Implementation: Progress and Promise.* Washington, DC: National Academies Press.

Jalsevac, J. 2006. International AIDS conference opens in Toronto: Gates booed for mentioning abstinence, faithfulness. *Life Site News.* August 14. http://www.lifesitenews.com/ldn/2006/aug/06081403.html (accessed September 13, 2010).

James, J. and J. Meyerding. 1977. Early sexual experience and prostitution. *American Journal of Psychiatry* 134:1381–85.

James, V. and R. Matikanya. 2006. Protective factors: A case study for Ngudzeni ADP (Swaziland), World Vision Australia/Swaziland. Central Statistical Office [Swaziland] and ORC Macro, unpublished.

Jana, M., M. Nkambule, and D. Tumbo. 2008. Multiple and concurrent sexual partnerships in southern Africa. Soul City: UNAIDS.

Janzen, J. and E.C. Green. 2003. Continuity, change, and challenge in African healing. In *Medicine Across Cultures*, H. Selin, ed., pp. 1–26. Dordecht, The Netherlands: Kluwer Academic Publishers.

Jewkes, R. 2007. Comprehensive response to rape needed in conflict settings. *The Lancet* 369:2140–41.

Jewkes, R., M. Nduna, J. Levin, et al. 2008. Impact of stepping stones on incidence of HIV and HSV-2 and sexual behaviour in rural South Africa: Cluster randomised controlled trial. *British Medical Journal* 337:a506. doi:10.1136/bmj.a506.

Jones, J. H. 1997. *Alfred C. Kinsey: A Public/Private Life*. New York: Norton.

Judson, F. N., T. A. Coburn, W. S. Smith, F. J. Payne. In press. Viral transmission in needle/syringe exchange programs. *Russian Journal of AIDS, Cancer and Public Health*.

Kaiser Daily HIV/AIDS Report. 2002. "Commercial Sex" down, condom use up in Cambodia, report says. Kaiser Family Foundation, May 24. http://dailyreports.kff.org/Daily-Reports/2002/May/24/dr00011349.aspx (accessed August 6, 2010).

Kajubi, P., M. R. Kamya, S. Kamya, et al. 2005. Increasing condom use without reducing HIV risk: Results of a controlled community trial in Uganda. *Journal of Acquired Immune Deficiency Syndromes* 40:77–82.

Kaleeba, N., J. Namulondo, D. Kalinki, et al. 2000. *Open Secret: People Facing up to HIV and AIDS in Uganda*, Strategies for Hope Series. London: Action AIDS.

Kalichman, S. C., L. C. Simbayi, M. Kaufman, D. Cain, and S. Jooste. 2007. Alcohol use and sexual risks for HIV/AIDS in Sub-Saharan Africa: Systematic review of empirical findings. *Prevention Science* 8(2):141–51.

Kalichman, S. C., E. A. Williams, C. Cherry, et al. 1998. Sexual coercion, domestic violence, and negotiating condom use among low-income African-American women. *Journal of Women's Health* 7:371–78.

Kamenga, M., R. W. Ryder, M. Jingu, et al. 1991. Evidence of marked sexual behavior change associated with low HIV-1 seroconversion in 149 married couples with discordant HIV-1 serostatus: Experience at an HIV counselling center in Zaire. *AIDS* 5:61–67.

Karim, Q. A., S.S. Karim, K. Soldan, and M. Zondi. 1995. Reducing the risk of HIV infection among South African sex workers: Socioeconomic and gender barriers. *American Journal of Public Health* 85(11):1521–25.

Katz, I. and D. Low-Beer. 2008. Why has HIV stabilized in South Africa, yet not declined further? Age and sexual behavior patterns among youth. *Sexually Transmitted Diseases* 35(1):837–42.

Kayirangwa, E., J. Hanson, L. Munyakazi, and A. Kabeja. 2006. Current trends in Rwanda's HIV/AIDS epidemic. *Sexually Transmitted Infections* 82(Suppl_1): i27–i31.

Kelly, R. J., R. H. Gray, N. K. Sewankambo, et al. 2003. Age differences in sexual partners and risk of HIV-1 infection in rural Uganda. *Journal of Acquired Immune Deficiency Syndromes* 32:446–51.

Kirby, D. 2003. Changing youth behaviors: Findings from U.S. and developing country research and their implications for A, B, and C. Paper presented at the meeting on HIV Prevention for Young People in Developing Countries, Washington, DC, July 24. http://www.fhi.org/en/Youth/YouthNet/NewsEvents/HIVprevenmeeting. htm (accessed July 30, 2010).

Kirby, D. 2008. Changes in sexual behavior leading to decline in the prevalence of HIV in Uganda: Confirmation from multiple sources of evidence. *Sexually Transmitted Infections* 84:35–41.

Kiwanuka, N., O. Laeyendecker, T. C. Quinn, et al. 2009. HIV-1 subtypes and differences in heterosexual HIV transmission among HIV-discordant couples in Rakai, Uganda. *AIDS* 23:2479–84.

Kocheleff, P. 2006. AIDS in Burundi and South Africa: A day-to-day experience. In *The HIV/AIDS Epidemic in Sub-Saharan Africa in a Historical Perspective*, P. Denis and C. Becker, eds., pp. 143–54. Published Online at Academia-Bruylant (Louvain-la-Neuve) and Karthala (Paris).

Koloko, P., B. Zokwe, E. C. Green, and J. D. Dupree. 1993. Ethnomedical practices of significance to the spread and prevention of HIV in southern Africa (1). 14ᵗʰ International Conference on AIDS and HIV/STD World Congress, Berlin, June 9. Abstract no. PO-C03-2610.

Kramer, L. 2004. The tragedy of today's gays: An address to the gay community. Speech made at The Cooper Union, New York on November 7, 2004, presented by the HIV Forum in conjunction with NYU's Office of LGBT Student Services, Broadway Cares/Equity Fights AIDS, Callen-Lorde, and the Gill Foundation.

Krige, E. 1936. *The Social System of the Zulu*. London: Longmans.

Kristof, N. 2005. When marriage kills. *New York Times*, March 30. http://www.nytimes.com/2005/03/30/opinion/30kristof.html (accessed July 28, 2010).

Langendam, M. W., G. H. van Brussel, R. A. Coutinho, et al. 1999. Methadone maintenance treatment modalities in relation to incidence of HIV: Results of the Amsterdam cohort study. *AIDS* 13:1711–16.

Le Blanc, M., D. Meintel, and V. Piche. 1991. The African sexual system: Comment on Caldwell et al. *Population and Development Review* 17:497–505.

Leclerc-Madlala, S. 2001. Virginity testing: Managing sexuality in a maturing HIV/AIDS epidemic. *Medical Anthropology Quarterly* 15:33–53.

Leclerc-Madlala, S. 2002. Prevention means more than condoms. *Johannesburg Mail & Guardian*, October 4, p. 19.

Leclerc-Madlala, S. 2003. Transactional sex and the pursuit of modernity. *Social Dynamics* 29:213–33.

Leclerc-Madlala, S. 2008. Age-disparate and intergenerational sex in southern Africa: The dynamics of hypervulnerability. *AIDS* 22:S17–S25.

Leonard, T. L. 1990. Male clients of female street prostitutes: Unseen partners in sexual disease transmission. *Medical Anthropology Quarterly* 4:41–55.

Lesbian and Gay Legislative Advocacy Network, The. 2006. "Gay statistics" in the Philippines by consensus. *HIV Trackback*, September 15. http://lagablab.word-press.com/2006/09/15/gay-statistics-in-the-philippines-by-consensus (accessed July 27, 2010).

Lloyd, S. and N. Taluc. 1999. The effects of male violence on female employment. *Violence Against Women* 5:370–92.

Long, L., M. Fox, I. Sanne, and S. Rosen. 2010. The high cost of second-line antiretroviral therapy for HIV/AIDS in South Africa. *AIDS* 24:915–19.

Longfield, K., S. Agha, T. Kusantha, et al. 2001. *Non-Use of Condoms: What Role Do Supply, Demand, and Acceptance Play in the 'Condom Gap'?* Presentation at the International Conference on AIDS and STDs in Africa, Ouagadougou, Burkina Faso, December.

Luadet, A. B. 2008. The impact of Alcoholics Anonymous on other substance abuse related Twelve Step programs. *Recent Developments in Alcoholism* 18:71–89. http://www.ncbi.nlm.nih.gov/pmc/articles/PMC2613294/ (accessed July 27, 2010).

Luke, N. 2003. Age and economic asymmetries in the sexual relationships of adolescent girls in sub-Saharan Africa. *Studies in Family Planning* 34:67–86.

Lyons, M. 1997. The point of view: Perspectives on AIDS in Uganda. In *AIDS in Africa and the Caribbean*, G. Bond, J. Kreniske, I. Susser, and J. Vincen, eds., pp. 133–49. Boulder, CO: Westview.

MacIsaac, V. n.d. Mechai renews crusade against the AIDS threat. *The Nation* [Thailand].http://www.nationmultimedia.com/search/read.php?newsid=120544 &keyword=nation (accessed July 19, 2010).

Mah, T. and D. T. Halperin. 2008. Concurrent sexual partnerships and the HIV epidemic in sub-Saharan Africa: The evidence to move forward. *AIDS and Behaviour*. doi:10.1007/s10461-008-9433-x.

Maharaj, P. and J. Cleland. 2004. Condom use within marital and cohabiting partnerships in KwaZulu-Natal, South Africa. *Studies in Family Planning* 35(2):116–24.

Maher, L. and W. Swift. 1997. *Heroin Use in Sydney's Indo-Chinese Communities: A Review of NDARC Research*. Monograph No. 33. National Drug and Alcohol Research Centre, University of New South Wales. http://ndarc.med.unsw.edu.au/NDARCWeb.nsf/resources/Mono_4/$file/Mono.33.PDF (accessed July 27, 2010).

Mahomva, A., S. Greby, S. Dube, et al. 2006. HIV prevalence and trends from data in Zimbabwe, 1997–2004. *Sexually Transmitted Infections* 82 (Suppl_1): i42–i47.

Malinowski, B. 1929. *The Sexual Life of Savages in North-western Melanesia: An Ethnographic Account of Courtship, Marriage, and Family Life among the Natives of the Trobriand Islands, British New Guinea*. New York: Harcourt, Brace & Company.

Maman, S., J. Campbell, M. D. Sweat, and A. C. Gielen. 2000. The intersections of HIV and violence: Directions for future research and interventions. *Social Science & Medicine* 50:459–78.

Manderson, L., L. R. Bennett, and M. Sheldrake. 1999. Sex, social institutions, and social structure: Anthropological contributions to the study of sexuality. *Annual Review of Sex Research* 10:184–209.

Marcus, A. 2001. Do some people "deserve" AIDS? One out of five think they do. *The Body: The Complete HIV/AIDS Resource*. http://www.thebody.com/content/art377.html (accessed July 31, 2010).

Marlatt, G. A. 1998. *Harm Reduction: Pragmatic Strategies for Managing High-Risk Behaviors*. New York: Guilford Press.

Marshall, P. A. and L. A. Bennett. 1990. Anthropological contributions to AIDS research. *Medical Anthropology Quarterly*, New Series, 4:3–5.

Mathur, S., M. Greene, and A. Malhotra. 2003. *Too Young to Wed: The Lives, Rights, and Health of Young Married Girls*. Washington, DC: International Center for Research on Women.

Matovu, J. K. B., G. Kigozi, and F. Nalugoda. 2003. Repetitive VCT, sexual risk behavior and HIV-incidence in Rakai, Uganda. Presented at the Uganda Virus Research Institute, Entebbe, Uganda, November 28.

Mattson, C. L., R. T. Campbel, R. C. Bailey, et al. 2008. Risk compensation is not associated with male circumcision in Kisumu, Kenya: A multi-faceted assessment of men enrolled in a randomized controlled trial. *PLoS ONE* 3:e2443. doi:10.1371/journal.pone.0002443.

Mayer, K. H. and H. F. Pizer. 2008. *HIV Prevention: A Comprehensive Approach.* London: Academic Press.

McGrath, J., C. B. Rwabukwali, D. A. Schumann, et al. 1993. Anthropology and AIDS: The cultural context of sexual risk behavior among urban Baganda women in Kampala, Uganda. *Social Science & Medicine* 36:429–39.

McKeganey, N., Z. Morris, J. Neale, et al. 2004. What are drug users looking for when they contact drug services: Abstinence or harm reduction? *Drugs: Education, Prevention and Policy* 11:423–35.

McKellar, J., E. Stewart, and K. Humphreys. 2003. Alcoholics Anonymous involvement and positive alcohol-related outcomes: Cause, consequence, or just a correlate? A prospective 2-year study of 2,319 alcohol-dependent men. *Journal of Consulting and Clinical Psychology* 71:302–8.

Mead, M. 1928. *Coming of Age in Samoa: A Psychological Study of Primitive Youth for Western Civilisation.* New York: American Museum of Natural History Press.

Mermin, J., J. Musinguzi, A. Opio, et al. 2008. Risk factors for recent HIV infection in Uganda. *Journal of the American Medical Association* 300:540–49.

Meyer, B. 2004. Christianity in Africa: From African independent to Pentecostal-charismatic churches. *Annual Review of Anthropology* 33:447–74.

Miller, A. M. and C. S. Vance. 2004. Sexuality, human rights, and health. *Health and Human Rights* 7:5–15.

Miller, N. and R. Rockwell, eds. 1988. *AIDS in Africa: The Social and Policy Impact.* New York: Mellen Press and the National Council for International Health.

Minnis, A. M., M. J. Steiner, M. F. Gallo, et al. 2009. Biomarker validation of reports of recent sexual activity: Results of a randomized controlled study in Zimbabwe. *American Journal of Epidemiology* 170:918–24.

Mishra, V. A. 2007a. HIV infection does not necessarily disproportionately affect the poorer in sub-Saharan Africa. *AIDS* 7:S17–S28.

Mishra, V. 2007b. Why do so many HIV discordant couples in sub-Saharan Africa have female partners infected, not male partners? Presentation at HIV/AIDS Implementers' Meeting, Kigali, Rwanda, June 18.

Mishra, V., S. Bignami-Van Assche, R. Greener, et al. 2007. HIV infection does not disproportionately affect the poorer in sub-Saharan Africa. *AIDS* 21 (Suppl_7):S17–S28.

Mishra, V., P. Agrawal, S. Alva, et al. 2009a. *Changes in HIV-related Knowledge and Behaviors in Sub-Saharan Africa.* DHS Comparative Reports No. 24. Calverton, MD, USA: ICF Macro.

Mishra, V., R. Hong, S. Bignami-Van Assche, and B. Barrere. 2009b. *The Role of Partner Reduction and Faithfulness in HIV Prevention in Sub-Saharan Africa: Evidence from Cameroon, Rwanda, Uganda, and Zimbabwe.* DHS Working Papers No. 61. Calverton, Maryland: Macro International Inc.

Mishra, V., R. Hong, Y. Gu, A. Medley, B. Robey. 2009c. *Levels and Spread of HIV Seroprevalence and Associated Factors: Evidence from National Household Surveys.* DHS Comparative Reports No. 22. Calverton, Maryland: Macro International Inc.

Mngadi, S., N. Fraser, H. Mkhatshwa, et al. 2009. *Swaziland HIV Prevention Response and Modes of Transmission Analysis*. Mbabane, Swaziland: National Emergency Council on HIV and AIDS [Swaziland], UNAIDS, and The World Bank.

Mogae, F. 2008. Opening session. Paper read at the 17th International AIDS Conference, Mexico City, August 3.

Mongeau, P. 1998. Another look at fear arousing messages. In *Persuasion: Advances through Meta-analysis*, M. Allen & R. Preis, eds., pp. 53–68. Cresskill, NJ: Hampton Press.

Moodie, R., A. Katahoire, and F. Kaharuza. 1991. An evaluation study of Uganda AIDS control programme's information education and communication activities. Kampala: AIDS Control Programme, Ministry of Health and Geneva, Switzerland: WHO.

Moos, R. H. and B. S. Moos. 2004. Long-term influence of duration and frequency of participation in Alcoholics Anonymous on individuals with alcohol use disorders. *Journal of Consulting and Clinical Psychology* 72:81–90.

Morgan, E. P. 2006. Social analysis, project development and advocacy in U.S. foreign assistance. *Public Administration and Development* 3:61–71.

Morris, M. A. 2002. Comparative study of concurrent sexual partnerships in the United States, Thailand and Uganda. *American Sociology Association Annual Meeting Published Abstracts*, Anaheim, California, August 18–21, Session 409.

Morris, M. A. and M. Kretzschmar. 1997. Concurrent partnerships and the spread of HIV. *AIDS* 11:641–48.

Motlalepula, K., R. Tshehlo, J. Nkonyana, et al. 2009. Lesotho HIV prevention response and modes of transmission analysis. March. Maseru, Lesotho: Lesotho National AIDS Commission, World Bank, and UNAIDS.

Motlogelwa, T. 2007. PSI pulls out controversial condoms adverts. *Mmegi Online*, May 10.

Muchini, B., C. Benedikt, S. Gregson, et al. 2010. Local perceptions of the forms, timing and causes of behavior change in response to the AIDS epidemic in Zimbabwe. *AIDS and Behavior*. doi: 10.1007/s10461-010-9783-z.

Mugyenyi, P. 2009. Flat-line funding for PEPFAR: A recipe for chaos. *The Lancet* 374:292.

Mukhopadhyay, M., M. Appel, N. Bandopadhyay, et al. 2005. *Operational Guide on Gender and HIV/AIDS: A Rights Based Approach*. Edited by UNAIDS Inter-Agency Task Team on Gender and HIV/AIDS. Amsterdam: UNAIDS.

Mulenga, O., H. Witola, C. Buyu, et al. 2009. *Zambia HIV Prevention Response and Modes of Transmission Analysis*. Lusaka: Zambia National HIV/AIDS/STI/TB Council, UNAIDS, and The World Bank.

Mullings, J. L., J. W. Marquart, and V. E. Brewer. 2000. Assessing the relationship between child sexual abuse and marginal living conditions on HIV/AIDS-related risk behavior among women prisoners. *Child Abuse and Neglect* 24:677–88.

Mulondo, M. 2009. Kabaka to visit northern Uganda. *Sunday Vision* (Kampala, Uganda), September 27, p. 1.

Murdock, G. P. 1980. *Theories of Illness*. Pittsburgh: University of Pittsburgh Press.

Murphy, E., M. E. Greene, and T. Duong. 2006. Defending the ABCs: A feminist perspective on AIDS prevention. Presentation at African Successes: Can

Behavior-Based Solutions Make a Crucial Contribution to HIV Prevention in sub-Saharan Africa? Munyonyo, Uganda, December 17–20.

Museveni, Y. K. 1991.VII International AIDS Conference, Florence, Italy. *The New Vision*, June 26.

Museveni, Y. K. 2000. *What Is Africa's Problem?* Minneapolis: University of Minnesota Press.

National Emergency Response Council on HIV/AIDS (NERCHA) [Swaziland], UNAIDS, and World Bank. 2009. *Swaziland HIV Prevention Response and Modes of Transmission Analysis*. Mbabane, Swaziland: NERCHA.

National Institute on Drug Abuse. 2005. Research Report Series: Heroin Abuse and Addiction. http://www.12steptreatmentcentres.com/Articles/Heroin.pdf (accessed July 31, 2010).

National Resistance Movement (NRM) (Uganda). n.d. *Guidelines for Resistance Committees on the Control of AIDS: Action for Survival*. Prepared by UNICEF Kampala with the approval of Directorate of Information and Mass Mobilisation, NRM Secretariat and the Health Education Division, Ministry of Health, Republic of Uganda.

Ngubane, H. 1977. *Body and Mind in Zulu Medicine*. London: Academic Press.

Nnko, S., J. T. Boerma, M. Urassa, et al. 2004. Secretive females or swaggering males? An assessment of the quality of sexual partnership reporting in rural Tanzania, *Social Science & Medicine* 59:299–310.

Ntozi, J. P. 1997. Widowhood, remarriage and migration during the HIV/AIDS epidemic in Uganda. *Health Transition Review* 7 (Suppl_1):125–44.

Nyanzi, S., R. Pool, and J. Kinsman. 2001. The negotiation of sexual relationships among school pupils in south-western Uganda. *AIDS Care* 13:83–98.

Nzima, M. 1995. Preliminary programmatic considerations questions and related analysis of the targeted intervention research (TIR) conducted in collaborative programs involving healers, Chimwemwe, Kitwe (June 13–24, 1994). Lusaka: Morehouse/Tulane AIDS Prevention Project.

Odets, W. 1994. AIDS education and harm reduction for gay men: Psychological approaches for the 21st century. *AIDS and Public Policy Journal* 9:3–15.

O'Farrell, N. 2001. Poverty and HIV in sub-Saharan Africa. *The Lancet* 357:636–37.

Okware, S., A. Opio, J. Musinguzi, et al. 2000. Fighting HIV/AIDS: Is success possible? *Bulletin of the World Health Organization* 79:1113–20.

Okware, S., S. Kinsman, S. Onyango, et al. 2005. Revisiting the ABC strategy: HIV prevention in Uganda in the era of antiretroviral therapy. *Postgraduate Medical Journal* 81:625–28.

Okyne, R. A. 2009. The great deception: The myth of a non-homosexual Africa: The Catholic Church and homosexuality in Africa. *Afrik News*, November 1, 2009. http://en.afrik.com/article16397.html (accessed July 30, 2010).

Onjoro, E. 2003. Cultural integration for effective AIDS prevention. *Anthropology News*, November:4, 8. http://www.aaanet.org/press/an/infocus/hivaids/0310_onjoroaids.htm (accessed July 26, 2010).

Open Society Institute. 2001. What is harm reduction? http://www.soros.org/initiatives/ health/focus/ihrd/articles_publications/articles/what_20010101 (accessed July 31, 2010).

Orubuloye, I. O., J. C. Caldwell, and P. Caldwell. 1991. Sexual networking in the Ekiti District of Nigeria. *Studies in Family Planning* 22:61–73.

Osborne, K. 2003. The ABCs of HIV: It's not that simple. *AIDSLink* 82, November 1. http://www.globalhealth.org/publications/article.php3?id=1061 (accessed August 2, 2010).

Oyeneye, O. 1985. Mobilizing indigenous resources for primary health care in Nigeria: A note on the place of traditional medicine. *Social Science & Medicine* 20:67–69.

PACHA (Presidential Advisory Council for HIV/AIDS). 2005. *Achieving an HIV-free Generation: Recommendations for a New American HIV Strategy*. Washington, DC: PACHA. www.aids.gov/federal-resources/policies/pacha/pacharev113005.pdf (accessed September 5, 2009).

Packard, R. M. and P. Epstein. 1991. Epidemiologists, social scientists, and the structure of medical research on AIDS in Africa. *Social Science & Medicine* 33:771–83.

Padian, N. S., S. I. McCoy, J. E. Balkus, and J. N. Wasserheit. 2010. Weighing the gold in the gold standard: Challenges in HIV prevention research. *AIDS* 24:621–35.

Page, J. B., D. D. Chitwood, P. C. Smith, N. Kane, and D. C. McBride. 1990. Intravenous drug use and HIV infection in Miami. *Medical Anthropology Quarterly* 4:56–71.

Paley, J. 2002. Toward an anthropology of democracy. *Annual Review of Anthropology* 31:469–96.

Parikh, A. 2007. The political economy of marriage and HIV: The ABC approach, "safe" infidelity, and managing moral risk in Uganda. *American Journal of Public Health* 97:1198–208.

Parker, R., D. di Mauro, B. Filiano, et al. 2004. Global transformations and intimate relations in the 21st century: Social science research on sexuality and the emergence of sexual health and sexual rights frameworks. *Annual Review of Sex Research* 15:362–98.

Parker, R. G. and D. Easton. 1998. Sexuality, culture, and political economy: Recent developments in anthropological and cross-cultural sex research. *Annual Review of Sex Research* 9:1–19.

Parker, R. G. and J. H. Gagnon, eds. 1995. *Conceiving Sexuality: Approaches to Sex Research in a Postmodern World*. New York: Routledge.

Pateguane, J. L. 1983. Tuberculos pulmonar e alguns factores culturais ao abandono do tratamento. *Trabalho Proposto as IV Jornadas de Saude Maputo*. Mozambique: Ministry of Health.

Pearson-Marks, J., S. Nakayiwa, B. Namande, et al. 1993. Anthropology and AIDS: The cultural context of sexual risk behavior among urban Baganda women in Kampala, Uganda. *Social Science & Medicine* 36:429–39.

Pelling, M. 1993. Contagion/germ theory/specificity. In *Companion Encyclopedia of the History of Medicine*, Vol. 1, W. F. Bynum and R. Porter, eds., 309–34. London: Routledge.

Pellow, D. 1977. *Women in Accra: Options for Autonomy*. Algonac, MI: Reference Publications.

Peltzer, K., N. Mngqundaniso, and G. Petros. 2006. A controlled study of an HIV/AIDS/STI/TB intervention with traditional healers in KwaZulu-Natal, South Africa. *AIDS and Behavior* 10:683–90.

Pen, M. 2008. Plenary session. Paper read at the 17th International AIDS Conference, Mexico City, August 4.

Peterson, J., S. G. Mitchell, Y. Hong, et al. 2006. Abstinência versus redução de danos: Questões conflitantes ou complementares entre usuários de drogas injetáveis

(Getting clean and harm reduction: Adversarial or complementary issues for injection drug users). *Cadernos de Saúde Pública* 22:733–40.

Philaretou, A. G. 2006. The social construction of erotophobia. *Journal of Sex Research* 43:293–95.

Phoolcharoen, W. 1998. HIV/AIDS prevention in Thailand: Success and challenges. *Science* 19:1873–74.

Pilcher, C. D., H. C. Tien, J. J. Eron, et al. 2004. Brief but efficient: HIV infection and the sexual transmission of HIV. *Journal of Infectious Diseases* 189:1785–972.

Pinkerton, S. D. 2007. Probability of HIV transmission during acute infection in Rakai, Uganda. *AIDS and Behavior* 12:677–84.

Piot, P. 2006. AIDS: From crisis management to sustained strategic response. *The Lancet* 368:526–30.

Piot, P. 2008. Opening session of the 17th International AIDS Conference, Mexico City, August 3.

Piot, P., M. Bartos, H. Larson, et al. 2008. Coming to terms with complexity: A call to action for HIV prevention. *The Lancet* 372:845–59.

Pisani, E. 2008. *The Wisdom of Whores: Bureaucrats, Brothels and the Business of AIDS*. New York: W. W. Norton.

PlusNews. 2007. Deadly cocktail: HIV and drug use. *IRIN/PlusNews Southern Africa*, November. http://www.plusnews.org/InDepthMain.aspx?InDepthId=67 &ReportId=75492&Country=Yes (accessed July 27, 2010).

PlusNews. 2009a. Condoms—the hole truth. *PlusNews*, September 10. http://www.plusnews.org/report.aspx?ReportID=86096 (accessed September 29, 2009).

PlusNews. 2009b. South Africa: Time to rethink testing. *PlusNews*, June 29. http://www.plusnews.org/Report.aspx?Reportid=85033 (accessed July 31, 2010).

PlusNews. 2009c. What of the female condom? *PlusNews*, September 10. http://www.plusnews.org/Report.aspx?ReportId=86081 (accessed September 29, 2009).

Potts, M., D. T. Halperin, D. Kirby, et al. 2008. Public health: Reassessing HIV prevention. *Science* 320:749–50.

Pronyk, P., J. R. Hargreaves, and J. C. Kim. 2006. Effect of a structural intervention for the prevention of intimate-partner violence and HIV in rural South Africa: A cluster randomised trial. *The Lancet* 368:1973–78.

Ramin, B. 2007. Anthropology speaks to medicine: The case of HIV/AIDS in Africa. *McGill Journal of Medicine* 10:127–32.

Rather, D. 2008. Both sides of the fence. HDnet. http://www.hd.net/transcript.html?air_mast-id=A5144 (accessed March 10, 2008).

Ratner, M. S., ed. 1993. *Crack Pipe as Pimp: An Ethnographic Investigation of Sex-for-Crack Exchanges*. New York: Lexington Books.

Reidpath, D. D. and K. Y. Chan. 2006. HIV, stigma, and rates of infection: A rumour without evidence. *PLoS Medicine* 3:1708.

Republic of Namibia Ministry of Health and Social Services. 2010. United Nations General Assembly Special Session (UNGASS) Country Report: Reporting Period 2008–2009. Windhoek, Namibia.

Reuee, E. 2002. *The Ills of Aid: An Analysis of Third World Development Policies*. Chicago: University of Chicago Press.

Ribaudu, N. 2009. Outspoken (interview). *The Washington Post*, May 24, p. B2.

Roberts, G., et al. 1998. How does domestic violence affect women's mental health? *Women's Health* 28:117–29.

Rotello, G. 1997. *Sexual Ecology: AIDS and the Destiny of Gay Men*. New York: Dutton.

Royce, R. A., A. Sena, W. Cates, and M. S. Cohen. 1997. Sexual transmission of HIV. *New England Journal of Medicine* 226:1072–80.

Ruark, A. 2008. HIV risk and marriage in Africa. Presentation at Global Health Council Annual Conference, Washington, DC, May 28.

Ruteikara, S., Rev. 2008. Let my people go, AIDS profiteers. *Washington Post*, June 30. http://www.washingtonpost.com/wp-dyn/content/article/2008/06/29/AR2008062901477.html (accessed July 26, 2010).

Saneka, M., S. Zondo, and S. LeClerc-Madlala. 2007a. Dangerous liaisons: When too much love can kill you. *Sunday Tribune* (Kwa-Zulu Natal, South Africa), June 3.

Saneka, M., S. Zondo, and S. LeClerc-Madlala. 2007b. Remaining faithful a fine idea, but is ... . *Sunday Tribune* (Kwa-Zulu Natal, South Africa), July 29.

Scarce, M. 1999. A ride on the wild side. *POZ*, February. http://www.poz.com/articles/211_1460.shtml (accessed July 27, 2010).

Schoepf, B. G. 1988. Women, AIDS, and economic crisis in Central Africa. *Canadian Journal of African Studies* 22:625–44.

Schoepf, B. G. 2001. International AIDS research in anthropology: Taking a critical perspective on the crisis. *Annual Review of American Anthropology* 30:335–61.

Schoepf, B. G. 2003. What happened in Uganda? *AIDS and Anthropology Bulletin* 15:13.

Schoofs, M. 1997. The law of desire. *The Village Voice*, April 15.

Second International Scientific–Practical Conference, The. 2008. HIV/AIDS in the developed countries. Moscow, Russian Federation, December 4–5.

Sepulveda, J., C. Carpenter, J. Curran, et al. 2007. *PEPFAR Implementation: Progress and Promise*. Washington, DC: National Academic Press.

Shelton, J. D. 2007. Ten myths and one truth about generalised HIV epidemics. *The Lancet* 371:1809–11.

Shelton, J. D. 2008. Counselling and testing for HIV prevention. *The Lancet* 372:273–75.

Shelton, J. D. 2009. Why multiple sexual partners? *The Lancet* 374(9687):367–69.

Shelton, J. D., D. T. Halperin, V. Nantulya, et al. 2004. Partner reduction is crucial for balanced "ABC" approach to HIV prevention. *British Medical Journal* 32:891–94.

Shelton, J. D., D. T. Halperin, and D. Wilson. 2006. Has global HIV incidence peaked? *The Lancet* 367:1120–22.

Shelton, J. D. and B. Johnston. 2001. Condom gap in Africa: Evidence from donor agencies and key informants. *British Medical Journal* 323:139.

Sherr, L., N. Lopman, M. Kakowa, et al. 2007. Voluntary counseling and testing: Uptake, impact on sexual behaviour, and HIV incidence in a rural Zimbabwean cohort. *AIDS* 21:851–60.

Shiffman, J., D. Berlan, and T. Hafner. 2009. Has aid for AIDS raised all health funding boats? *Journal of Acquired Immune Deficiency Syndromes* 52:S45–S48.

Shilts, R. 1987. *And The Band Played On: Politics, People and the AIDS Epidemic*. New York: St. Martin Press.

Shisana, O., T. Rehle, L. Simbayi, et al. 2005. *South African National HIV Prevalence, HIV Incidence, Behavior and Communication Survey*. Cape Town, South Africa: Human Science Research Council Press.

Sidibé, M. and K. Buse. 2010. Fomenting a prevention revolution for HIV. *The Lancet* 375:533–35.

Singer, M. 1990. Reinventing medical anthropology: Toward a critical realignment. *Social Science & Medicine* 30:179–87.

Smith, J. D. 2007. Modern marriage, men's extramarital sex, and HIV risk in south-eastern Nigeria. *American Journal of Public Health* 97 :997–1005.

Smyth, B., V. Hoffman, J. Fan, and Y.-I. Hser. 2007. Years of potential life lost among heroin addicts 33 years after treatment. *Preventive Medicine* 44:369–74.

Sopheab, H., G. Morineau, J. J. Neal, et al. 2008. Sustained high prevalence of sexually transmitted infections among female sex workers in Cambodia: High turnover seriously challenges the 100% condom use programme. *BMC Infectious Diseases* 8:167. doi:10.1186/1471-2334-8-167.

Southern African Development Community (SADC). 2006. *Expert Think Tank Meeting on HIV Prevention in High-prevalence Countries in Southern Africa: Report.* Gaborone, Botswana: SADC. http://www.sadc.int/downloads/news/ SADCPrevReport.pdf (accessed August 6, 2010).

Sapa. 2010. Health minister won't make his HIV test results public. *Times Live* (South Africa), March 17. http://www.timeslive.co.za/local/article361564.ece (accessed August 6, 2010).

Spark-du Preez, N., B. Zaba, C. Nyamukapa, et al. 2004. *Kusvika raparadzaniswa nerufu* (Until death do us part). *African Journal of AIDS Research* 3:81–91.

Specter, M. 2005. Higher risk. *The New Yorker*, May 23. http://www.newyorker. com/archive/2005/05/23/050523fa_fact?currentPage=all (accessed July 27, 2010).

Spiegel, P., A. R. Bennedsen, J. Claass, et al. 2007. Prevalence of HIV infection in conflict-affected and displaced people in seven sub-Saharan African countries: A systematic review. *The Lancet* 369:2187–95.

Steinglass, M. 2001. It takes a village healer. *Lingua Franca* 11. http://linguafranca. mirror.theinfo.org/print/0104/cover_healer.html (accessed August 6, 2010).

Stoneburner, R. L. and D. Low-Beer. 2003. Behaviour and communication change in reducing HIV: Is Uganda unique? *African Journal of AIDS Research* 2:9–21.

Stoneburner, R. L. and D. Low-Beer. 2004. Population-level HIV declines and behavioral risk avoidance in Uganda. *Science* 304:714–18.

Strathdee, S., N. Galai, M. Safaeian, et al. 1997. Gender differences in risk factors for HIV seroconversion among injection drug users: A ten year perspective. *Archives of Internal Medicine* 161:1281–88.

Sutton, S. R. 1982. Fear-arousing communications: A critical examination of theory and research. In *Social Psychology and Behavioral Medicine*, J. R. Eiser, ed., pp. 303–37. London: Wiley.

Suwannawong, P. 2004. The agony of Bangkok: Thai activist exhorts conference crowd to stand firm against U.S. Patent regime and "masks of fake concern." *The Body: The Complete HIV/AIDS Resource.* http://www.thebody.com/content/art1525.html (accessed August 1, 2010).

Swezey, T. and M. Tietelbaum. 2008. HIV/AIDS and the context of polygyny and other marital and sexual unions in Africa. In *AIDS, Culture, and Africa*, D. A. Feldman, ed., pp. 220–38. Gainesville: University Press of Florida.

Tangwa, G. B. 2005. The HIV/AIDS pandemic, African traditional values and the search for a vaccine in Africa. In *Ethics of AIDS in Africa: The Challenge to Our*

Thinking, A. A. Van Niekirk and L. M. Kopelman, eds., pp. 179–89. Claremont, South Africa: David Philip Publisher.

Tapiwanashe, H. 2008. Moving beyond prevention of HIV transmission to prevention of HIV progression: ABC versus SAVE. *Safaids News* 14:10–11.

Tawfik, L. and S. C. Watkins. 2007. Sex in Geneva, sex in Lilongwe, and sex in Balaka. *Social Science & Medicine* 64:1090–101.

Timberg, C. 2006. How AIDS in Africa was overstated; Reliance on data from urban prenatal clinics skewed early projections. *The Washington Post*, April 6. http://www. washingtonpost.com/wp-dyn/content/article/2006/04/05/AR2006040502517. html (accessed August 6, 2010).

Timberg, C. 2007. In Zimbabwe, fewer affairs and less HIV. *Washington Post*, July 13. http://www.washingtonpost.com/wp-dyn/content/article/2007/07/12/ AR2007071202369.html (accessed July 26, 2010).

Tonigan, J. S., R. Toscov, and W. R. Miller. 1996. Meta-analysis of the literature on Alcoholics Anonymous: Sample and study characteristics moderate findings. *Journal of Studies on Alcohol* 57:65–72.

Turner, C. F. and H. G. Miller. 1997. Zenilman's anomaly reconsidered: Fallible reports, ceteris paribus, and other hypotheses. *Sexually Transmitted Diseases* 24:522–27.

Twa-Twa, J., I. Nakanaabi, and D. Sekimpi. 1997. Underlying factors in female sexual partner instability in Kampala. *Health Transition Review* Suppl_7:83–88.

Tylor, E. B. 1958 [1871]. http://www.anthrobase.com/Dic/eng/def/culture.htm (accessed January 18, 2010).

Ubuntu Planning Meeting for SADC Four Country Research Project. 2008. Mbabane, Swaziland, November 11.

Uganda AIDS Commission (UAC). 2003. *And Banana Trees Provided the Shade: The Story of AIDS in Uganda*. Kampala: UAC.

UNAIDS. 2005a. *AIDS Epidemic Update 2005*. Geneva: UNAIDS. http://www. unaids.org/ Epi/2005/ (accessed January 3, 2006).

UNAIDS. 2005b. *Evidence for HIV Decline in Zimbabwe: A Comprehensive Review of the Epidemiological Data*. Geneva: UNAIDS. http://data.unaids.org/Publications/ IRCpub06/Zimbabwe_Epi_report_ Nov05_en.pdf (accessed March 2, 2006).

UNAIDS. 2006. Collaborating with traditional healers for HIV prevention and care in sub-Saharan Africa: Suggestions for programme managers and field workers. Geneva: Joint United Nations Programme on HIV/AIDS (UNAIDS).

UNAIDS. 2008a. Mozambique Country Analysis. July 2008. http://data.unaids.org/ pub/FactSheet/2008/sa08_moz_en.pdf (accessed July 31, 2010).

UNAIDS. 2008b. *Report on the Global AIDS Epidemic*. Geneva: UNAIDS (Joint UN Programme on HIV/AIDS).

UNAIDS. 2009a. Consultation on concurrent sexual partnerships: Recommendations from a meeting of the UNAIDS Reference Group on Estimates, Modelling and Projections held in Nairobi, Kenya, April 20–21, 2009. http://www.epidem. org/Publications/Concurrency%20meeting%20recommendations_Final.pdf (accessed August 21, 2010).

UNAIDS. 2009b. *Meeting Report: Addressing Multiple and Concurrent Partnerships in Southern Africa: Developing Guidance for Bold Action*. http://www.unaidsrstesa. org/files/u1/MCP_Meeting_Report_Gabarone_28-29_Jan_2009.pdf (accessed August 3, 2010).

UNAIDS/UNFPA/UNIFEM. 2004. *Women and HIV/AIDS: Confronting the Crisis.* Geneva: UNAIDS. http://www.unfpa.org/upload/lib_pub_file/308_filename_women_aids1.pdf (accessed April 11, 2007).

UNGASS/UNAIDS. 2010. *Monitoring the Declaration of Commitment on HIV/AIDS: Guidelines on Construction of Core Indicators, 2010 Reporting.* Geneva, Switzerland: UNAIDS.

United Nations Development Programme (UNDP). 2004. *Thailand's Response to HIV/AIDS: Progress and Challenges.* Bangkok: UNDP.

United Nations Development Programme (UNDP). 2007. *Swaziland Human Development Report: HIV and AIDS and Culture.* Mbabane, Swaziland: UNDP. http://planipolis.iiep.unesco.org/upload/Swaziland/Swaziland_NHDR_2008.pdf (accesed August 6, 2010).

USAID. n.d. Social Soundness Analysis (ADS Supplementary Reference 202). http://www.usaid.gov/policy/ads/200/2026s7.pdf (accessed March 16, 2010).

Vance, C. S. 1991. Anthropology rediscovers sexuality: A theoretical comment. *Social Science & Medicine* 33:875–84.

Van Den Berg, C., C. Smit, I. G. Van Brusse, et al. 2007. Full participation in harm reduction programmes is associated with decreased risk for human immunodeficiency virus and hepatitis C virus: Evidence from the Amsterdam Cohort Studies among drug users. *Addiction* 102:1454–62.

Van Griensven, G., J. P. Robert, A. P. Tielman, et al. 1987. Risk factors and prevalence of HIV antibodies in homosexual men in the Netherlands. *American Journal of Epidemiology* 125:1048–57.

van Haastrecht, II. J. A., E. J. C. van Ameijden, J. A. R. van den Hoek, et al. 1996. Predictors of mortality in the Amsterdam cohort of human immunodeficiency virus (HIV)-positive and HIV-negative drug users. *American Journal of Epidemiology* 143:380–91.

Velimirovic, B. 1984. Traditional medicine is not primary health care: A polemic. *Curare* 7:61–79.

Ventevogel, P. 1992. Aborofodee (Whiteman's things): Effects of training programme for indigenous healers in the Techiman District, Ghana. Master's Thesis, Free University of Amsterdam, The Netherlands.

Wabwire, F., N. Asingwire, A. Opio, and P. Bukuluku. 2006. *Rapid Assessment of Trends and Drivers of the HIV Epidemic and Effectiveness of Prevention Interventions in Uganda: A Synthesis Report.* Kampala: Uganda AIDS Commission. http://www.aidsuganda.org/yeah/n3.pdf (accessed August 1, 2010).

Wabwire-Mangen, F., M. Odiit, W. Kirungi, et al. 2009. *Uganda HIV Prevention Response and Modes of Transmission Analysis.* Kampala: Uganda AIDS Commission.

Wagner, B. G., J. S. Kahn, and S. Blower. 2010. Should we try to eliminate HIV epidemics by using a "Test and Treat" strategy? *AIDS* 24:775–76.

Warren, D. M. 1979. The role of emic analysis in medical anthropology: The case of the Bono of Ghana. In *African Therapeutic Systems*, D. M. Warren, Z. Ademuwagun, J. Ayoade, and I. Harrison, eds., pp. 36–42. Los Angeles: Crossroads Press for the African Studies Association.

Warren, D. M., G. S. Bova, M. A. Tregoning, and M. Kliewer. 1982. Ghanaian national policy towards indigenous healers: The case of the primary health training for indigenous healers (PRHETIH) program. *Social Science & Medicine* 16:1873–81.

Watson-Jones, D., K. Baisley, H. A. Weiss, et al. 2009. Risk factors for HIV incidence in women participating in an HSV suppressive treatment trial in Tanzania. *AIDS* 23:415–22.

Weatherford, J. M. 1985. *Tribes on the Hill.* New York: Bergin & Garvey.

Weatherford, J. M. 1986. *Porn Row.* New York: Arbor House.

Weinhardt, L. S., M. P. Carey, B. T. Johnson, and N. L. Bickham. 1999. Effects of HIV counseling and testing on sexual risk behavior: A meta-analytic review of published research, 1985–1997. *American Journal of Public Health* 89:1397–405.

Weiss, H. A., D. Halperin, R. C. Bailey, et al. 2008. Male circumcision for HIV prevention: From evidence to action? *AIDS* 22:567–74.

Weller, S. and K. Davis. 2002. Condom effectiveness in reducing heterosexual HIV transmission (Cochrane Methodology Review). *The Cochrane Library,* Issue 4. Chichester, UK: John Wiley & Sons.

Whelehan, P. 2009. *The Anthropology of AIDS: A Global Perspective.* Gainesville: University Press of Florida.

White, R., J. Cleland, and M. Caraël. 2000. Links between premarital sexual behaviour and extramarital intercourse: A multi-site analysis. *AIDS* 14:2323–31.

Wilson, D. A. 2005. *Monitoring and Evaluation Framework for Concentrated Epidemics and Vulnerable Populations.* Washington, DC: The World Bank.

Winstanley, J. 2008. Rallying for harm reduction in Thailand. http://www.huffingtonpost.com/jennifer-winstanley/rallying-for-harm-reducti_b_113116.html (accessed April 26, 2010).

Witte, K. 1992. Putting the fear back into fear appeals: The extended parallel process model. *Communication Monographs* 59:329–49.

Witte, K. 1998. How to motivate protective action. *Health Risk Communicator* 2:1–2.

Witte, K. and M. Allen. 2000. A meta-analysis of fear appeals: Implications for effective public health campaigns. *Health Education & Behavior* 27:608–32.

Wojcicki, J. M. and J. Malala. 2001. Condom use, power and HIV/AIDS risk: Sex-workers bargain for survival in Hillbrow/Joubert Park/Berea, Johannesburg. *Social Science & Medicine* 53:99–121.

World Bank, UNAIDS. 2009. *The Global Economic Crisis and HIV Prevention and Treatment Programmes: Vulnerability and Impact.* http://siteresources.worldbank.org/INTHIVAIDS/Resources/375798-1103037153392/TheGlobalEconomicCrisisandHIVfinalJune30.pdf (accessed June 30, 2009).

World Health Organization (WHO). 2004. *Effectiveness of Sterile Needle and Syringe Programming in Reducing HIV/AIDS among Injecting Drug Users: Evidence for Action Technical Papers.* Geneva: World Health Organization.

World Health Organization (WHO). 2006. *Addressing Violence against Women in HIV Testing and Counseling: A Meeting Report.* Geneva: Department of Gender, Women, and Health (GWH) and Department of HIV/AIDS, World Health Organization.

Zeelie, C. 2002. Uganda hails HIV success. *BBC News,* August 2.

Zenilman, J., C. S. Weisman, A. M. Rompalo, et al. 1995. Condom use to prevent incident STDs: The validity of self-reported condom use. *Sexually Transmitted Diseases* 22:15–21.

Zierler, S., L. Feingold, D. Laufer, et al. 1991. Adult survivors of childhood sexual abuse and subsequent risk of HIV infection. *American Journal of Public Health* 81:572–75.

DHS REFERENCES

Cote d'Ivoire 2005: Institut National de la Statistique (INS) and Ministère de la Lutte contre le Sida [Côte d'Ivoire] and ORC Macro. 2006. *Enquête sur les Indicateurs du Sida, Côte d'Ivoire 2005.* Calverton, Maryland, USA: INS and ORC Macro.

Cote d'Ivoire 1998–99: Institut National de la Statistique [Côte d'Ivoire] et ORC Macro. 2001. *Enquête Démographique et de Santé, Côte d'Ivoire 1998–1999.* Calverton, Maryland USA: Institut National de la Statistique et ORC Macro.

Ethiopia 2005: Central Statistical Agency [Ethiopia] and ORC Macro. 2006. *Ethiopia Demographic and Health Survey 2005.* Addis Ababa, Ethiopia, and Calverton, Maryland, USA: Central Statistical Agency and ORC Macro.

Haiti 2005: Cayemittes, Michel, Marie Florence Placide, Soumaïla Mariko, Bernard Barrère, Blaise Sévère, Canez Alexandre. 2007. *Enquête Mortalité, Morbidité et Utilisation des Services, Haïti, 2005–2006.* Calverton, Maryland, USA: Ministère de la Santé Publique et de la Population, Institut Haïtien de l'Enfance and Macro International Inc.

Kenya 2003: Central Bureau of Statistics (CBS) [Kenya], Ministry of Health (MoH) [Kenya], and ORC Macro. 2004. *Kenya Demographic and Health Survey 2003.* Calverton, Maryland, USA: CBS, MoH, and ORC Macro.

Lesotho 2004: Ministry of Health and Social Welfare (MoHSW) [Lesotho], Bureau of Statistics (BoS) [Lesotho], and ORC Macro. 2005. *Lesotho Demographic and Health Survey 2004.* Calverton, Maryland, USA: MoH, BoS, and ORC Macro.

Liberia 2007: Liberia Institute of Statistics and Geo-Information Services (LISGIS) [Liberia], Ministry of Health and Social Welfare [Liberia], National AIDS Control Program [Liberia], and Macro International Inc. 2008. *Liberia Demographic and Health Survey 2007.* Monrovia, Liberia: Liberia Institute of Statistics and Geo-Information Services (LISGIS) and Macro International Inc.

Malawi 2004: National Statistical Office (NSO) [Malawi], and ORC Macro. 2005. *Malawi Demographic and Health Survey 2004.* Calverton, Maryland, USA: NSO and ORC Macro.

Mozambique 2003: Instituto Nacional de Estatística [Mozambique], Ministério da Saúde [Mozambique], and ORC Macro. *Moçambique Inquérito Demográfico e de Saúde 2003.* Calverton, Maryland, USA: Instituto Nacional de Estatística [Mozambique], Ministério da Saúde [Mozambique], and ORC Macro.

Namibia 2006: Ministry of Health and Social Services (MoHSS) [Namibia] and Macro International Inc. 2008. *Namibia Demographic and Health Survey 2006–07.* Windhoek, Namibia, and Calverton, Maryland, USA: MoHSS and Macro International Inc.

Rwanda 2005: Institut National de la Statistique du Rwanda (INSR) and ORC Macro. 2006. *Rwanda Demographic and Health Survey 2005.* Calverton, Maryland, USA: INSR and ORC Macro.

Senegal 2005: Ndiaye, Salif, et Mohamed Ayad. 2006. *Enquête Démographique et de Santé au Sénégal 2005.* Calverton, Maryland, USA: Centre de Recherche pour le Développement Humain [Sénégal] and ORC Macro.

South Africa 2003: Department of Health, Medical Research Council, OrcMacro. 2007. *South Africa Demographic and Health Survey 2003*. Pretoria: Department of Health.

Swaziland 2006–07: Central Statistical Office (CSO) [Swaziland], and Macro International Inc. 2008. *Swaziland Demographic and Health Survey 2006–07*. Mbabane, Swaziland: Central Statistical Office and Macro International Inc.

Tanzania 2007–08: Tanzania Commission for AIDS (TACAIDS), Zanzibar AIDS Commission (ZAC), National Bureau of Statistics (NBS), Office of the Chief Government Statistician (OCGS), and Macro International Inc. 2008. *Tanzania HIV/AIDS and Malaria Indicator Survey 2007–08*. Dar es Salaam, Tanzania: TACAIDS, ZAC, NBS, OCGS, and Macro International Inc.

Uganda 2000–01: Uganda Bureau of Statistics (UBoS) and ORC Macro. 2001. *Uganda Demographic and Health Survey 2000–2001*. Calverton, Maryland, USA: UBOS and ORC Macro.

Uganda 2004–05: Ministry of Health (MoH) [Uganda] and ORC Macro. 2006. *Uganda HIV/AIDS Sero-behavioural Survey 2004–2005*. Calverton, Maryland, USA: Ministry of Health and ORC Macro.

Uganda 2006: Uganda Bureau of Statistics (UBoS) and Macro International Inc. 2007. *Uganda Demographic and Health Survey 2006*. Calverton, Maryland, USA: UBOS and Macro International Inc.

Zambia 2007: Central Statistical Office (CSO), Ministry of Health (MoH), Tropical Diseases Research Centre (TDRC), University of Zambia, and Macro International Inc. 2009. *Zambia Demographic and Health Survey 2007*. Calverton, Maryland, USA: CSO and Macro International Inc.

Zimbabwe 2005–06: Central Statistical Office (CSO) [Zimbabwe] and Macro International Inc. 2007. *Zimbabwe Demographic and Health Survey 2005–06*. Calverton, Maryland: CSO and Macro International Inc.

Index

Notes: Italicized page numbers indicate boxes, figures, and tables. Notes are indicated by the letter "n" and note number following the page number.

About the Authors

Edward C. Green, PhD, is an anthropologist and, until recently, a senior research scientist at Harvard University and director of the AIDS Prevention Research Project at the Harvard Center for Population and Development Studies. He has worked for over 30 years in international health. Much of his work since the latter 1980s has been in AIDS and sexually transmitted diseases, primarily in Africa, but also in Asia, Latin America, and the Caribbean. He served as a public health advisor to the governments of both Mozambique and Swaziland. He is also well known for his studies of African indigenous health belief systems and for pioneering programs of collaboration between African indigenous healers and medically trained practitioners, to achieve mutually agreed upon public health goals. He is the author of six previous books, including *Broken Promises* (in press), *Rethinking AIDS Prevention* (2003), *Indigenous Theories of Contagious Disease*, and *AIDS and STDs in Africa* (1994).

Allison Herling Ruark is a doctoral student at the Johns Hopkins Bloomberg School of Public Health. Prior to this, she spent four years as a research fellow at the Harvard AIDS Prevention Research Project, where she wrote and published on HIV prevention in Africa.